Development of the Central Nervous System in Vertebrates

NATO ASI Series

Advanced Science Institutes Series

A series presenting the results of activities sponsored by the NATO Science Committee, which aims at the dissemination of advanced scientific and technological knowledge, with a view to strengthening links between scientific communities.

The series is published by an international board of publishers in conjunction with the NATO Scientific Affairs Division

A	**Life Sciences**	Plenum Publishing Corporation
B	**Physics**	New York and London
C	**Mathematical and Physical Sciences**	Kluwer Academic Publishers
D	**Behavioral and Social Sciences**	Dordrecht, Boston, and London
E	**Applied Sciences**	
F	**Computer and Systems Sciences**	Springer-Verlag
G	**Ecological Sciences**	Berlin, Heidelberg, New York, London,
H	**Cell Biology**	Paris, Tokyo, Hong Kong, and Barcelona
I	**Global Environmental Change**	

Recent Volumes in this Series

Series A: Life Sciences

Development of the Central Nervous System in Vertebrates

Edited by

S. C. Sharma

New York Medical College
Valhalla, New York

and

A. M. Goffinet

Université Notre Dame de la Paix
Namur, Belgium

Plenum Press
New York and London
Published in cooperation with NATO Scientific Affairs Division

Proceedings of a NATO Advanced Study Institute on
Development of the Central Nervous System in Vertebrates,
held June 23–July 6, 1991,
in Maratea, Italy

NATO-PCO-DATA BASE

The electronic index to the NATO ASI Series provides full bibliographical references (with key-words and/or abstracts) to more than 30,000 contributions from international scientists published in all sections of the NATO ASI Series. Access to the NATO-PCO-DATA BASE is possible in two ways:

—via online FILE 128 (NATO-PCO-DATA BASE) hosted by ESRIN, Via Galileo Galilei, I-00044 Frascati, Italy.

—via CD-ROM "NATO-PCO-DATA BASE" with user-friendly retrieval software in English, French, and German (© WTV GmbH and DATAWARE Technologies, Inc. 1989)

The CD-ROM can be ordered through any member of the Board of Publishers or through NATO-PCO, Overijse, Belgium.

Library of Congress Cataloging-in-Publication Data

NATO Advanced Study Institute on Development of the Central Nervous
  System in Vertebrates (1991 : Maratea, Italy)
    Development of the central nervous system in vertebrates / edited
  by S. C. Sharma and A.M. Goffinet.
        p.   cm. -- (NATO ASI series. Series A, Life sciences ; vol.
  234)
    "Proceedings of a NATO Advanced Study Institute on Development of
  the Central Nervous System in Vertebrates, held June 23-July 6,
  1991, in Maratea, Italy."--T.p. verso.
    "Published in cooperation with NATO Scientific Affairs Division."
    Includes bibliographical references and index.
    ISBN 0-306-44304-X
    1. Central nervous system--Growth--Congresses. 2. Developmental
  neurology--Congresses.   I. Sharma, S. C. (Sansar C.), 1938-
  II. Goffinet, A. III. Title. IV. Series.
    [DNLM: 1. Central Nervous System--embryology--congresses.   WL 300
  N279d 1991]
  QP356.25.N35   1991
  DNLM/DLC
  for Library of Congress   92-49267
                                                         CIP

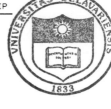

ISBN 0-306-44304-X

© 1992 Plenum Press, New York
A Division of Plenum Publishing Corporation
233 Spring Street, New York, N.Y. 10013

Printed in the United States of America

PREFACE

The major theme of this book is the development of the vertebrate central nervous system. This volume contains summaries of most of the invited participants at the NATO advanced study institute entitled "Development of central nervous system in vertebrates" held in Maratea, Italy, from June 23-July 5, 1991. In order to address this topic, we have drawn upon a selection of current studies dealing with molecular, cellular and system analysis which specifically pertain to the general principles of the development. The major aim of this institute was to bring together a select group of investigators who would present their views on the current issues in their respective fields and to foster extensive discussions amongst participants in smaller groups. Such interactions brought together the exchanges of ideas amongst participants and helped clarify the intricate details and formulate new vistas and collaborations.

Since the study of nervous system development has focused mostly on the origin of neuron and glia cells, the area of current research was represented by talks on early cellular events including effects of growth factors, HOX and other gene expressions and cell lineage of specific cell type(s). Formation of specific cell types and the specific neuronal connections have been a major theme in the study of the nervous system development. Recent technical advances has resulted in new information at both cellular and molecular levels which have provided new details. Current research was represented by "selective" topics discussed at the meeting.

The intensive discussions by both lecturers and students throughout the meeting, were indicative of the level of participation. Every one apparently benefited from such discussions which clarified the points to non-experts in the field and helped bring a clearer understanding of the subject. In their attempt to link molecular, cellular and morphological events during neural development, the diversity of topics discussed at the institute will, it is hoped, be evident in the book.

I am deeply indebted to the organizing committee for the help provided during the course of the meeting and to the management of Hotel Villa del Mare who catered to every conceivable problem and were gracious hosts.

Sincere thanks are also due to the National Science Foundation U.S. for partial funding of the travel expenses of six students. A special grant to supplement the expenses was provided by the Maratea Regione Basicalata, Italy. NATO Scientific Affairs Division provided the major funding for this meeting. I am deeply thankful to the Director of the ASI programme Mr. L.V. da Cunha for his keen interest and his willingness to help at every stage of this meeting. Thanks are due to every member of my research team who willingly provided time to assist in the organization of

the meeting. Special thanks to Laura Rendine for her patience and
technical expertise in typing the manuscripts and help in the organization
of the meeting.

S.C. Sharma
New York Medical College

CONTENTS

REGULATION OF THE EARLY DEVELOPMENT OF THE NERVOUS

SYSTEM BY GROWTH FACTORS

Perry F. Bartlett, John Drago, Trevor J. Kilpatrick,
Linda J. Richards, Peter Wookey and Mark Murphy

The Walter and Eliza Hall Institute of Medical Research, and
The Cooperative Research Centre for Cellular Growth Factors
Parkville, Victoria 3050, Australia

INTRODUCTION

The nervous system of vertebrates begins as a thickening of the
dorsal ectoderm early in embryogenesis which subsequently involutes to
form the neural tube consisting of a single layer of epithelium
(neuroepithelium); from this develops the entire central nervous sytem
(CNS). Another population of cells bud off from the dorsal portion of the
tube just prior to closure, the neural crest; these cells give rise to all
the cells of the peripheral nervous system (PNS), and to many structures
in the facial and branchial regions of the developing embryo.

At the simplest level, neural development can be considered as a
process whereby epithelial like cells proliferate and ultimately
differentiate into cells of the nervous sytem: neurons and glia. The
magnitude of this process is best illustrated by the fact that the 100
billion neurons found in the human brain are derived from approximately
125 thousand primitive cells present at the early stage of neural tube
formation. The regulation of this process of growth and differentiation
has been thought of as being both intrinsic, genetically predetermined
within individual cells, and to be due to enviromental or epigenetic
factors. The distinction between the two types of regulation is often not
clear and cell phenotype, as will be discussed, may often depend on their
interplay.

Beyond understanding how individual cells are regulated to divide
and differentiate lies the question of how organisation and pattern
formation occurs in the nervous system. This question has been examined
in detail in invertebrates, especially in the fruit fly, Drosophila. Here
it has been elegantly shown, mainly by the use of developmental mutants,
that the segmentation observed in both the nervous system and body
compartments are regulated by a family of genes (homeobox), which code for
proteins sharing a common amino acid sequence (homeodomain) that bind to
regulatory elements in DNA (See Ingham, 1988 for review). Similar genes
have been identified in most vertebrate species, including man, and their
distribution within the developing nervous system has suggested that they
may play a part in determining segmentation. However, segmentation is not
at all obvious in the developing neural tube of animals such as chicken or
mice, and that which does occur in the spinal cord is secondary to somite
formation.

Development of the Central Nervous System in Vertebrates
Edited by S.C. Sharma and A.M. Goffinet, Plenum Press, New York, 1992

Recently, it has been shown by Lumsden et al., (1989, 1990) that the series of folds that appear in the developing hindbrain of chicks, called rhombomeres, does indeed represent true segmentation of the neuroepithelium. They have shown that rhombomere boundaries restrict the migration of clones of neurons and demarcate the origin of the nerve roots of many of the cranial nerves. Pairs of rhombomeres also correspond to the branchial arches that give rise to head and neck structures. The significance of this latter observation is that neural crest cells give rise to much of the mesenchyme of this region and these crest cells have been shown to migrate within these boundaries suggesting that they carry preexisting information concerning their ultimate cellular phenotype.

Of particular interest is that boundaries of rhombomeres correspond to boundaries of expression of many of the homeobox genes as well as other genes coding for DNA binding proteins such as Krox-20 (See Wilkinson and Krumlauf, 1990 for review), implying that these genes are directly responsible for the observed segmentation. The importance of this gene expression to neural development in higher vertebrates awaits gene knockout experiments. Early results indicate that gene ablation leads to developmental defects which do not correspond to the extent of gene expression: loss of Hox-1.5 does not interfere with cranial nerve development even though it is expresed in all rhombomeres (Chisaka and Capechi, 1991). Thus, it may be that the system is degenerate in higher vertebrates, with no single gene determining regional specificity. Recent experiments favour another interpretation, that families of homeobox genes share the same distribution within the hindbrain but may determine the fate of only some of the cells within that region (Hunt et al., 1991). This would account for the loss of only some of the derivatives of a particular rhombomere.

It is notable that expression of genes coding for growth factors such as FGF like molecules (Int-2) and Steel factor are also regionally restricted in the nervous system (Matsui et al., 1990). It could be argued that these two categories of regionally distributed genes represent the two possible mechanisms that influence neural development: one acting directly as a DNA binding proteins that influence cell growth and phenotype within a particular area, and the second, also regionally expressed, influencing the same characteristics by regulating the cell through receptor-ligand interactions. How one type of interaction influences the other and in what sequence are major questions for the 90s.

This review details the evidence, principally gained from in vitro cell culture, in favor of the concept that the regulation of proliferation of precursor cells in the developing CNS and PNS is largely due to growth factors produced within the nervous system. It also suggests that there are quite separate signals for precursor proliferation from those which are required for differentiation.

EARLY EVENTS IN THE FORMATION OF THE CNS

From studies primarily carried out in amphibians it appears that neural induction begins at the time of gastrulation and is due to interactions with the underlying mesoderm. The classical studies of Mangold (1933) also indicated that mesoderm was important in specifying the subsequent phenotype of the neurectoderm: anterior mesoderm induced forebrain whereas posterior produced spinocaudal structures. Although it has been suggested that soluble factors mediate induction their indentity remains unclear. Recent experiments have shown that protein kinase activators such as phorbol ester can act as inducing agents (Davids et al., 1987).

Once induced the number of cells in the neural plate does not change appreciably as the process of tube formation proceeds. Proliferation commences after tube closure in the midline and gives the neuroepithelium of the neural tube a columnar appearance. At a macroscopic level swellings begin to appear in the rostral region of the tube that represent the three major areas of the brain: the forebrain (cerebral cortex and basal ganglia), the midbrain, and the hindbrain (medulla, pons and cerebellum). As mentioned earlier within the hindbrain there are additional folds called rhombomeres which have been shown to represent segmental areas of the neuroepithelium. the remainder of the neural tube gives rise to the spinal cord.

As the stratification of the cells proceeds, cell division is primarily restricted to the neuroepithelium adjacent to the cavities that will ultimately form the ventricles, although mitotically active cells can also be found in the other areas including the external granular layer of the cerebellum.

There appear to be two distinct phases of proliferation in the CNS: the first peaking some 3 to 4 days after neural tube closure in the mouse (Angevine and Sidman, 1961) and which correlates with the neuronal precursor division; and the second which occurs later and is associated with glial cell formation.

The major questions that arise when examining these early events are: What controls the proliferation of the neuroepithelial cells? What regulates the generation of cell lineages? If the cells of the neuroepithelium are multipotential, can subsequent differentiation be influenced by epigenetic factors?

REGULATION OF PRECURSOR PROLIFERATION IN THE CNS

One of the hallmarks of early neural development is the enormous degree of proliferation that occurs in the neuroepithelium. We have endeavored to explore the possibility that this could be regulated by epigenetic factors including soluble growth factors and components of the extra-cellular matrix. In order to examine this, new in vitro assays were developed in which pure populations of neuroepithelial cells (Drago et al., 1991a), prepared from mouse neural tubes at the time of closure, were cultured in the presence or absence of a wide range of soluble growth factors. It was found that both acidic and basic fibroblast growth factors (a,bFGF) were unique as they were potent stimulators of neuroepithelial cell division as assessed by tritiated thymidine incorporation (Murphy et al., 1990). Other factors including nerve growth factor (NGF), epidermal growth factor (EGF) and insulin-like growth factors (IGF-I,II), previously shown to be associated with embryonic neural tissue (Nexo et al., 1980; Sara et al., 1981), were ineffective in stimulating cell division. It was subsequently shown that FGF stimulation was dependent on the presence of IGF-I and especially the truncated form of IGF-1, which is primarily found in developing brain (Drago et al., 1991b). These studies demonstrated that FGF acted predominantly as a proliferative agent (see later for discussion on differentiation), whereas IGF-I was primarily a survival agent for the precursors. Recent experiments using clones of neuroepithelial cells support this conclusion, as they continue to proliferate in the presence of FGF without overt signs of differentiation. Differentiation can be induced in these populations by specific signals (Kilpatrick et al. manuscript in preparation).

What relevance does this in vitro data have to the regulation of precursors in vivo? To answer this question directly would require the ablation of these growth factors in the tissue at the relevant time. Although such technologies as gene ablation by homologous recombination, anti-sense mRNA or ribozyme provide potential tools to answer the question directly they are still at an early stage of development. We can determine, however, whether the factors are present in the tissue at the appropriate time. mRNA for both BFGF and IGF-I was detectable in freshly isolated neuroepithelial cells, implying that these factors are produced endogenously by the precursor populations (Drago et al., 1991).

This idea was compatible with the observation that the requirement for growth factors in vitro could be largely overcome if the cells were plated at high cell density; implying that there was a limiting amount of factors produced by the cells. This proved to be correct as blocking antibodies specific for either bFGF or IGF-I totally inhibited the survival or growth of the precursor population (Drago et al., 1991b). Thus, it appears that the neuroepithelial cells may be regulated by an autocrine or paracrine mechanism, which is in stark contrast to that previously postulated as the mechanism for neurotrophic factor action on developing neurons; where it has been largely attributed to external or target derived factors.

If precursor cells produce their own stimulatory factors then how is the system regulated? One likely regulatory mechanism is the binding of FGF to heparan sulphate proteoglycans which are known to be present in the basement membrane with which the dividing precursors are all in contact. Recently, we have shown that there is FGF bound to the ECM of neuroepithelial cells and that there is an enormous excess capacity of the low affinity FGF receptor, provided by a heparan sulphate proteoglycan, compared to the high affinity receptor on the neuroepithelial cells (Nurcombe and Bartlett, manuscript submitted). This would result in the vast majority of the secreted FGF (the exact mode of secretion is still unclear because FGF does not have a leader sequence) being bound to the ECM and only accessible after cleavage of the core protein.

Another molecule to which FGF can bind via its attachment to heparin is the laminin molecule. Laminin is a large multidomain molecule expresssed early in development and is found in abundance in the basal lamina next to the proliferating neuroepithelial cells (Tuckett and Morris-Kay, 1986). It has been shown to promote survival and neurite extension in cultured neuronal cells (Cohen et al., 1986) and to be involved in the transdifferentiation of cultured retinal pigment cells into neurons (Reh et al., 1987). It was also found to stimulate the survival and proliferation of neuroepithelial cells in vitro and to be additive with FGF (Drago et al., 1991c). However, in contrast to FGF, the action of laminin was dependent on cell aggregation, a response which laminin promoted. It therefore appears that laminin responsiveness may result from its ability to promote cell-cell contacts that may in turn upregulate other endogenous stimulatory molecules.

ARE NEURAL PRECURSORS IN THE CNS MULTIPOTENTIAL?

As much of the data, until recently, relies on in vitro cultures to answer the above question it is important to establish how accurately the system reflects the in vivo situation. It has been shown that the spectrum of cell phenotypes cen indeed be generated from neuroepithelial cells in vitro (Abney et al., 1981; Bailey et al., 1987). More surprisingly, perhaps, is the finding that in high density cultures the appearance of specific phenotypic markers coincides temporally with their appearance in vivo (Saleh and Bartlett, 1989; Abney et al., 1981). This has given rise to the concept of an inbuilt biological clock that is

independent of its enviroment. However, it should be noted that this
phenomenon has been largely established with high density cell culture and
there is evidence from our laboratory using neuroepithelial clones that
this mechanism does not operate without exogenous stimuli. Another
example is the precursor cell in the optic nerve, termed the 0-2A
precursor, which has the capability of differentiating into either an
oligodendrocyte or a type II astrocyte in vitro, but does not recapitulate
the in vivo sequence unless the appropriate growth factors are present
(Raff, 1989). This observation again stresses the importance of the
interrelationship between intrinsic and extrinsic factors in the
development of the nervous system and highlights the difficulty in
interpreting ill-defined culture systems.

Beside the 0-2A precursor cited above, there are several in vitro
studies that strongly suggest that cells of developing CNS can give rise
to cells of various phenotypes. It was shown in clonal assay of blast
cells obtained from the rat hippocampus that about one fifth of the clones
contained cells of the two major types in the CNS: neurons and glia
(Temple, 1989). Recent work in our laboratory also suggests that some of
the clones derived from neuroepithelial cells also have the ability to
differentiate into neurons and astrocytes (Kilpatrick and Bartlett,
manuscript in preparation).

A recently devised method based on the ability of retroviruses to
insert into dividing cells and act as a marker of their progeny has led to
the fate mapping in several vertebrate CNS systems. Two groups have shown
that in the developing retina a single precursor can give rise to an array
of glial and neuronal types (Turner and Cepko, 1987; Wetts and Fraser,
1988). In contrast, workers using a similar approach in the cortex of
mice and rats failed to observe mixed progeny. This may indicate either
that there are no multipotential cells in the cortex or that there is
heirarchy whereby cells become progressively more committed with
developmental age. The latter explanation appears more likely from studies
that use markers to distinguish committed precursor populations.

It has been known for some time that the brain is unique as it does
not express Class I MHC molecules constitutively. It was subsequently
shown that this molecule could be induced by the lymphokine, interferon
gamma (Wong et al., 1984). However, it is now known that neurons do not
express this molecule under any circumstances (Bartlett et al., 1989) and
it was established that cells in the developing neuroepithelium that were
not inducible with the lymphokine gave rise to neurons exclusively when
selected by cell sorting and were cultured (Bartlett et al., 1990). These
committed precursors were not found, however, when the earliest precursor
cells were examined, implying that commitment only began to occur after
proliferation of the neuroepithelium was underway. From this type of
phenotype study it was possible to construct a heirachy of commitment
which originates with the multipotential cell, flows into the restricted
glia or neuronal precursor and ends with the fully differentiated cell.

Another approach to investigating the differentiation potential of
cells in the developing CNS is to generate cell lines from the precursor
populations. This was first achieved by infecting neuroepithelium with a
retrovirus containing the c-myc gene, chosen for its ability to promote
proliferation rather than differentiation (Bartlett et al., 1988). One of
the lines generated, 2.3D, grew as a stable neuroepithelial cell line and
was found not to spontaneously differentiate. Subsequently, it was found
to respond to FGF by rounding up and putting out neurite-like processess
that stained with the neuron specific intermediate filament marker,
neurofilament. Some of the cells in this cloned cell line expressed the
glial specific marker, glial fibrillary acidic protein (GFAP) (Bartlett et

al., 1988). Thus, there can be no doubt that epithelial cells thus immortalised retain the ability to differentiate down both major CNS pathways.

FACTOR REGULATION OF NEURAL DIFFERENTIATION IN THE CNS

One of the problems in identifying factors that may act as differentiating agents is trying to separate them from the agents that stimulate survival and proliferation. As has been noted, cells cultured at sufficiently high cell density or with factors such as FGF proceed to differentiate, but it is far from clear exactly what signals are driving that differentiation. Originally we had thought that FGF was a differentiating agent (Murphy et al., 1990). However, even in spite of the observation with the cell line 2.3D, this conclusion is less clear. Recent experiments indicate that when precursors were plated at low cell density on monolayers of astrocytic cells and grown in serum-free medium, fewer neurons differentiated in the presence of FGF than in medium alone (Kilpatrick and Bartlett, manuscript in preparation). This implies that there are positive signals for differentiation that are quite separate from proliferative stimuli. Some of these signals are being identified in the neural crest (see below). However, in the CNS such factors remain uncharacterised.

THE PERIPHERAL NERVOUS SYSTEM

The peripheral nervous system is distinguished from the central nervous system on the basis of both anatomical and developmental criteria. Anatomically, the PNS neuronal cell bodies lie outside the brain and spinal cord and can be divided functionally into three major systems: sensory, autonomic and enteric. The autonomic nervous system can be further subdivided on the basis of anatomical, physiological, and pharmacological grounds into the sympathetic and parasympathetic subgroups. The enteric nervous system is considered a separate entity as it can function independently of the central nervous system.

Developmentally, all these structures have the same embryonic origin, the neural crest. As discussed above, the neural crest forms as a group of cells at the dorsal aspect of the neural plate, and just prior to neural tube closure, they bud off from the plate and migrate to specific locations in the embryo. At these locations, the neural crest cells then differentiate into the component ganglia of the PNS. The PNS is almost exclusively derived from the neural crest, except for some cranial ganglia which are derived from a related structure, the ectodermal placodes. The cell types derived from the neural crest are not restricted to neural cells but also include mesenchymal elements of the head and face, melanocytes of the skin, the adrenal medulla, meninges in the pro- and mesencephalon, corneal endothelium and the large arterial walls from the aortic arches (see Le Douarin and Smith, 1988). The generation of such an array of different phenotypes raises questions fundamental not only to neurobiology but to the field of vertebrate development in general. Are the crest cells a homogeneous population of pluripotent precursor cells or are they a heterogeneous population of committed progenitors? If there is evidence for commitment of these cells, what determined that commitment initially? How do the neural crest cells migrate through the embryo to their correct location? What controls the proliferation of the neural crest cells enabling their numbers to increase from a few thousand cells to a few million? What controls the subsequent differentiation of these crest cells into their differentiated phenotypes? As will become evident below, some of these questions have been investigated extensively, whereas others have hardly been touched upon.

COMMITMENT AND MULTIPOTENTIALITY OF THE NEURAL CREST

One of the early problems in the study of neural crest ontogeny was to determine where regional populations of crest cells migrate to, and then to identify the phenotype of their progeny. This was achieved by the use of chick-quail chimeras: regions of the chick neural tube were replaced with quail neural tube, including the neural crest, taken from the same region at a similar stage of development (Le Douarin, 1982; 1986; Le Douarin and Smith, 1988). These chimeras remain viable at least until after birth and the quail cells could be distinguished from the host by its nuclear heterochromatin pattern. Over a period of ten years or more this approach led to the construction of a fate map of the neural crest. This map showed that there were defined regions of the crest which gave rise to particular ganglia and other neural crest derived structures. The fate map generally supports the idea that most neural crest cell migration is lateral and therefore the resultant neural crest derivatives reflect their position along a rostro-caudal axis. For example, the adrenal medullary cells originate from the spinal neural crest between the level of somites 18-24; the spinal neural crest caudal to somite 5 gives rise to the ganglia of the sympathetic chains; and the ciliary ganglion is derived from the mesencephaic neural crest; all of the meso-ectodermal derivatives are derived from the rostral regions of the neural crest and are mainly located in the head and neck.

The fate map described above only addresses questions of normal development as all grafting experiments were placed isotopically, and thus only identical regions of the crest were grafted. To ask whether neural crest cells were lineage restricted according to regional placement, experiments were performed using heterotopically placed grafts. It was found that it was the location of the grafted cells within the chimeric embryo, and not their origin, that ultimately determined their developmental fate. For example, vagal crest cells (which normally show parasympathetic innervation of the gut) grafted to the level of somites 18-24, differentiated into sympathetic ganglia and adrenal medulla - the normal derivatives of this region of the crest. The reverse experiment, where the adrenomedullary level neural crest was transplanted into the vagal region, gave rise to enteric ganglia containing cholinergic and peptidergic neurons. Such experiments not only established that in most cases it was the embryonic environment of the neural crest cells that determined their differentiated phenotype but it also implied that the crest cells were multipotential, at least at the population level.

There appear to be, however, some significant exceptions to the concept that neural crest cells are multipotential. The major exception is in the cephalic regions of the crest, which are unique in that they alone can give rise to the ectomesenchymal derivatives such as bone, smooth muscle, adipose tissue, meninges and endothelial cells- all crest derivatives being exclusively located in the head and upper body. In addition, there are some differences in the capacity of different regions of the crest to duplicate the normal crest region. Replacement of the mesencephalon with the trunk neural crest results in the development of an abnormal trigeminal ganglion (Noden, 1978), whereas the potential of the trunk for adrenergic differentiation is geater in the trunk than in the cephalic crest (Newgreen et al., 1980). Alternatively, when cephalic crest is transplanted to the trunk region, the neural crest cells migate into the dorsal mesentery and colonize the gut, which does not normally happen (Le Douarin & Teillett, 1973).

It is these exceptions which lead one to the view that there are indeed local differences in the composition of the crest different propensities of the various regions of the crest to be committed to different cell types. With respect to the PNS, this commitment is not extensive at least at the population level, but with respect to the mesectoderm, there is a complete restriction to the cephalic levels of the crest. The final decision, however, as to what the cells differentiate into appears to be primarily left to the environment. The identities of the environmental factors which influence these decisions are unknown and have been the object of recent study in our laboratory (see below).

In order to dissect out the events which determine neural crest development it is necessary to turn to in vitro culture techniques as described above. Under these conditions the environment of the neural crest cells can be influenced or manipulated relatively simply by adjusting the components of the medium. Thus it may be possible to determine which factors influence the development of the crest derivatives. In addition, the question of multipotentiality versus commitment can be directly asked in clonal cultures of the cells. A number of workers have begun to develop these clonal cultures and their results suggest that there is both commitment and multipotentiality in the neural crest.

Sieber-Blum and Cohen (1980) first used this approach in the clonal analysis of quail neural crest cells. They grew clones from single neural crest cells and found that some contained both catecholaminergic and pigmented cells. More recently, Sieber-Blum (1989) extended these studies using antibodies specific for the sensory lineage and found three classes of clones: clones committed to the melanogenic lineage, clones that were unpigmented and clones containing both pigmented and non-pigmented cells. The unpigmented and mixed clones all contained both catecholaminergic and sensory neurons. Thus, in this system there is evidence for tripotent cells, cells restricted to two cell lineages and fully committed cells.

Studies from the laboratory of Le Douarin also found evidence for a similarly heterogeneous range of clones (Barofflo et al., 1988; Dupin et al., 1990). In these studies, multipotent clones comprising neurons, pigmented cells and non-neuronal cells were found as well as more restricted clones of Schwann cells, satellite cells and neurons. There was also evidence of some segregation of pigment cells from neurons. In a very few cases there were clones containing cartilage, a marker for the ectomesenchymal lineage. The cartilage containing cells were not associated with neurons or pigmented cells.

These studies support the idea that both multipotentiality and commitment reside within the neural crest cells at the migratory stage. The observation of considerable heterogeneity in the clones is not necessarily a proof that there is intrinsic heterogeneity in the neural crest cells. It may be that at the time the cells are isolated they are at different stages of differentiation: some of the cells may already have gone through a number of steps down a commitment pathway and so may look to be restricted, whereas others may be a little "younger" and so may still be more multipotent. If this is the case, then the actual lineage pathways, or commitment steps, may be inferred from the segregation of the different cell types. Thus, pigment cells appear to segregate from other cell types frequently, as do non-neuronal cells from mixed clones containing both neurons and non-neuronal cells. Cartilage cells are only found in clones with non-neuronal cells including Schwann cells.

As analyses of the clones are normally undertaken after a number of weeks when there can be thousands of cells in each clone, the microenvironment of each clone might itself vary; there might be endogenous production of different growth factors. This raises the question of which factors are required for neural crest differentiation. A possible result of this is that no clones are found which are solely neuronal. Until the conditions have been found which allow for the unrestricted growth of the neural crest derivatives, these clonal analyses will be limited.

One in vivo approach which has been used to determine the degree of multipotentiality or commitment of the neural crest cells is that of Bronner-Fraser and Fraser (1988), who microinjected single neural crest cells with a fluorescent dye prior to migration from the neural tube. The progeny of these cells were traced after two days and in some cases were found to be distributed in all of the regions to which neural crest cells normally migrate. The phenotype of these cells could not be definitively ascribed. However on the basis of morphology and antibody binding, individual clones containing sensory neurons, presumptive melanoblasts, satellite cells in dorsal root ganglia, adrenomedullary cells and neural tube cells were found. Thus, these findings support the idea that there are multipotential neural crest cells in vivo.

In mammals, very little is known about cell lineage and commitment of the neural crest. The isolation of large numbers of neural crest cells from mammals is difficult and they have a limited life span in vitro. In order to overcome these restrictions, we have developed cell lines representative of migratory neural crest cells and their progeny in order to study cell lineage associations as well as to characterize environmental factors which influence the developmental fate of neural crest cells (Murphy et al., 1991a). Previous work from our laboratory and others has shown that retrovirus mediated proto-oncogene transduction of the neural precursor cells from mouse neuroepithelium results in the production of stable neuroepithelial cell lines (Bartlett et al., 1988; Bernard et al., 1989; reviewed in Cepko, 1988, 1989). These cell lines have similar characteristics to primary neuroepithelial cells and, like their primary culture cell counterparts, they differentiate in response to fibroblast growth factor (FGF).

We have immortalized mouse neural crest cultures using retroviruses bearing the c-myc or the N-myc proto-oncogenes and have cloned a series of cell lines (Murphy et al., 1991a). In order to classify these cell lines as being linked to a particular neural crest lineage, the cell lines were examined for the expression of some lineage specific or lineage related antigenic markers which are found on neural crest derived cells. We used antibodies to glial fibrillary acidic protein (GFAP), neurofilament (NF) and the A2B5 antibody. GFAP is specific for mature glia in the central nervous system and has also been found in the glia of the enteric nervous system (Jessen and Mirsky, 1983) as well as in a subpopulation of non-myelinating Schwann cells (Yen and Fields, 1981). A2B5 reacts with a ganglioside present on neurons and probably their precursors in avian neural crest cultures (Girdlestone and Weston, 1985). It also recognizes some glial cells and their precursors in the rat central nervous system (Raff et al., 1983 and 1984).

The results of this analysis showed patterns of staining consistent with individual cell lines being at different stages of differentiation. Eleven cell lines were selected as being representative of the different types of cells which emerged from the neural crest immortalization. RNA from these 11 cell lines was analyzed for the expression of neural specific mRNAs. We examined the expression of nerve growth factor (NGF) and its receptor (NGF-R), which are expressed by cells in the peripheral nervous system, myelin basic protein (MBP) and the proteolipid (PLP) of myelin which, in the peripheral nervous system, are specific to Schwann cells. A neuron specific gene SCG-10 (superior cervical ganglion, see Anderson and Axel, 1985) was also used in the analysis.

A major question arising from the establishment of the neural crest cell lines is whether they possess characteristic features of migrating crest cells and their differentiated progeny. Morphologically, the cell lines had a variety of appearances from flat cells resembling migrating neural crest cells through to multi-processed cells reminiscent of neurons or Schwann cells. One group of cell lines not only morphologically resembled migrating neural crest cells, but this group also was largely devoid of phenotypic markers, both antigenic and mRNA expressed by mature neural cells. These observations are consistent with the idea that some of the migrating neural crest cells are not yet committed to a single developmental pathway and probably represent stem-cells. These stem cells have presumably been frozen at this stage by the immortalization process.

Some of the cell lines also displayed a bipotential nature, a major characteristic of the neural crest. Particular cell lines expressed their bipotentiality in the expression of markers associated with two lineages. In one case a cell line, NC14.9.1, appeared to be bipotential since in a cloned population these cells expressed neurofilament as well as MBP and PLP, showing that it had characteristics of both neurons and Schwann cells. Likewise another cell line, NC14.4.9D, expressed both PLP mRNA and SCG-10 mRNA and all the cells expressed neurofilament. Similarly, multipotent neural cell lines have been isolated from newborn brain (Fredericksen et al., 1988; Ryder et al., 1990). These cell lines also share some other characteristics of our cell lines in that some of the antigenic markers examined were expressed on a small proportion of cells in particular cell lines.

The multipotential nature of the neural crest cells which were originally infected with either c-myc or N-myc containing viruses was also demonstrated by the observation that cell lines which have the same myc integration pattern, and thus must have originated from the same cell, can have quite different phenotypes. It is possible that an immortalized multipotential cell divided a number of times before differentiation of the progeny cells into the different phenotypes took place. Thus, a single crest cell can give rise to a neural crest-like line, Schwann cell progenitor and a bipotential cell line.

In addition to stem-like activities there is evidence that some of the lines also represent progenitor populations that can differentiate in culture. For example NC14.4.8 cells contained cells that differentiated after 1-2 weeks in culture, into Schwann-like cells. Further, these older cultures expressed MRNA for MBP, PLP, NGF and NGF-R. All these observations are consistent with this cell line comprising Schwann cell progenitors.

Finally, one of the cell lines appears to represent a neuronal cell line. This cell line (NC14.4.6E cells) has fine processes which contain neurofilament. In addition, the cells from this line express mRNA for the neuronal protein SCG-10, as well as for NGF, but not NGF-R or other non-neuronal markers. The cells do express vimentin, but this is not surprising since vimentin is present in neural crest cells up until neuronal differentiation.

Although cell lines representative of both neurons and Schwann cells have been characterized there is no evidence that other neural crest derived cells are represented. None of the lines contain melanin pigments or resembled melanocytes, and this is in contrast to the finding in quail

neural crest transformed by Rous sarcoma virus in which the cell lines
gave rise to melanocytes (Pessac et al., 1985). However, avian and mouse
neural crest appear to differ markedly in their capacity to give rise to
mature melanocytes: the mouse neural crest appears to require phorbol
ester (see below) to induce melanin formation in vitro; whereas melanin
formation occurs spontaneously in primary avian neural crest cultures.
Preliminary experiments using phorbol ester on our cell lines have shown
no evidence for melanocyte differentiation. The particular viruses and
oncogenes used in these experiments must also have an influence on the
phenotypes of the resultant cell lines (see Cepko, 1989).

Many of the neuroepithelial cell lines responded to growth factors
such as FGF (Bartlett et al., 1988) which is known to affect neural
proliferation and differentiation of freshly isolated neuroepithelial
cells (Murphy et al., 1990). Likewise, most of the neural crest cell
lines in this study respond to FGF by proliferating and by changes in
morphology, including the group 1 crest-like cells. The significance of
these morphological changes in terms of differentiation is currently being
investigated. In addition high cell density and foetal calf serum are
often required to ensure continued growth of some of the immortalized
lines. Thus, these cell lines may be very useful in assaying for factors
which are important in differentiation, eg FGF, serum factors (see Ziller
et al., 1983). It is possible, therefore, that the cells could be pushed
down different differentiative pathway by the addition of particular
factors in a similar manner to that shown for the neural crest derived
sympathoadrenal cell types (see Doupe et al., 1985a and b, Anderson and
Axel, 1986). In addition, mixing experiments between the cell lines and
other cell types may help to uncover the importance of cell-cell
interaction in neural crest development. Such experiments are effectively
impossible to do with primary neural crest cultures because they rapidly
become a heterogeneous population of cells.

WHAT EPIGENETIC FACTORS INFLUENCE THE DEVELOPMENT OF THE NEURAL CREST?

FGF

The observation that FGF stimulates the proliferation of most of the
neural crest cell lines might be indicative of its activity on primary
neural crest cells. There are a number of other indications that FGF may
have an important role in neural crest development at various stages.
At the migratory stage of neural crest development, FGF has been reported
to have a survival role for neural crest cells (Kalcheim, 1989). If
silastic membranes were inserted between the neural tube and the neural
crest cells of the dorsal root ganglion anlage, there was a selective
death of the neural crest cells which were distally located with respect
to the silastic implants. This suggests that there are factors in the
neural tube which are necessary for the survival of the migrated neural
crest cells. If these silastic membranes were implanted with laminin and
bFGF there was significant survival of the neural crest cells for a period
of over 30 hr after grafting.

In addition to these in vivo studies, the effects of bFGF were
examined in mixed cultures of avian trunk neural crest cells and somite
cells or in pure cultures of neural crest cells (Kalcheim, 1989). Under
the conditions of the assay, that is in a serum-free defined medium, bFGF
was found to act as a survival agent for non-neuronal cells of neural
crest origin (which were identified using the HNK-I antibody).

These studies were followed by a study of the location of FGF in
culture and in situ at the time of neurogenesis and neural crest migration

(Kalcheim and Neufeld, 1990). In quail neural tube cells from E2, which
had been cultured for one day, bFGF was found by immunocytochemistry.
Staining for bFGF was also found in sensory neurons and in some non-
neuronal cells in neural crest cultures. Staining was detected in spinal
cord and ganglionic neurons in situ at E6 and increased towards E10. In
addition bFGF was detected in mesodermal tissues dorsal to the neural
tube as well as in other mesoderm-derived structures. These in situ
immunohistochemical observations were supported by radio-immunoassays
which showed levels of bFGF in spinal cords from as early as E3 and which
increased to a maximum at E10.

    The location of bFGF in situ is entirely consistent with an action
for it in the development of the neural crest. Its reported action as a
survival factor in vivo and in vitro on a subpopulation of non-neuronal
crest cells thus probably reflects this action. However, it is not clear
whether FGF may have other actions on the neural crest cells at the
migratory stage, perhaps in conjunction with other growth factors, given
that it has such a strong proliferative activity on the neuroepithelial
cells of the neural tube, as described above, and that it stimulates the
proliferation of most of the neural crest lines. We are currently
investigating this possibility and have preliminary evidence that the
actions of FGF may be more extensive and that it is probably acting as a
proliferative agent for the majority of neural crest cells.

    Perhaps the best characterized cell lineage within the neural crest
is the sympathoadrenal lineage. There are three cell types in this
lineage, the sympathetic neuron, the adrenal chromaffin cell and a third
cell of an intermediate phenotype, the so called small, intensely
fluorescent cell (SIF cell) (see Patterson, 1990; Anderson, 1989).
Although progenitors of this lineage have not been isolated from neural
crest cultures, they have have been isolated from embryonic adrenal
medulla as well as both embryonic and neonatal sympathetic ganglia. These
progenitors will differentiate into either chromaffin cells or sympathetic
neurons depending on culture conditions (Doupe et al., 1985a & b; Anderson
& Axel, 1986).

    FGF will initiate neuronal differentiation as well as a dependency
of the cells on nerve growth factor (NGF) for their survival.
Glucocorticoids will stimulate the cells to differentiate into mature
chromaffin cells. The evidence for the presence of FGF in the embryo
around the neural tube has been presented above. In addition, FGF has
been located in extracts of nervous tissue such as embryonic brain (Risau
et al., 1988). The possibility that the developing sympathetic neuron
precursors will find a supply of this factor at the site of ganglia is
thus quite reasonable. In the adrenal medulla, on the other hand, when
the precursors migrate into the adrenal gland they are probably subject to
a high concentration of steroids produced in the adrenal cortex.

NGF

    The role of NGF as a survival factor for the sympathetic neurons has
been demonstrated over the past forty years using numerous experimental
systems (see Levi-Montalcini & Angeletti, 1968). It is one of the few
molecules to be shown to have a critical role in vivo for the survival of
sympathetic neurons. The injection of anti-NGF antibodies into newborn
mice results in the destruction of the sympathetic nervous system.
Studies of the mechanism of action of NGF have resulted in it being the
model factor which demonstrates the importance of target derived
neurotrophic factors. In this scheme, the newly differentiated neurons
sprout axons to their target fields, where there is a limited supply of a
target derived survival factor. Only those neurons which have made the

right connections to the target field will obtain this factor and survive. This model provides a part of a mechanism for the control of the development of the nervous system into a three dimensional network.

A number of other factors have been implicated in the development of the sympathoadrenal lineage and in particular the development of sympathetic neurons. IGF-1 stimulates the proliferation of neurons or their precursors in cultures of rat sympathetic ganglia (DiCicco-Bloom et al., 1990). Whether this is a direct effect of IGF-1 on the proliferation of the neuronal precursor cells or whether the IGF-1 is acting principally as a survival agent and there are endogenous proliferative factors in these cultures, as described above for the neuroepithelial cells, is unclear at present. Ciliary neurotrophic factor, conversely, inhibits the proliferation of the neuroblasts and may provide a signal to initiate the differentiation of the cells (Ernsberger et al., 1989).

Other factors have been described which influence the transmitter phenotype of the sympathetic neurons. Most of the sympathetic neurons are adrenergic, except for those which innervate the sweat glands, which are cholinergic. One of the factors which may influence the switching of phenotype of these neurons to cholinergic has recently been purified and is equivalent to LIF (Yamamori et al., 1989). As discussed below, it is beginning to emerge that LIF has multiple activities within the nervous system as well as outside it.

LIF

The factors which control the development of sensory neurons from their precursor cell are not well defined. We have recently shown that leukemia inhibitory factor (LIF) a protein with multiple activities (Gearing et al., 1987; Abe et al., 1986; Yaniamori et al., 1989; Williams et al., 1988; Baumann & Wong, 1989, see above) stimulates the generation of sensory-like neurons in the mouse neural crest (Murphy et al., 1991b). This stimulation of neuron numbers in the neural crest is due either to a stimulation of differentiation of these precursor cells and/or a selective survival of the neuronal precursors.

The total number of neural crest cells in the cultures was increased in the presence of LIF. There were two to three fold more cells in the LIF treated cultures compared to controls. This suggests that LIF is acting as a survival factor for the neural crest cells, as there is no stimulation of proliferation by LIF. We further examined whether LIF may have been influencing the whole population of neural crest cells, by looking at the expression of the marker A2B5 on these cells. As stated above, A2B5 is expressed on a variety of cells in the neural lineage, in particular neural crest derived neurons and their precursors (Girdleston & Weston, 1985), although it is unclear how many of the A2B5 positive cells differentiate into neurons. In mouse neural crest cultures grown in the presence of 10% fetal calf serum alone, 5% of the cells are A2B5 positive, whereas when the cells are grown in the presence of LIF, the number of A2B5 cells increases to 40% of the whole population. This infers that LIF may be influencing a significant proportion of the whole neural crest population, perhaps down a neuronal differentiation pathway. Whether all of these cells are capable of forming neurons is another question. However this finding implies that there is still significant plasticity in the neural crest cells.

LIF does not act only on the sensory precursors, but also on maturing and mature sensory neurons as well. In cultures of dorsal root ganglia isolated at various times through sensory development up until birth, a high proportion of neurons survived in the presence of LIF. Thus

LIF is also a neuron survival factor, like NGF. Binding studies on the DRG cultures from P2 mice showed that greater than 60% of the neurons bound significant amounts of ^{125}I-LIF, which was completely inhibited by the addition of cold LIF. Furthermore, there was negligible cold-inhibitable binding of ^{125}I-LIF to non-neuronal cells in the culture. Thus, at this age, the only cells capable of responding to LIF in the DRG are the sensory neurons.

These results indicate that LIF can act throughout embryonic sensory neuron development in vitro. In neural crest cultures, it may act to stimulate neuronal differentiation and/or survival of the sensory precursors. As stated above, the effects of LIF on the bulk population of neural crest cells in the induction of the A2B5 antigen suggest that it may be acting directly to stimulate the differentiation of the neural crest cells, whether or not it is acting as a survival agent for the sensory precursors.

NGF also has a clear role in the development of sensory neurons but probably at a later stage of development. The observation that anti-NGF given via the placenta results in almost complete ablation of the sensory nervous system is proof enough of this. NGF is most likely acting as a target derived neurotrophic factor (Purves et al., 1988) in the same fashion as described for the development of the sympathetic nervous system. An alternate or additional explanation is that both NGF and LIF are required or act synergistically during development and the removal of either results in the neuronal loss. Evidence for this concept has recently been derived from in vitro experiments that indicate that endogenous NGF is required for maximum survival of embryonic sensory neurons in the presence of LIF.

One of the essential criteria to be fulfilled by a neurotrophic factor is that there appears to be a requirement for factors taken up by the nerve terminals to be retrogradely transported back to the neural perikarya. The transport of the neurotrophic factor is the signal from the target tissue to the neuron that results in neuronal survival (Hendry et al., 1974). Having demonstrated the presence of LIF receptors on sensory neurons in vitro, we investigated whether receptor mediated uptake of LIF would result in retrogade transport to the sensory neuron soma.

Adult mice were injected in the skin or muscle and in those animals injected in the skin of the foot, there was a significant accumulation of radioactivity in the sensory ganglia centered on lumbar ganglion 4 (L4). In newborn mice there was a greater accumulation of radioactivity after both leg and foot injections. The accumulation of radioactivity after skin injection again was centered on L4. Autoradiographic examination of histological sections through L4 ganglia from both adult and newborn animals injected with ^{125}I-LIF into the footpad revealed the presence of radioactive material in a subpopulation of neurons. The number of neurons with significant number of grains is between 5-10% of the population. Again there is no evidence of radioactivity associated with non-neuronal cells.

STEEL FACTOR

The melanocyte lineage is apparently determined early in development in the mouse and there is evidence that thirty-four primordial melanoblasts are lined up in pairs longitudinally during neural crest formation (Mintz, 1967). From related studies in the chick, the melanoblasts then undergo rapid proliferation and migrate laterally to the skin (Rawles, 1944; Weston, 1963) where they differentiate into mature melanocytes. The processes which control the proliferation, migration and differentiation of these melanocyte precursors are not clearly understood. However two classes of mouse mutants point the way for the involvement of a newly characterised growth factor in this process. These are the White dominant-spotting (W) and Steel (Sl) mice. Phenotypically, mice homozygous at either of these alleles are blacked-eyed white, anaemic and sterile; some of the mutations result in lethality (reviewed in Silvers, 1979; Russel, 1979; Geissler et al., 1981).

An analysis of the mutations in these mice has revealed a complementary molecular relationship between the two alleles. Firstly, it was found that W allele coded for a growth factor receptor-like tyrosine kinase and which was identical to the proto-oncogene c-kit (Geissler et al., 1988; Chabot et al., 1988). Subsequently, the ligand for c-kit was purified and cloned and was found to be encoded by the Sl locus (Anderson et al., 1990; Williams et al., 1990; Martin et al., 1990; Zsebo et al., 1990a & b; Huang et al., 1990). Thus, this Sl factor and the c-kit receptor are strongly implicated in melanogenesis as well as germ cell production and in haemopoiesis. Because of this range of involvement the Sl factor has been variously called mast cell gowth factor, stem cell factor, and the c-kit ligand.

We tested whether Sl factor could stimulate the production of melanocytes in our neural crest cultures by adding it at the time of plating of the neural tubes. However the presence of Sl factor had no observable effect on the cultures and in particular no melanocytes arose in these cultures. Thus, it must concluded that Sl factor alone is not sufficient to stimulate the differentiation of melanocytes from their precursors in the neural crest.

In other studies, the phorbol ester drug, TPA, has been shown to influence the development of melanocytes. Human melanocytes will grow for long periods when stimulated with TPA (Eisenger & Marko, 1982; Halaban et al., 1983). Further, TPA appears to stimulate the development of melanocytes in cultures of avian dorsal root ganglia (Ciment et al., 1986). Thus, we investigated the effects of TPA on the development of melanocytes in mouse neural crest cultures after a period of two weeks. Invariably, the melanocytes appeared on the neuroepithelial sheet which grew out from the neural tube.

Given that TPA stimulates melanocyte differentiation in the neural crest cultures, it was possible that this differentiation could be influenced by Sl factor. We added Sl factor and TPA to the neural crest cultures to test this and found an approximately 10 fold increase in melanocyte numbers compared to cultures with TPA alone. Thus Sl factor is acting with TPA in the induction of melanocytes.

The synergy between TPA and Sl factor in the production of melanocytes may be a direct synergistic effect of the two factors acting on the same cell to produce melanocytes. Alternatively, Sl factor may act on the melanocyte precursors to stimulate division and/or survival but not act as a differentiating agent. These possibilities could partially be tested by pulsing the cultures first with Sl factor, then washing it out and adding TPA to separate temporally the activities of Sl factor and TPA. The results of these experiments indicate Sl factor is mainly acting on the melanocyte precursors but not as a differentiation agent. That there is a requirement for added Sl factor early in the culture period in these pulsing experiments indicates that Sl factor is acting as a survival agent for the melanoblasts. The reason that melanocytes arise in cultures containing TPA from the start might be that there is a limited amount of endogenous Sl factor in the cultures. This is quite possible as there is

expression of S1 factor in the neural tube during this time in vivo
(Matsui et al., 1990).

Presumably, TPA is mimicking a function normally found in vivo at
the time and place of melanocyte differentiation, which is postnatally in
the skin. TPA activates the protein kinase C pathway and so may be
activating any number of growth factors, hormones, cell surface molecules
or other types of cell activation pathways. One possible hormone
implicated in melanocyte differentiation is melanocyte stimulating
hormone. However, we have found no activity of MSH in the neural crest
cultures either in the presence or absence of S1 factor.

CONCLUDING REMARKS

Clearly, there must be many factors involved in the neural crest
differentiation process. The factors described so far are only a few of
all the factors which are required to determine this specificity. What
factors influence the enteric nervous system, the parasympathetic nervous
system, glial cells in the PNS, and the myriad of cells arising in the
facial regions? While there are suggestions that these cell types are
also influenced by soluble peptide growth factors, the identity of these
factors is not known. Perhaps, some of these factors are already purified
and cloned, but their roles in this system have yet to be elucidated. In
addition, cell surface molecules, extracellular matrix molecules and
steroids, such as retinoic acid, are also likely to contribute to this
process. The other key questions which have not been addressed here are:
How do these factors work? What genes are being regulated by the factors?
How do they interact with genes that regulate DNA binding proteins? The
search for the key regulatory genes in this process is just beginning. It
is this interaction between growth factors and the transcriptional
regulators that probably leads to the harmony of cell differentiation.

ACKNOWLEDGEMENTS

The work cited from our laboratory was supported by grants from the
National Health and Medical Research Council of Australia, the A.L.S
Society, Australia, the M.S Society, Australia, the A.M.R.A.D corporation
and the Australian Government Cooperative Research Centres Scheme.

REFERENCES

Abe, E., Tanaka, H., Ishimi, Y., Miyaura, C., Hayashi, T., Nagasawa, H.,
    Tomida, M., Yamaguchi, Y., Hozumi, M. and Suda, T. (1986)
    Differentiation-inducing factor purified from conditioned medium of
    mitogen-treated spleen cell cultures stimulates bone resorption.
    Proc. Natl. Acad. Sci. USA. 83:5958-5962.
Abney, E.R., Bartlett, P.F. and Raff, M.C. (1981) Astrocytes, ependymal
    cells, and oligodendrocytes develop on schedule in dissociated cell
    cultures of embryonic rat brain. Dev. Biol. 83:301-310.
Anderson, D.J. (1989) The neural crest cell lineage problem:
    Neuropoiesis? Neuron. 3:1-12.
Anderson, D.J. and Axel, R. (1985) Molecular probes for the development
    and plasticity of neural crest derivatives. Cell 42: 649-662.
Anderson, D.J. and Axel, R. (1986) A bipotential neuroendocrine precursor
    whose choice of cell fate is determined by NGF and glucocorticoids.
    Cell 47:1079-1090.
Anderson, D.M., Lyman, S.D., Baird, A., Wignall, J.M., Eisenman, J.,
    Rauch, D., March, C.J., Boswell, H.S., Gimpel, S.D., Cosman, D.,

Williams, D.E. (1990) Molecular cloning of mast cell growth factor, a hematopoietin that is active in both membrane bound and soluble forms. <u>Cell</u> 63:235-243.

Anderton, B.H., Breinburg, D., Downes, M.J., Green, P.J., Tomlinson, B.E., Ulrich, J., Wood, J.N., Kahn, J. (1982) Monoclonal antibodies show that neurofibrillary tangles and neurofilaments share antigenic determinants. <u>Nature</u> 298:84-86.

Angevine, J.B. and Sidman, R.L. (1961) Autoradiographic study of cell migration during histogenesis of cerebral cortex in the mouse. <u>Nature</u> 192:766-768.

Bailey, K.A., Wycherley, K and Bartlett, P.F. (1987) Identification of neural precursor cells by their ability to express histocompatability antigens. <u>Neurosci. Letts</u> 27:51.

Barbin, G., Manthorpe, M. and Varon, S.J. (1984) Purification of the chick eye ciliary neuronotrophic factor. <u>J. Neurochem.</u> 43:1468.

Barde, Y. (1989) Trophic factors and neuronal survival. <u>Neuron.</u> 2: 1525-1534.

Baroffio, A., Dupin, E. and Le Douarin, N.M. (1988) Clone forming ability and differentiation potential of migratory neural crest cells. <u>Proc. Natl. Acad. Sci. USA</u> 85:5325-5329.

Bartlett, P.F., Noble, M.D., Pruss, R.M., Rat, M.C., Rattray, S. and Willimas, C.A. (1981) Rat neural antigen-2 (Ran-2): A cell surface antigen on astrocytes, ependymal cells, Mueller cells and lepto-meninges defined by a monoclonal antibody. <u>Brain Res.</u> 204: 339-351.

Bartlett, P.F., Reid, H.H., Bailey, K.A. and Bernard, O. (1988) Immortalization of mouse neural precursor cells by the c-myc oncogene. <u>Proc. Natl. Acad. Sci. USA</u> 85:3255-3259.

Bartlett, P.F., Kerr, R.S.C. and Bailey K.A. (1989) Expression of NMC antigens in the central nervous system. <u>Transp. Proc.</u> 21:3163-3165.

Bartlett, P.F., Rosenfeld J.V., Harvey, A. and Kerr R.S.C. (1990) Allograft rejection overcome by immunoselection of neuronal precursor cells. <u>Prog. in Brain Res.</u> 82:153-160.

Baumann, H. and Wong, G.G. (1989) Hepatocyte-stimulating factor IH shares structural and functional identity with leukemia-inhibitory factor. <u>J. Immunol.</u> 143:1163-1167.

Bernard, O., Reid, H.H. and Bartlett, P.F. (1989) The role of c-myc and N-myc proto-oncogenes in the immortalisation of neural precursors. <u>J. Neurosci. Res.</u> 24:9-20.

Bronner-Fraser, M. and Fraser, S.E. (1988) Cell lineage analysis reveals multipotency of some avian neural crest cells. <u>Nature</u> 335:161-164.

Cepko, C. (1988) Retrovirus vectors and their applications in neurobiology. <u>Neuron.</u> 1:345-353.

Cepko, C.L. (1989) Immortalisation of neural cell lines via retrovirus-mediated oncogene transduction. <u>Ann. Rev. Neurosci.</u> 12:47-55.

Chabot, B., Stephenson, D.A., Chapman, V.M., Besmer, P. and Bemstein, A. (1988) The proto-oncogene c-kit encoding a transmembrane tyrosine kinase receptor maps to the mouse W locus. <u>Nature</u> 335: 88-89.

Chisaka, O. and Capechi, M. (1991) Regionally resticted developmental defects resulting from targeted disruption of the mouse homeobox gene Hox-1.5. <u>Nature</u> 350:473-479.

Ciment, G., Glimelius, B., Nelson, D.M. and Weston, J.A. (1986) Reversal of a developmental restriction of neural crest-derived cells of avian embryos by a phorbol ester drug. <u>Dev. Biol.</u> 118: 392-398.

Cohen, J., Burne, J.F., Winter, J. and Bartlett, P.F. (1986) Retinal ganglion cells lose response to laminin with maturation. <u>Nature</u> 322:465-467.

Copeland, N.G., Gilbert, D.J., Cho, B.C., Donovan, P.J., Jenkins, N.A., Cosman, D., Anderson, D., Lyman, S.D. and Williams, D.E. (1990) Mast cell gowth factor maps near the steel locus on mouse chromosome 10 and is deleted in a number of steel alleles. <u>Cell</u> 63:175-183.

Davids, M., Loppnow, B., Tiedemann, H. and Tiedemann, H. (1987) Rouxs
    Arch. Dev. Biol. 196:137-140.
Dicicco-Bloom, E., Townes-Anderson, E. and Black, I.B. (1990) Neuroblast
    mitosis in dissociated culture: Regulation and relationship to
    differentiation. J. Cell. Biol. 110:2073-2086.
Doupe, A.J., Patterson, P.H. and Landis, S.C. (1985a). Environmental
    influences in the development of neural crest derivatives:
    Glucocorticoids, growth factors and chromaffin cell plasticity. J.
    Neurosci. 5:2119-2142.
Doupe, A.J., Patterson, P.H. and Landis, S.C. (1985b) Small intensely
    fluorescent (SEF) cells in culture: Role of glucocorticoids and
    growth factors in their development and phenotypic interconversions
    with other neural crest derivatives. J. Neurosci. 5:2143-2160.
Drago, J., Murphy, M., Bailey, K.A. and Bartlett, P.F. (1991) A method
    for the isolation of purified muiine neuroepithelial cells from the
    developing mouse brain. J. Neurosci. Methods. 37:251-256.
Drago, J., Murphy, M., Carroll, S.M., Harvey, R.P. and Bartlett, P.F.
    (1991) Fibroblast growth factor-mediated proliferation of central
    nervous system precursors depends on endogenous production of
    insulin-like gowth factor 1. Proc. Natl. Acad. Sci. USA 88:2199-
    2203.
Drago, J., Nurcombe, V. and Bartlett, P.F. (1991c) Neural cell
    differenfiation is mediated through the long arm of the laminin
    molecule. Exp. Cell. Res. 192:256-265.
Dupin, E., Barofflo, A., Dulac, C., Cameron-Curry, P. and Le Douarin, N.M.
    (1990) Schwann-cell differentiafion in clonal cultures of the
    neural crest, as evidenced by the anti-Schwann cell myelin protein
    monoclonal antibody. Proc. Natl. Acad. Sci. USA 87:1119-1123
Eisenger, M. and Marko, O. (1982) Selective proliferation of normal human
    melanocytes in vitro in the presence of phorbol ester and cholera
    toxin. Proc. Natl. Acad. Sci. USA 79:2018-2022.
Emsberger, U., Sendtner, M. and Rohrer, H. (1989) Proliferation and
    differentiation of embryonic chick sympathetic neurons: Effects of
    ciliary neurotrphic factor. Neuron. 2:1275-1284.
Frederiksen, K., Jat, P.S., Levy, D. and McKay, R. (1988) Immortalization
    of precursor cells from the mammalian CNS. Neuron. 1:439-448.
Furness, J.B., Costa, M.C. Gibbons, I.L., Lewellyn-Smith, I.J. and Oliver
    J.R. (1985) Neurochemically similar myenteric and subraucous
    neurons directly traced to the mucosa of the small intestine. Cell
    Tiss. Res. 241:155-163.
Gearing, D.P., Gough, N.M., King, J.A., Hilton, D.J., Nicola, N.A.,
    Simpson, R.J., Nice, E.C., Kelso, A. and Metcalf, D. (1987)
    Molecular cloning and expression of CDNA encoding a murine myeloid
    leukaemia inhibitory factor (LIF). EMBO J. 6:3995-4002.
Geissler, E.N., McFarland, E.C. and Russell, E.S. (1981) Analysis of the
    pleiotropism at the dominant white-spotting (W) locus of the house
    mouse: A description of ten new W alleles. Genetics 97: 337-361.
Geissler, E.N., Ryan, M.A. and Housman, D.E. (1988) The dominant-white
    spotting (W) locus of the mouse encodes the c-kit proto-oncogene.
    Cell 55:185-192.
Girdleston, J. and Weston, J.A. (1985) Identification of early neuronal
    subpopulations in avian neural crest cell cultures. Dev. Biol.
    109:274-287.
Halaban, R., Pomerantz, S.H., Marshall, S, Lambert, D.T. and Lemer, A.B.
    (1983) The regulation of tyrosinase in human melanocytes gown in
    culture. J. Cell. Biol. 97:480-488.
Halaban, R., Langdon, R, Birchall, N., Cuono, C., Baird, A., Scott, G.,
    Moellman, G. and McGuire, J. (1988) Basic fibroblast growth factor
    from human keratinocytes is a natural mitogen for melanocytes. J.
    Cell. Biol. 107:1611-1619.
Hendry, I.A., Stockel, K., Thoenen, H. and Iversen, L.L. (1974) The

retrograde axonal transport of nerve growth factor. <u>Brain Res.</u> 68:103-121.

Hilton, D.J., Nicola, N.A. and Metcalf, D. (1988) Purification of a murine leukemia inhibitory factor from Krebs Ascites cells. <u>Analytical Biochem.</u> 173:359-367.

Huang, E., Nocka, K., Beier, D.R., Chu, T-Y., Buck, J., Lahm, H-W., Wellner, D., Leder, P. and Besmer, P. (1990) The haematopoietic growth factor KL is encoded by the SL locus and is the ligand of the c-kit recptor, the gene product of the W locus. <u>Cell</u> 63:225-233.

Hunt, P., Gulisano, M., Cook, M., Sham, H-H., Faiella, A., Wilkinson, D., Boncinelli, E. and Krurfflauf, R. (1991) A distinct Hox code for the branchial region ot the vertebrate head. <u>Nature</u> 353:861-864.

Ingham, P.W. (1988) The molecular genetics of embryonic pattern formation in Drosophila. <u>Nature</u> 335:25-34.

Ito, K. and Takeuchi, T. (1984) The differentiation of the neural crest cells of the mouse embryo. <u>J. Embryol. Exp. Morph.</u> 84:49-62.

Jessen, K.R and Mirsky (1983) Astrocyte like glia in the peripheral nervous system: An immunohistochemical study of enteric glia. <u>J. Neurosci.</u> 3:2206-2218.

Kalcheim, C. (1989) Basic fibroblast growth factor stimulates survival of non-neuronal cells developing from trunk neural crest. <u>Dev. Biol.</u> 134:1-10.

Kalcheim, C. and Gandreau, M. (1988) Brain-derived neurotrophic factor stimulates survival and neuronal differentiation in cultured avian neural crest. <u>Dev. Brain Res.</u> 41:79-86.

Kalcheim, C. and Neufeld, G. (1990) Expression of basic fibroblast growth factor in the nervous system of developing embryos. <u>Development</u> 109:203-215.

Kessler, J.A. and Black, I.B. (1980) Nerve growth factor stimulates the development of substance P in the sensory ganglia. <u>Proc. Nad. Acad. Sci. USA</u> 77:649-652.

Le Douarin, N.M. (1982) The Neural Crest. Cambridge Univ. Press.

Le Douarin, N.M. (1986) Cell line segregation during peripheral nervous system ontogeny. <u>Science</u> 231:1516-1522.

Le Douarin, N.M. and Smith, J. (1988) Development of the peripheral nervous sytem from the neural crest. <u>Ann. Rev. Cell. Biol.</u> 4:375-404.

Le Douarin, N.M. and Tiellett (1973) Migration of neural crest cells to the wall of the digestive tract in avian embryo. <u>J. Embryol. Exp. Morphol.</u> 30:31-48.

Levi-Montalcini R. and Angeletti, P.U. (1968) The nerve growth factor. <u>Physiol. Rev.</u> 48:534-569.

Lumsden, A. and Keynes, R (1989) Segmental patterns of neuronal development in the chick hindbrain. <u>Nature</u> 337:424-428.

Lumsden, A (1990) The cellular basis of segmentation in the developing hindbrain. <u>Trends in Neurosci.</u> 13:329-334.

Mangold, O. (1933) <u>Naturwissenschaften</u> 21:761-766.

Martin, F.H., Suggs, S.V., Langley, K.E., Lu, H.S., Ting, J., Okino, K.H., Monis, C.F., Mc Niece, I.K., Jacobsen, F.W., Mendiaz, E.A., Birkett, N.C., Smith, K.A., Johnson, M.J., Parker, V.P., Flores, J.C., Patel, A.C., Fisher, E.F., EferjavecJ, H.O, Herrers, C.J., Wypych, J., Sachdev, R.K., Pope, J.A., Leslie, I., Wen, D., Lin, C-H., Cupples, R.L. and Zsebo, K.M. (1990) Primary structure and functional expression of rat and human stem cell factor DNA'S. <u>Cell</u> 63:203-211.

Matsui, Y., Zsebo, K.M. and Hogan, B.M. (1990) Embryonic expression of a haematopoietic growth factor encoded by the S1 locus and the ligand for c-kit. <u>Nature</u> 347:667-669.

Mintz, B. (1967) Gene control of mammalian pigmentary differentiation. 1. Clonal origin of melanocytes. <u>Proc. Natl. Acad. Sci. USA</u> 58:344-351.

Murphy, M., Drago, J. and Bartlett P.F. (1990) Fibroblast growth factor stimulates the proliferation and differentiation of neural precursor cells in vitro. J. Neurosci. Res. 25:463-475.

Murphy, M., Bernard, O., Reid, K. and Bartlett, P.F. (1991). Cell lines derived from mouse neural crest are representative of cells at various stages of differentiation. J. Neurobiol. 22:522-535.

Murphy, M., Reid, K., Hilton, D.J. and Bartlett, P.F. (1991) Generation of sensory neurons is stimulated by leukemia inhibitory factor. Proc. Natl. Acad. Sci. USA 88:3498-3501.

Newgeen, D.F., Jahnke, I., Allan, I.J. and Gibbons, I.L. (1980) Differentiation of sympathetic and enteric neurons of the fowl embryo in grafts to the chorio-allantoic membrane. Cell. Tissue Res. 208:1-19.

Nexo, E., Hollenberg, M.D., Figuero, A. and Pratt, R.M. (1980) Detection of epidertnal growth factor-urogastrone and its receptor during fetal mouse development. Proc. Nat. Acad. Sci. USA 77:2782-2785.

Noden, D.M. (1978) The control of avian cephalic neural crest cytodifferentiation. Dev. Biol. 67:296-312.

Patterson, P.H. (1990) Control of cell fate in a vertebrate neurogenic lineage. Cell 62:1035-1038.

Pessac, B., Ziller, C., Vautrion, J., Girard, A. and Calothy, G. (1985) Quail neural crest cells transformed by Rous sarcoma virus can be established into differentiating permanent cell cultures. Dev. Brain Res. 20:235-239.

Purves, D., Snyder, W.D., Voyvodic, J.T. (1988) Trophic regulation of nerve cell morphology and innervation in the autonomic nervous system. Nature 336:123-128.

Raff, M.C. (1989) Glial cell diversification in the rat optic nerve. Science 243:1450-1455.

Rat, M.C., Abney, E.R. and Miller, R.H. (1984) Two glial cell lineages diverge prenatally in rat optic nerve. Dev. Biol. 106: 53-64.

Raff, M.C., Miller, R.H. and Noble, M. (1983) A glial progenitor cell that develops in vitro into an astrocyte or an oligodendrocyte depending on culture medium. Nature 303:390-396.

Rawles M.E. (1944) The migration of melanoblasts after hatching into pigment-free skin grafts of the common fowl. Physiol. Zool. 17: 167-183.

Reh, T.A., Nagy, T. and Gretton, H. (1987) Retinal pigmented epithelial cells induced to transdifferentiate to neurons by laminin. Nature 330:68-71.

Risau, W., Gautschi-Sova, P. and Bohlen, P. (1988) Endothelial cell growth factors in embryonic and adult chick brain are related to human acidic fibroblast growth factor. EMBO J. 7:959-962.

Russel, E.S. (1979) Hereditary anemias of the mouse: A review for geneticists. Adv. Genet. 20:357-459.

Ryder, E.F., Snyder, E.Y. and Cepko, C.L. (1990) Establishment and characterization of multipotent neural cell lines using retrovirus vector-mediated oncogene transfer. J. Neurobiol. 21: 356-375.

Saleh, M. and Bartlett P.F. (1989) Evidence from neuronal heterokaryons for a transacting factor suppressing Thy-I expression during neuronal development. J. Neurosci. Res. 23: 406-415.

Sara, V.R., Hall, K., Rodeck, C.H. and Wetterberg, L. (1981) Human embryonic somatomedin. Proc. Nat. Acad. Sci. USA 78:3175-3179.

Sieber-Blum, M. (1989) Commitment of neural crest cells to the sensory lineage. Science 243:1608-1610.

Sieber-Blum, M and Cohen, A.M. (1980) Clonal analysis of quail neural crest cells: They are pluripotent and differentiate in vitro in the absence of noncrest cells. Dev. Biol. 80:96-106.

Silvers, W.K. (1979) White-spotting, patch and rump-white; steel, flexed tail, splotch and variant-waddler. In the coat colors of mice: A model for gene action and interaction (New York: Springer-Verlag), pp. 206-241.

Temple, S. (1989) Division and differentiation of isolated CNS blast
    cells in microculture. Nature 340:471-473.
Tuckett, S.F. and Morriss-Kay, G.M. (1986) The distribution of
    fibronectin, laminin and entactin in the neurulating rat embryo
    studied by indirect immunoflourescence. J. Embryol. Exp. Morph.
    94:95-112.
Tumer, D.L. and Cepko, C.L. (1987) A common progenitor for neurons and
    glia persists in rat retina late in development. Nature 328: 131-
    136.
Weston, J.A. (1963) A radioautographic analysis of the migration and
    localization of trunk neural crest cells in the chick. Dev. Biol.
    6:279-310.
Weston, J.A. (1986) Phenotypic diversification in neural crest-derived
    cells: The time and stability of commitment during early
    development. Current Topics in Developmental Biol. 20:195-210.
Wetts, R. and Fraser, S.S. (1988) Multipotent precursors can give rise to
    all major cell types in the frog retina. Science 239: 1142-1145.
Wilkinson, D.G. and Krumlauf, R. (1990) Molecular approaches to the
    segmentation of the hindbrain. Trends in Neurosci. 13:335-339.
Williama, D.E., Eisenman, J., Baird, A., Rauch, C., Van Ness, K.V., March,
    C.J., Park, L.S., Martin, U., Mochizuki, D.Y., Boswell H.S.,
    Burgess, G.S., Cosman, D. and Lyman, S.D. (1990) Identification of
    a ligand for the c-kit proto-oncogene. Cell 63:167-174.
Williams, R.L., Hilton, D.J., Pease, S., Willson, T.A., Stewart, C.L.,
    Gearing, D.P., Wagner, E.F., Metcalf, D., Nicola, N.A. and Gough,
    N.M. (1988). Myeloid leukaemia inhibitory factor maintains the
    developmental potential of embryonic stem cells. Nature 336:684-
    687.
Wong, G.H.W., Bartlett, P.F., Clark-Lewis, I. and Schrader, J.W. (1984)
    Inducible expression of H-2 and la antigens on brain cells. Nature
    310:688-691.
Yamamori, T., Fukada, K., Aebersold, R., Korsching, S., Fann, M-J. and
    Patterson, P.H. The cholinergic neuronal differentiation factor
    from heart cells is identical to leukemia inhibitory factor.
    Science 241:1412-1416.
Yen, S-H. and Fields, K.L. (1981) Antibodies to neurofilament, glial
    filament and fibroblast intermediate filament proteins bind to
    different cell types of the nervous system. J. Cell. Biol. 88: 115-
    126.
Ziller, C., Dupin, E., Brazeau, P., Paulin, D. and Le Douarin, N.M. (1983)
    Early segregation of a neuronal precursor cell line in the neural
    crest as revealed by culture in a chemically defined medium. Cell
    32:627-638.
Ziller, C., Fauquet, M., Kalcheim, C., Smith, J. and Le Douarin, N.M.
    (1987) Cell lineages in peripheral nervous system ontogeny:
    Medium-induced modulation of neuronal phenotypic expression in
    neural crest cell cultures. Dev. Biol. 120:101-111.
Zsebo, K.M., Williams, D.A., Geissler, E.N., Broudy, V.C., Martin F.H.,
    Atkins, H.L., Hsu, R.Y., Birkett, N.C., Okino, K.H., Murdock, D.C.,
    Jacobsen, F.W., Langley, K.E., Smith, K.A., Takeishi, T., Cattanach,
    B.M., Galli, S.J. and Suggs, S.V. (1990a) Stem cell factor is
    encoded at the S1 locus of the mouse and is the ligand for the c-kit
    tyrosine kinase receptor. Cell 63:213-223.
Zsebo, K.M., Wypych, J., McNiece, I.K., Lu, H.S., Smith., K.A., Karkare,
    S.B., Sachdev, R.K., Yuschenkoff, V.N., Birkett, N.C., Williams,
    L.R., Satyagal, V.B., Tung, W., Bosselman, R.A., Mendiaz, E.A. and
    Langley, K.E. (1990b) Identification, purification and biological
    characterization of Haematopoietic stem cell factor from Buffalo rat
    liver-condtioned medium. Cell 63:195-201.

POLYSIALIC ACID AS A REGULATOR OF CELL-CELL INTERACTIONS

DURING MUSCLE INNERVATION

Urs Rutishauser

Department of Genetics
Case Western Reserve University
School of Medicine
Cleveland OH 44106

INTRODUCTION

The study of cell-cell interactions in tissue formation has spanned several decades, with particularly rapid progress in recent years (for review see Rutishauser and Jessell, 1988). A fundamental hypothesis throughout has been that these interactions reflect specific molecular complementarity mediated by distinct components at the cell surface. In addition, it is generally assumed that the developmental control of interactions occurs through regulation of expression of the molecules directly involved. Thus many studies have interpreted the function of a particular cell interaction molecule on the basis of where and when it is detected in an embryo. That is, the burden of regulating cell-cell interactions is largely given to the control of genes that encode the relevant receptors.

Regulation of cell-cell interactions by NCAM and PSA

Is control of such genes sufficient to explain the exquisite pattern of cell-cell interactions that occurs during the formation of a tissue or the guidance and targeting of axons? Recent work from our laboratory on the neural cell adhesion molecule (NCAM) and its unusual polysialic acid moiety (PSA), suggest that regulation of specific ligands is only one aspect of the developmental control of cell-cell interactions. These studies suggest that at least some cell contact-dependent phenomena are a multistep process in which the specific or recognition event requires a prior permissive adhesion event, mediated by a general adhesion system, which brings the two membranes into intimate apposition. We have represented this idea in the form of a model (Figure 1) by which NCAM and its PSA can serve respectively as positive and negative regulators of cell apposition, and thereby affect a wide variety of interactions (Rutishauser et al., 1988).

In this chapter, we will focus on the dual role of NCAM and PSA during the innervation of muscle. These studies suggest that while adhesions mediated by NCAM and another adhesion molecule called L1 are important factors in innervation, it is the

Development of the Central Nervous System in Vertebrates
Edited by S.C. Sharma and A.M. Goffinet, Plenum Press, New York, 1992

Changes in PSA expression are linked to normal patterns of innervation in vivo (Landmesser et al., 1990)

As described above, the patterns of innervation are distinct for fast and slow muscle regions. If NCAM and L1 are major factors in establishing these patterns, one would expect that differences could be detected in the function of these two molecules. However, the relative levels of NCAM and L1 expression within and between fast and slow regions are not detectably different. On the other hand, there is considerably more PSA on axons in the fast region than in the slow.

A straightforward interpretation of this correlation is that high levels of PSA limit axon-axon interactions and thereby allow environmental cues to attract fibers toward the fast region and to branch out over the muscle surface. Conversely, the lower levels of PSA on slow fibers produces thick fascicles that continue to grow along muscle fibers, with new growth cones occasionally sprouting off into surrounding areas. To test this hypothesis, a PSA-specific endoneuraminidase (Rutishauser et al., 1985) was infused into developing limbs, thereby removing all detectable PSA from the tissue. As predicted, in the absence of PSA, all axons grew with in the manner characteristic of the slow region.

Another change in fasciculation during development is a progressive tightening of bundles. This increase in fiber-fiber interaction also is correlated with a loss of axonal PSA rather than with altered NCAM or L1 expression, and can be mimicked in vivo by infusion of endoneuraminidase.

Blockade of neuromuscular synaptic activity causes both sprouting and up-regulation of PSA (Landmesser et al., 1990)

The ability of synaptic activity to remodel the morphology of presynaptic elements is a property of many neural systems. A frequent feature of this plasticity is the formation of numerous axonal sprouts and branchings upon exposure to a neurotoxin, for example curare in the neuromuscular system. As above, the question is raised as to the molecular mechanism underlying the increased sprouting. Once again the relevant component appears to be PSA. That is, curare causes a dramatic increase in PSA levels without a significant change in NCAM or L1 expression.

The causal relationship between activity-dependent sprouting and PSA is further indicated by the fact that co-adminstration of curare and the PSA-specific neuraminidase results in a nearly complete reversal of the changes produced by activity blockade. Consistent with the mechanisms proposed in Figs. 1(bottom) and 2, The inhibition of axon-axon interaction with antibodies against L1 (but not against NCAM) both mimics the effects of curare and reverses the effects of the neuraminidase.

Summary and implications. Figure 3 depicts the relationship between elements and events that influence muscle innervation. This schematic illustrates the pivotal role played by PSA, and the common basis for understanding both developmental and neurotoxin-induced differences in the pattern of axon growth, bundling and sprouting.

26

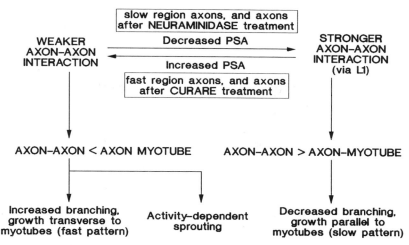

Figure 3. Relationships between cellular and molecular events that contribute to muscle innervation.

How general is this overall mechanism? All of the work reviewed here work was carried out on the neuromuscular system of the chick hindlimb. Although L1 is widely expressed on axonal surfaces and NCAM is present on many neuronal and non-neuronal cells, different axons are likely to be influenced by a variety of other positive (and negative) cell-cell interactions. Thus the specific players may change, and the consequences may even be reversed.

However, the abundance of PSA on many types of growing vertebrate axons, and its widespread influence on cell-cell interactions, suggests that this parameter may be common to many types of axonal behavior. Furthermore, PSA-mediated regulation may be applicable not only to development, but also to repair and possibly some functions of the adult nervous system. With respect to the latter, it must be noted that PSA is in general lost from the vertebrate nervous system as it matures. The questions are raised, therefore, whether the ability to effect repair is in part related to the ability to reexpress this carbohydrate, and why certain parts of the brain (such as olfactory bulb and hypothalamus) maintain its presence.

REFERENCES

Landmesser, L., Dahm, L., Schultz, K. and Rutishauser, U., 1988, Distinct roles for adhesion molecules during innervation of embryonic chick muscle., Dev. Biol., 103:645-670.
Landmesser, L., Dahm, L., Tang J. and Rutishauser, U., 1990, Polysialic acid as a regulator of intramuscular nerve branching during embryonic development., Neuron, 4:655-667.
Rutishauser, U., Watanabe, M., Silver, J., Troy, F.A. and Vimr, E.R., 1985, Specific alteration of NCAM-mediated cell adhesion by an endoneuraminidase., J. Cell Biol., 101:1842-1849.

Rutishauser, U., Acheson, A., Hall, A.K., Mann, D.M. and Sunshine, J., 1988, The neural cell adhesion molecule (NCAM) as a regulator of cell-cell interactions, Science 240:53-57.

Rutishauser, U. and Jessell, T. 1988. Cell adhesion molecules in vertebrate neural development, Physiological Reviews, 68(3):819-857.

THE O-2A CELL LINEAGE: CELLULAR INTERACTIONS INFLUENCING THE
CHOICE OF THE DIFFERENTIATION ROUTE OF BIPOTENTIAL GLIAL
PROGENITORS

Giulio Levi and Cristina Agresti

Istituto Superiore di Sanità, Neurobiology Section
Laboratory of Pathophysiology
Viale Regina Elena, 299 – 00161 Roma, Italy

INTRODUCTION

In the present report we would like to discuss some
recent data, part of which from our laboratory, on the origin
of macroglial cells. In particular, we would like to deal
with the concept that epigenetic factors may play a crucial
role in determining the differentiation destiny of immature
glial progenitor cells, and that among the epigenetic factors
cell-cell interactions seem to have a critical importance.

Before discussing this, however, I must make a short
introduction for those of you who are not familiar with the
field. Up to until recently, the prevailing idea (which is
still held by a discrete group of investigators) was that
astrocytes, oligodendrocytes and neurons have completely
separate lineages (see: Wood and Bunge, 1984, for review of
older studies; Luskin et al., 1988 and Vaysse and Goldman for
more recent approaches to the problem). Each of them would
derive from progenitor cells which, in turn, derive from
pluripotent stem cells. In the present report I will deal
with the alternative idea, supported by other investigators,
that one subpopulation of astrocytes and oligodendrocytes
share a common progenitor cell, different from the progenitor
of the major astrocytes population (Raff et al., 1983a).
Before entering into the topic of glial cell lineage, however, I think that it is useful to spend some time in the
description of the above mentioned astrocytes subpopulations.
This will also help to better understand the cell lineage
problem.

TYPE-1 AND TYPE-2 ASTROCYTES

Cell culture studies published in the last 8 years,
first by the group of Martin Raff, then by our own group and
then by others, have provided evidence for the existence, in
the rat CNS, of two subpopulations of astrocytes, characterized by distinct morphological, antigenic and functional
features (Raff et al., 1983b, Johnstone et al., 1986; Levi et

Development of the Central Nervous System in Vertebrates
Edited by S.C. Sharma and A.M. Goffinet, Plenum Press, New York, 1992

29

al., 1986). The concept that has been more easily absorbed by the literature is that type-1 astrocytes have a flat, epithelioid morphology, while type-2 astrocytes have a stellate shape. However, this concept is elusive, and its validity is restricted to defined experimental conditions. For example, in serum-free media type-1 astrocytes have an elongated, process bearing morphology and are not easily distinguishable from type-2 astrocytes on morphological grounds (Levi et al., 1986). Even in serum containing media morphology can be a dangerous criterion. For example, it has been shown that type-2 astrocytes may lose their stellate shape when they come in contact with type-1 astrocytes (Wilkin et al., 1983). Moreover, type-2 astrocytes tend to lose their stellate shape after prolonged time in culture (Aloisi et al., 1988a). On the other hand, type-1 astrocytes can acquire a stellate shape in certain experimental conditions, such as exposure to ß-adrenergic agonists or to cAMP (e.g. see Lim et al., 1973).

A more reliable criterion seems to be the expression of certain antigens, although none of the antigens that have been studied is specific for astrocytes. Since the earlier studies it has been reported that type-2 astrocytes express some surface gangliosides not expressed by type-1 astrocytes, such as those recognized by A2B5 (Raff et al., 1983a, b) or by anti-GD3 (Levi et al., 1986, 1987; Aloisi et al., 1988a; Curtis et al., 1988) monoclonal antibodies (mAbs). It has been also reported that type-2 astrocytes express the receptors for tetanus toxin (Raff et al. 1979, 1983a), previously considered as typical of neurons, while type-1 astrocytes express the antigen recognized by the mAb Ran 2 (Bartlett et al., 1981). Later it was found that type-2 astrocytes may express the antigens recognized by another mAb, O4 (Levi et al., 1987; Trotter and Schachner, 1989; Armstrong et al., 1990) which was originally thought to be typical of oligodendrocytes (Schachner, 1982). Type-1 and 2 astrocytes have been also shown to differ in the expression and production of extracellular matrix molecules. While type-2 astrocytes exhibit intracellular and extracellular immunoreactivity for chondroitin sulfate (Gallo et al., 1987; Levine and Stallcup, 1987), type-1 astrocytes have been shown, in some cases, to express laminin and fibronectin (see Gallo and Bertolotto, 1990 also for previous references).

However, also these antigenic criteria are not absolute. Not only, as already mentioned, the antigen described are not astrocytes-specific, but some degree of overlap between the two astrocytes populations has been recognized. So, a small but consistent proportion of type-1 astrocytes has been shown to bind the mAbs A2B5 (Raff, 1983a) and anti-GD3 (Goldman et al., 1986) and type-2 astrocytes kept in culture for a long time have been shown to bind the mAb Ran-2 (Lillien and Raff, 1990). Moreover, A2B5 and GD3 immunoreactivity is lost with prolonged time in culture, and the same is true for chondroitin sulfate positivity (Aloisi et al., 1988a). On the other hand, we noted that a certain proportion of type-2 astrocytes may acquire intracellular immunoreactivity for fibronectin in long term cultures (Aloisi et al., 1988a). It has to be added that none of these antigenic features has been useful for distinguishing type-2 astrocytes in vivo. Whether this means that type-2 astrocytes do not normally exist in vivo is still an open question.

Are other discrimination criteria less elusive? In cultures of rat brain cells type-2 astrocytes have been shown to express a high affinity uptake system for GABA that is not shared by type-1 astrocytes (Levi et al., 1983; Johnstone et al., 1986; Levi et al., 1986). Incidentally, this uptake system has structural requirements that are more similar to those of a "neuronal" than of a glial GABA transport system. It has to be mentioned, however, that also GABA uptake tends to be lost with time in culture (Aloisi et al., 1988a).

Other properties of type-2 and type-1 astrocytes are more difficult to evaluate, and do not lend themselves to performing rapid discrimination tests that may be required to ascertain the purity of a given type of culture. For example, in serum containing cultures, type-1 astrocytes proliferate rapidly, while type-2 astrocytes tend to rapidly cease proliferating (Wilkin et al., 1983). Biochemical, pharmacological and electrophysiological studies agree in showing that type-2 astrocytes, but not type-1 astrocytes, express the non-NMDA subtypes of excitatory amino acid receptors. The activation of such receptors stimulates the release of preloaded ^{3}H-GABA (Gallo et al., 1986, 1989, 1991) and of a number of endogenous amino acids (Levi and Patrizio, 1991) from type-2, but not from type-1 astrocytes and patch-clamp studies have shown that non-NMDA receptor-linked cationic channels are highly expressed in type-2, but not in type-1 astrocytes (Usowicz et al., 1989; Wyllie et al., 1991). The presence of such channels, however, has been described also in cultures presumably enriched in type-1 astrocytes (Kettenmann and Schachner, 1985; Cornell-Bell et al., 1990; see also review by Barres et al., 1990a).

To make the picture more complete, I must mention that other functional differences have been described between type-1 and type-2 astrocytes. The endogenous levels of various amino acids, some of which are neuroactive, are significantly higher in type-1 than in type-2 astrocytes (Levi and Patrizio, 1991). In autoradiographic studies it was reported that ß-adrenergic receptors are mainly present on type-1 astrocytes (Trimmer et al., 1984), and we confirmed this by measuring the ß-adrenergic stimulation of cAMP formation (Levi and Patrizio, unpublished). There are several differences in the expression of ionic channels between the two types of astrocytes (Barres et al., 1988). Finally, the immunocompetent properties (expression of class II antigens and antigen presentation) of type-1 and type-2 astrocytes also show some differences (Aloisi, 1991; Sazaki et al., 1989).

THE O-2A GLIAL CELL LINEAGE

The surface antigenic features of type-2 astrocytes have been instrumental for the discovery that type-1 and type-2 astrocytes derive from different progenitor cells and that type-2 astrocytes share a common progenitor with oligodendrocytes, at least in the rat CNS (Raff et al., 1983a). The cell lineage in question has been named O-2A. In fact, double immunofluorescence studies allowed to detect, first in cultures from optic nerve (Raff et al., 1983a) and then also in other brain areas (Levi et al., 1986; Behar et al., 1988), the presence of cells with the same surface features of type-

2 astrocytes, but lacking differentiated glial antigens, such as glial fibrillary acidic protein (GFAP), the major glial intermediate filament protein, or galactocerebroside (GalC), the major myelin glycolipid. The latter antigens were progressively acquired by maturing astrocytes or oligodendrocytes, respectively, and the type of antigen acquired was found to depend on the composition of the culture medium, and in particular on the presence or absence of fetal calf serum (FCS) (Raff et al., 1983a). The undifferentiated cells carrying the type-2 astrocytes surface antigens could be selectively killed by immunocytolysis with a mAb and complement. This procedure led to the disappearance from the cultures of the putative progenitor cells and prevented the appearance of type-2 astrocytes or of oligodendrocytes with time in vitro (Raff et al., 1983a; Levi et al., 1986; Behar et al., 1988).

Even if the antigenic properties of type-2 astrocytes and of their progenitors were instrumental for the discovery of the O-2A cell lineage, subsequent observations showed that the bipotential progenitors share with type-2 astrocytes also a number of functional features, such as ability to accumulate GABA (Levi et al., 1986), to synthesize chondroitin sulfate (Gallo et al., 1987), to express non-NMDA receptors (Gallo et al., 1989) and other membrane properties such as type of ionic channels (Barres et al., 1990b). One may wonder whether the progenitors express a number of properties of differentiated cells, or whether apparently differentiated type-2 astrocytes retain a number of properties characteristic of more immature cells and are, in fact, poorly differentiated. The question is not easy to answer. As already mentioned, type-2 astrocytes tend to lose several of their characteristic properties with time in culture (Aloisi et al., 1988a). Is this a sign of differentiation or of dedifferentiation? It is known that astrocytes tend to lose even GFAP positivity upon repeated passages (Vernadakis et al., 1986), and this is generally considered a sign of dedifferentiation. On the other hand, although with a different timing, O-2A progenitors tend to lose a set of functional and antigenic properties as they acquire differentiated oligodendrocytes markers (Levi et al., 1987; Gallo et al., 1987; Reynolds et al., 1987). In conclusion, we would favor the idea that the above mentioned properties of the progenitors, such as GABA uptake, excitatory amino acid receptors, synthesis of chondroitin sulfate, reflect particular requirements and functions of the progenitors themselves, rather than being early manifestations of the properties of the mature progeny.

THE LINEAGE DECISION

Several studies have been, and still are, devoted to the understanding of the factors that influence the lineage decision of O-2A progenitors. Understanding these factors has obviously an interest that goes beyond the limits of pure developmental neurobiology and spans in the field of repair and remyelination in the adult CNS. In fact, bipotential glial progenitors have been described also in the adult rat CNS (ffrench-Constant and Raff, 1986; Wolswijk and Noble, 1989), and may be involved not only in the normal turnover of oligodendrocytes, but also in the replacement of injured oligodendrocytes.

Martin Raff and coworkers have first shown that O-2A progenitors differentiate into oligodendrocytes by default, namely following their constitutive pathway (see Raff, 1989 for review). In culture they do so when grown in a chemically defined, serum-free medium. On the other hand, the differentiation of the progenitors into type-2 astrocytes seems to require exogenous, astrocytes-inducing factors (Raff et al., 1983a). Classically, it has been reported that FCS contains such factors, and it has been suggested that seral factors mimic factors present in the living brain at critical developmental stages. The most recent studies of the group of Raff have been focused on the identification and characterization of the signals capable of promoting the astroglial differentiation of the progenitor cells and of diverting them from their constitutive pathway (Lillien et al., 1990). Our studies, instead, have been directed at understanding what exogenous factors can induce an oligodendroglial differentiation of the progenitors when these are grown in the presence of astrocyte-inducing factors. Interestingly, both lines of study indicate that the differentiation destiny of O-2A progenitors is greatly influenced by specific cellular interactions.

Before mentioning these studies, however, I would like to recall another set of studies initiated by the groups of Noble and Raff and then extended also by the group of M. Dubois-Dalcq, which already revealed the importance of cell interactions for the proliferation and differentiation of O-2A progenitors. These authors have in fact shown that the progenitors respond to a growth factor secreted by type-1 astrocytes, PDGF (Raff et al., 1988; Richardson et al., 1988). In serum-free cultures, it has been reported that PDGF prevents the premature differentiation of the progenitors into oligodendrocytes and stimulates their proliferation (Noble et al., 1988). After a defined number of cell cycles, however, the progenitors differentiate into non-dividing oligodendrocytes. On the other hand, if also bFGF is present in the medium in addition to PDGF, the progenitors continue to proliferate and do not differentiate (Bögler et al., 1990). This seems to be due on one hand to a mitogenic effect of bFGF itself, on the other hand to an increased expression of PDGF-α receptors induced by bFGF (McKinnon et al., 1990).

In addition to PDGF, however, Raff's group has shown that type-1 astrocytes secrete another growth factor, CNTF, which can initiate the astroglial differentiation of the progenitors grown in serum-free conditions (Lillien et al., 1988). This initial differentiation (GFAP expression) is only transient, and can be stabilized if other factors collaborate with CNTF. Such factors, although not yet identified, have been shown to be present in the extracellular matrix produced by a non-neural cell type, leptomeningeal cells (Lillien et al., 1990). The activity of the extracellular matrix could be removed by a high salt concentration and restored by the addition of an optic nerve extract. Thus, two different cell types co-operate to induce O-2A progenitors to differentiate into type-2 astrocytes, even if the cells are cultured in conditions under which, by default, they would differentiate into oligodendrocytes.

Our approach has been in a way specular to that of

Lillien and Raff. We started from the observation, made using cerebellar mixed glial cultures grown in the presence of 10% FCS, that the proportion of progenitors differentiating into oligodendrocytes rather than into type-2 astrocytes increased as the plating cell density was increased. We also provided some evidence that direct contact between the progenitor cells and type-1 astrocytes (the major cell population in the cultures) was important in facilitating the oligodendroglial differentiation route of the progenitors (Aloisi et al., 1988b). This finding was reminiscent of a previous observation of Keilhauer et al. (1985). However, we soon realized that working with mixed cell populations was not an ideal condition for drawing sure conclusions. For example, in the mixed cultures or cocultures it was impossible to prevent the secretion of mitogens such as PDGF by type-1 astrocytes, and it was difficult to assess whether the facilitated differentiation of the progenitors into oligodendrocytes was related to direct interactions with molecules present on the surface of type-1 astrocytes or to increased proliferation.

We then subcultured purified populations of O-2A progenitors in conditions (low density, presence of FCS, poly-L-lysine substrate) in which they by and large differentiate into type-2 astrocytes (Aloisi et al., 1988a) and studied the cellular interactions that can induce the progenitors to change their lineage decision and to differentiate into oligodendrocytes (Agresti et al., 1991). In order to study the type-1 astrocyte-O-2A progenitor interactions independently of the mitogenic effect of PDGF, we subcultured the progenitors on a substrate of type-1-astrocytes killed by air drying. In the control subcultures most of the progenitors differentiated into GFAP+ type-2 astrocytes and very few of them expressed the oligodendrocytes marker GalC. When the progenitor cells were cultured at the same density and in the same medium on a substrate of killed astrocytes, they preferentially differentiated into GalC+ oligodendrocytes rather than into GFAP+ type-2 astrocytes (Agresti et al., 1991).

In addition to this shift in antigenic profile, we noted that the progenitors achieved a higher cell density on the killed astrocyte substrate, which was due to greater proliferative activity. These results suggested a possible correlation between the density achieved by the progenitor cells on killed astrocytes and their lineage decision. In order to try to circumvent the problem of cell density, we analyzed the phenotype of cells grown at much lower density, a density at which they survived on killed astrocytes, but not on poly-L-lysine. Also in these conditions, the progenitors preferentially differentiated into oligodendrocytes, although the differentiation was delayed. However, since after a few days of culturing the progenitors were often present in clones of increasing size, the results obtained were again not sufficiently clear to establish whether the preferential differentiation into oligodendrocytes was related to direct interactions with the killed astrocytes or to the density achieved, even though at a later stage.

In order to determine what was responsible for the increased proliferation of the progenitors grown on killed astrocytes, we performed a series of [3H]thymidine incorporation studies to characterize the proliferative activity.

First we noted that not only a substrate of killed astrocytes, but also a cell free substrate of extracellular matrix produced by type-1 astrocytes had a mitogenic effect on O-2A progenitors. The mitogenic effect of type-1 astrocytes derived substrates appeared to be specific, since killed leptomeningeal or microglial cells or extracellular matrix produced by these cells had scarce or no effect on O-2A cell proliferation. Several experiments were performed to determine the nature of the mitogen(s) present on killed astrocytes or astrocyte extracellular matrix which, for this purpose, were treated with antibodies, enzymes and physico-chemical agents. Only drastic treatments with proteases, heat and low pH inhibited the mitogenic activity, suggesting that the mitogen has a polypeptide nature (Agresti et al., 1991).

To sum up, the experiments presented seem to indicate that type-1 astrocytes promote the proliferation of O-2A progenitors through mitogens present in their extracellular matrix or on their surface and facilitate the oligodendroglial differentiation of the progenitors. They do not answer the question of whether the two phenomena are related. Further experiments seem to indicate that the enhanced oligodendroglial differentiation of the progenitors is at least partly related to the higher density they achieve on the killed astrocyte substrate.

In fact, when the same number of cells was plated on coverslips at low and high density and cultured in identical culture dishes in the same volume of FCS-containing medium on a poly-L-lysine substrate, the proportion of progenitors differentiating into oligodendrocytes was much greater when the cells were at high density (Levi et al., 1991). The fact that this result was obtained with the same number of cells seems to exclude that it was due to inactivation by the cells at high density of serum factors inhibiting oligodendrocytes differentiation. Two other possibilities should then be considered. One is that homotypic cell interactions among the progenitors trigger some event promoting oligodendrocyte differentiation. The second is that the progenitors secrete autocrine differentiation factors into the culture medium. Obviously, the two possibilities are not mutually exclusive since homotypic cell contacts might trigger the secretion of autocrine factors.

That autocrine factors may indeed be involved is supported by the observation that a medium conditioned by high density O-2A cell cultures induced a rapid oligodendroglial differentiation of the progenitors cultured at low density. The conditioned medium was not mitogenic for the progenitors, and the differentiating activity could be recovered in high molecular weight components (Levi et al., 1991).

In conclusion we can say that multiple and at times competing cellular interactions influence the proliferation and differentiation of O-2A progenitors. If similar interactions occurred in the living brain, they might be important not only during normal brain development, but also in the course of remyelination processes in the adult animal. Indirect evidence suggests that reactive astrocytes in vivo belong to the type-1 astrocyte subpopulation (Miller et al., 1986). Thus reactive astrocytes may fulfil the role of expanding the limited population of oligodendrocyte precursors present in the adult CNS (Wolswijk and Noble, 1989) through the secretion of known mitogens such as PDGF (Noble et al., 1988; Raff et al., 1988; Richardson et al., 1988) and of a mitogenic extracellular matrix (Agresti et al., 1991). The expanded progenitor cell population could then respond to differentiation signals (if any) provided by astrocytes, as well as to autocrine differentiation factors (Levi et al., 1991).

REFERENCES

Agresti, C, Aloisi, F., and Levi, G., 1991, Heterotypic and homotypic cellular interactions influencing the growth and differentiation of bipotential oligodendrocyte type-2 astrocyte progenitors in culture, Dev.Biol., 144:16.

Aloisi, F., 1991, In vitro studies on the interactions between antigenic specific T line cells and CNS glial cells, Cytotechnology, 5:S166.

Aloisi, F., Agresti, C., and Levi, G., 1988a, Establishment, characterization, and evolution of cultures enriched in type-2 astrocytes, J.Neurosci.Res., 21:188.

Aloisi, F., Agresti, C., D'Urso, D. and Levi, G., 1988b, Differentiation of bipotential glial precursors into oligodendrocytes is promoted by interaction with type-1 astrocytes in cerebellar cultures, Proc.Natl.Acad.Sci.USA, 85:6167.

Armstrong, R., Friedrich, V.L. jr., Holmes, K.V., and Dubois-Dalcq, M., 1990, In vitro analysis of the oligodendrocyte lineage in mice during demyelination and remyelination, J.Cell Biol., 111:1183.

Barres, B.A., Chun, L.L.Y., and Corey, D.P., 1988, Ion channel expression by white matter glia: I. Type 2 astrocytes and oligodendrocytes, Glia, 1:10.

Barres, B.A., Chun, L.L.Y., and Corey, D.P., 1990a, Ion channels in vertebrate glia, Annu.Rev.Neurosci., 13:441.

Barres, B.A., Koroshetz, W.J., Swartz, K.J., Chun, L.L.Y., and Corey, D.P., 1990b, Ion channel expression by white matter glia: the O-2A glial progenitor cell, Neuron, 4:507.

Bartlett, P.F., Noble, M.D., Pruss, R.M., Raff, M.C., Rattray, S., and Williams, C.A., 1981, Rat neural antigen-2 (Ran-2): a cell surface antigen on astrocytes, ependymal cells, Müller cells and leptomenginges defined by a monoclonal antibody, Brain Res., 204:339.

Behar, T., McMorris, F.A., Novotny', E.A., Barker, J.L., and Dubois-Dalcq, M., 1988, Growth and differentiation properties of O-2A progenitors purified from rat cerebral hemispheres, J.Neurosci.Res., 21:168.

Bögler, O., Wren, D., Barnett, S.C., Land, H., and Noble, M., 1990, Co-operation between two growth factors promotes extended self-renewal and inhibits differentiation of oligodendrocyte-type-2 astrocyte (O-2A) progenitor cells, Proc.Natl.Acad.Sci. USA, 87:6368.

Cornell-Bell, A.H., Finkbeiner, S.M., Cooper, M.S., and Smith, S.J., 1990, Glutamate induces calcium waves in cultured astrocytes: long-range glial signalling, Science, 24:470.

Curtis, R., Cohen, J., Fok-Seang, J., Hanley, M.R., Gregson, N.A., Reynolds, R., and Wilkin, G.P., 1988, Development of macroglial cells in rat cerebellum. I. Use of antibodies to

follow early in vivo development and migration of oligodendrocytes, <u>J.Neurocytol.</u>, 17:43.
ffrench-Constant, C., and Raff, M.C., 1986, Proliferating
bipotential glial progenitor cells in adult rat optic
nerve, <u>Nature</u>, 319:499.
Gallo, V., and Bertolotto, A., 1990, Extracellular matrix of
cultured glial cells: selective expression of chondroitin
4-sulfate by type-2 astrocytes and their progenitors,
<u>Exp.Cell Res.</u>, 187:211.
Gallo, V., Suergiu, R., and Levi, G., 1986, Kainic acid stimulates GABA release from a subpopulation of cerebellar
astrocytes, <u>Eur.J.Pharmacol.</u>, 133:319.
Gallo, V., Bertolotto, A., and Levi, G., 1987, The proteoglycan chondroitin sulfate is present in a subpopulation of
cultured astrocytes and in their precursor, <u>Dev.Biol.</u>,
123:282.
Gallo, V., Giovannini, C., Suergiu, R., and Levi, G., 1989,
Expression of excitatory amino acid receptors by cerebellar
cells of the type-2 astrocyte cell lineage, <u>J.Neurochem.</u>,
52:1.
Gallo, V., Patrizio, M., and Levi, G., 1991, GABA release
triggered by the activation of neuron-like non-NMDA
receptors in cultured type 2 astrocytes is carrier-
mediated, <u>Glia</u>, 4:245.
Goldman, J.E., Geier, S.S., and Hirano, M., 1986, Differentiation of astrocytes and oligodendrocytes from germinal
matrix cells in primary culture, <u>J.Neurosci.</u>, 6:52.
Johnstone, S.R., Levi, G., Wilkin, G.P., Schneider, A., and
Ciotti, M.T., 1986, Subpopulations of rat cerebellar astrocytes in primary culture: Morphology, cell surface antigens
and ^{3}H-GABA transport, <u>Dev.Brain Res.</u>, 24:63.
Keilhauer, G., Meier, D.H., Kuhlmann-Krieg, S., Nieke, J.,
and Schachner, M., 1985, Astrocytes support incomplete
differentiation of oligodendrocyte precursor cell, <u>EMBO J.</u>,
4:2499.
Kettenmann, H., and Schachner, M., 1985, Pharmacological properties of -aminobutyric acid-, glutamate-, and
aspartate-induced depolarizations in cultured astrocytes,
<u>J.Neurosci.</u>, 5:3295.
Levi, G., and Patrizio, M., 1991, Astrocyte heterogeneity:
endogenous amino acid levels and release evoked by non-NMDA
receptor agonists and by potassium-induced swelling in
type-1 and type-2 astrocytes, submitted.
Levi, G., Wilkin, G.P., Ciotti, M.T., and Johnstone, S.,
1983, Enrichment of differentiated, stellate astrocytes in
cerebellar interneuron cultures as studied by GFAP immunofluorescence and autoradiographic uptake patterns of ^{3}H-D-
aspartate and ^{3}H-GABA, <u>Dev.Brain Res.</u>, 10:227.
Levi, G., Gallo, V., and Ciotti, M.T., 1986, Bipotential precursors of putative fibrous astrocytes and oligodendrocytes
in rat cerebellar cultures express distinct surface
features and "neuron-like" GABA transport,
<u>Proc.Natl.Acad.Sci.USA</u>, 83:1504.
Levi, G., Aloisi, F., and Wilkin, G.P., 1987, Differentiation
of cerebellar bipotential glial precursors into oligodendrocytes in primary culture: developmental profile of
surface antigens and mitotic activity, <u>J.Neurosci.Res.</u>,
18:407.
Levi, G., Agresti, C., D'Urso, D., and Aloisi, F., 1991, Is
the oligodendroglial differentiation of bipotential oligo-

dendrocyte-type 2 astrocyte progenitors promoted by autocrine factors?, Neurosci.Lett., 128:37.

Levine, J.M., and Stallcup, W.B., 1987, Plasticity of developing cerebellar cells in vitro studied with antibodies
against the NG2 antigen, J.Neurosci., 7:2721.

Lillien, L.E., and Raff, M.C., 1990, Analysis of the cell-
cell interactions that control type-2 astrocyte development
in vitro, Neuron, 4:525.

Lillien, L.E., Sendtner, M., Rohrer, H., Hughes, S.M., and
Raff, M.C., 1988, Type-2 astrocyte development in rat brain
cultures is initiated by a CNTF-like protein produced by
type-1 astrocytes, Neuron, 1:485.

Lillien, C.E., Sendtner, M., and Raff, M.C., 1990, Extracellular matrix-associated molecules collaborate with ciliary
neurotrophic factor to induce type-2 astrocyte development,
J.Cell Biol., 111:635.

Lim, R., Mitsunobu, K., and Li, W.K.P., 1973, Maturation-
stimulating effect of brain extract and dibutyryl cyclic
AMP on dissociated embryonic brain cells in culture,
Exp.Cell Res., 79:243.

Luskin, M.B., Pearlman, A.L., and Sanes, J.R., 1988, Cell
lineage in the cerebral cortex of the mouse studied in vivo
and in vitro with a recombinant retrovirus, Neuron, 1:635.

McKinnon, R.D., Matsui, T., Dubois-Dalcq, M., and Aaronson,
S.A., 1990, FGF modulates the PDGF-driven pathway of oligodendrocyte development, Neuron, 5:603.

Miller, R.H., Abney, E.R., David, S., ffrench-Constant, C.,
Lindsay, R., Patel, R., Stone, J., and Raff, M.C., 1986, Is
reactive gliosis a property of a distinct subpopulation of
astrocytes?, J.Neurosci., 6:22.

Noble, M., Murray, K., Stroobant, P., Waterfield, M.D., and
Riddle, P., 1988, Platelet-derived growth factor promotes
division and motility and inhibits premature differentiation of the oligodendrocyte/type-2 astrocyte progenitor
cell, Nature, 333:560.

Raff, M.C., 1989, Glial cell diversification in the rat optic
nerve, Science, 243:1450.

Raff, M.C., Fields, K.L., Hakomori, S.-L., Mirsky, R., Pruss,
R.M., and Winter, J., 1979, Cell-type-specific markers for
distinguishing and studying neurons and the major classes
of glial cells in culture, Brain Res., 174:283.

Raff, M.C., Miller, R.H., and Noble, M., 1983a, A glial progenitor cell that develops in vitro into an astrocyte or an
oligodendrocyte depending on culture medium, Nature,
303:390.

Raff, M.C., Abney, E.R., Cohen, J., Lindsay, R., and Noble,
M., 1983b, Two types of astrocytes in cultures of developing rat white matter differences in morphology, surface
gangliosides, and growth characteristics, J.Neurosci.,
3:1289.

Raff, M.C., Lillien, L.E., Richardson, W.D., Burne, J.F., and
Noble, M.D., 1988, Platelet-derived growth factor from
astrocytes drives the clock that times oligodendrocyte
development in culture, Nature, 333:562.

Reynolds, R., Steffen, C., and Herschkowitz, N., 1987, High-
affinity uptake of -[³H]aminobutyric acid by isolated
mouse oligodendrocytes in culture, Neurochem.Res., 12:885.

Richardson, W.D., Pringle, N., Mosley, M.J., Westermark, B.,
and Dubois-Dalcq, M., 1988, A role for platelet-derived
growth factor in normal gliogenesis in the central nervous
system, Cell, 53:309.

Sasaki, A., Levison S.W., and Ting, J.P.-Y., 1989, Comparison and quantitation of Ia antigen expression on cultured macroglia and ameboid microglia from Lewis rat cerebral cortex: analyses and implications, J.Neuroimmunol., 25:63.

Schachner, M., 1982, Cell type-specific surface antigens in the mammalian nervous system, J.Neurochem., 39:1.

Trimmer, P.A., Evans, T., Smith, M.M., Harden, T.K., and McCarthy, K.D., 1984, Combination of immunocytochemistry and radioligand receptor assay to identify ß-adrenergic receptor subtypes on astroglia in vitro, J.Neurosci., 4:1598.

Trotter, J., and Schachner, M., 1989, Cells positive for the O4 surface antigen isolated by cell sorting are able to differentiate into astrocytes or oligodendrocyte, Dev.Brain Res., 46:115.

Usowicz, M.M., Gallo, V., Cull-Candy, S.G., 1989, Multiple conductance channels in type-2 cerebellar astrocytes activated by excitatory amino acids, Nature, 339:380.

Vaysse, P.J.-J., and Goldman, J.E., 1990, A clonal analysis of glial lineages in neonatal forebrain development in vitro, Neuron, 5:227.

Vernadakis, A., Davies, D., Sakellaridis, N., and Mangoura, D., 1986, Growth patterns of glial cells dissociated from newborn and aged mouse brain with cell passage, J.Neurosci.Res., 15:79.

Wilkin, G.P., Levi, G., Johnstone, S., and Riddle, P.N., 1983, Cerebellar astroglial cells in primary culture: expression of different morphological appearances and differential ability to take up ^{3}H-D-aspartate and ^{3}H-GABA, Dev.Brain Res., 10:265.

Wolswijk, G., and Noble, M., 1989, Identification of an adult-specific glial progenitor cell, Development, 105:387.

Wood, P., and Bunge, R.P., 1984, The biology of the oligodendrocyte, In "Oligodendroglia", W.T. Norton, ed., Plenum Press, New York.

Wyllie, D.J.A., Mathie, A., Symonds, C.J., and Cull-Candy, S.G., 1991, Activation of glutamate receptors and glutamate uptake in identified macroglial cells in rat cerebellar cultures, J.Physiol., 432:235.

CELL FATE IN THE CEREBRAL CORTEX

Jack Price

National Institute for Medical Research
Mill Hill, London, NW7 1AA, UK

INTRODUCTION

In part, the process of development is the determination of cell
fate. Different cells in the adult animal have different phenotypes, that
is they have taken on different fates. Somehow during embryogenesis,
cells have to be channelled so that they take on a fate appropriate to
their position in the body. The problem of how the body achieves this is
in principle no different in the brain than in any other somatic tissue.
Yet the complexity of the brain makes the problem more daunting than it
appears in apparently simpler structures.

In this article I shall be considering the acquisition of cell fate
in one part of the brain, the cerebral cortex, and there, as elsewhere, we
can think of cell fate as having two components. The first is cell type
in the classic histological sense: cells become one of the many types of
either neurons or glia that make up the cortex. Second, cells take on a
positional identity, that is a cell in one part of the structure will
behave differently and have different relationships from a similar cell in
another part of the structure. In the cerebral cortex, we can break this
aspect of fate down into two components: lamina and cytoarchitectonic
area. The sheet of gray matter that comprises the cerebral cortex is
laminated, and the allocation of a neuron to a particular lamina is an
important component of its fate determination. Similarly , different
areas of the cortical sheet have evolved to take on different functions –
motor, somatosensory, visual, etc. – so the cytoarchitectonic area to
which a cell is allocated is, again, an important aspect of its fate.

In considering how fate allocation is brought about in the cerebral
cortex, my colleagues and I have posed a particular question. We have
asked which aspects of fate are determined before a cell leaves the
germinal zone, and which are determined later? All the neuronal and
macroglial cell types of the adult cortex are derived from the germinal
cells in a region of embryonic cortex called the ventricular zone. These
germinal cells are indistinguishable under the microscope, but our
question was whether there were different populations among them, each
dedicated in one or other aspect of cortical cell fate. It was possible
that no fate decisions had been taken among these germinal cells. Were
that the case, each of the cells would be of equal developmental
potential, and each able to give rise to any of the cells of the cortex.

Development of the Central Nervous System in Vertebrates
Edited by S.C. Sharma and A.M. Goffinet, Plenum Press, New York, 1992

Alternatively, there could be subpopulations among the germinal cells, each generating either a single cell type, or contributing to a single lamina or area. If we could work out which of these alternatives were true, we would know whether fate decisions were made early, before cells were generated in the ventricular zone, or late, after they had migrated into the cortex itself.

In order to address these issues, ourselves and others have developed a means of using retroviral vectors as lineage markers (Sanes et al., 1986; Price et al., 1987). Briefly, this approach allows individual germinal cells to be genetically labelled with a retroviral vector, such that their fate can be followed. By the expression of a histochemical marker gene encoded by the virus, all the progeny of an infected cell can be identified. We have mostly used the BAG virus, which encodes the ß-galactosidase gene, lac-Z (Price et al., 1987). In this construct lac-Z is driven from the endogenous retroviral promoter elements, but to control for promoter effects we have also used the pIRV vector, which also encodes lac-Z, but driven off the rat ß-actin promoter (Beddington et al., 1988).

CORTICAL CELL LINEAGE

When we virally-labelled ventricular zone cells during the period of cortical neurogenesis, and analyzed the marked clones sometime after the birth of the injected animal, we discovered four distinct types of clones (Price & Thurlow, 1988). Three of these were simple, being composed apparently of a single cell type; the fourth was more complex being composed of at least two types of cells.

One type of clone was composed entirely of neurons. They were small, the majority having one or two cells. They were confined to the gray matter, as would be expected of neurons. Mostly, they were also confined to the supragranular layers. Again this is as one would expect as most of our viral injections were made at postnatal day 16 (E16), by which time most of the infragranular layers would have already been generated.

The second type of clone was also confined to the gray matter, but was composed entirely of astrocytes. These clones were larger, frequently having as many as forty or fifty cells and seldom fewer than twenty. They also occupied more space, spreading from the pial surface through to the deepest layers of lamina VI. Despite this dispersion, related cells were often found in small clusters of two to four cells, as if after migrating into the gray matter, cells had gone on to divide once or twice more. These labelled astrocytes often had blood vessel or pial endfeet and labelled with glial fibrillary acidic protein (GFAP), the archetypal astrocyte marker (unpublished observations).

The third simple type of clone was composed entirely of white matter cells. In our original experiments, we analyzed the labelled tissue 14 days after birth. At that stage of development, the white matter cells were for the most part undifferentiated morphologically. This made them very difficult to identify, but we concluded that they had to be glial. This was largely a process of elimination. They neither looked neuronal, nor were they in a region that contains more than an occasional neuronal cell body. Moreover, they were horizontally oriented in a fashion similar to intrafasicular oligodendrocytes in the mature nerve, albeit without the extensive processes of such nerves. Consequently, we tentatively identified them as glial precursor cells (Price and Thurlow, 1988). Our subsequent studies have confirmed that many of these cells turn into either oligodendrocytes or astrocytes if left to develop longer. We are

42

still investigating the question of whether clones include both of these white matter cell types or just one.

The fourth type of clone was, as I have said, more complex. It was composed both of neurons, indistinguishable from the neurons found in the simple neuronal clones, and of white matter glial cells, again indistinguishable from those cells found in the clones composed only of this cell type. Spatially, these clones were arranged with the neuronal component of the clone occupying the cortical gray matter immediately superficial to the white matter containing the glial component. Although the least common of all the clonal types, these mixed neuronal-white matter glial clones comprised between 6 and 9% of the total of clones observed when we injected virus at E16 and analyzed on postnatal day 14 (P14).

We interpreted these data to mean that there were at least three different precursor cell types in the ventricular zone at E16: one each for neurons, gray matter astrocytes, and white matter glia. Moreover, there was a relationship between the precursors that generated neurons and those that generated white matter glia, although from these data we could not be certain what that relationship was. I will return to this point later.

THE DISTRIBUTION OF NEURONAL CLONES

The data I have described so far provide <u>prima facie</u> evidence that one aspect of cell fate, namely cell type, is already determined before cells have left the germinal zone. In fact, these data have alternative interpretations that I shall discuss later. What of the positional aspects of cell fate; are they also determined?

I have already mentioned that most neuronal clones tended to be confined to the supragranular layers. Neurogenesis in the cerebral cortex works by an 'inside-out' temporal sequence, that is the deepest neurons are the first generated and subsequent cohorts of neurons lie more and more superficially (Berry and Rogers, 1965; Miller, 1986). However even viral injections as late as E16 would be expected to label some infragranular neurons, and so it proved. Consequently, we could address two questions. First, did clones with infragranular neurons also include supragranular cells; second, were supragranular clones confined entirely to one supragranular layer or did they contribute to more than one lamina?

In both cases, neuronal clones failed to respect lamina boundaries (Price et al., 1991). Clones that had cells in layers V or VI also frequently had cells in more superficial layers. Clones confined to layers IV, III, and II often contributed to more than one, or to all three of these layers. Thus there was no evidence that neuronal precursors were restricted in the laminae to which they could contribute. Without a more systematic analysis, it is difficult to be certain that there is no bias at all in this distribution data; and indeed, unless we can be sure that there is only one type of neuronal precursor cell, we cannot discount the possibility that different subsets of the neuronal precursors might have some positional bias. Nonetheless, there is no evidence for such a bias, whereas we have clear evidence that precursors can contribute to more than one lamina.

What of the second positional aspect of cell fate, that associated with cytoarchitectonic area? If we ask whether germinal cells are already restricted in terms of the area to which they can contribute, we are really asking two questions. First, whether the boundaries that exist between areas in the adult cortex are already to be found in the ventricular zone before the cortical gray matter begins to form. Second, do neurons respect these boundaries as they migrate radially into the cortical plate? These questions have become particularly pertinent recently since it became clear that in the hindbrain there are lineage restriction boundaries that arise prior to neurogenesis (Fraser et al., 1990). There is no such direct evidence for boundaries in the embryonic cortex. However, it has been suggested that one function of cortical radial glial cells is to direct the migration of neurons strictly radially, hence preventing the neurons destined for one area from wandering into adjacent regions of cortex (Rakic, 1988). This suggestion does not necessarily presuppose boundaries between cortical regions in the embryo, but it does assume that neurons already have their areal identities prior to migration.

The initial retroviral studies of cortical lineage did not specifically address the question of boundaries between areas. However, all of these studies made the observation that there was considerable tangential spread of clones, including neuronal clones (Price & Thurlow, 1988; Luskin et al., 1988; Walsh & Cepko, 1988). The limit to this dispersion has not yet been ascertained, but it certainly seems to be at least several hundred micrometers. This did not disprove the existence of boundaries, but it did raise the possibility that clones could contribute to more than one cytoarchitectonic area.

We have recently studied this issue in the part of the cortical mantle that generates the hippocampal formation (Grove et al., 1992). This part of the cortex had two features that made it particularly suitable for this study. First, the boundaries between hippocampal fields are easily distinguished histochemically unlike the area boundaries in rodent neocortex. Second, we observed that neuronal clones dispersed much more regularly than they did in the neocortex. Thus the boundaries to clonal dispersion were much more easily defined in the hippocampal formation.

Our first result was that if we injected virus at E16 and analyzed hippocampal clones in the young adult, we found the same four types of clones that we had observed in the neocortex. Second, we looked at the distribution of the neuronal clones with respect to the boundaries between hippocampal fields. We discovered that none of these boundaries were respected by hippocampal neuronal precursor cells. Clones could contribute to any two neighbouring CA fields, and even to CA1, CA2, and CA3. They could contribute to CA1, the prosubiculum, and the subiculum. Moreover, this was not the behavior of a few aberrant clones. We were able to show statistically that the degree of dispersion of the clones that crossed boundaries was no greater than that of those that did not. Also, the number of border-crossing clones in our sample was about what would be expected were all clones free to disperse unhindered across boundaries. Thus, the border-crossing clones are not the result of some uninhibited set of precursor cells that are disregarding borders that others respect. So just as precursor cells are not restricted in the cortical laminae to which they can contribute in the neocortex, neither are they restricted in the fields to which they can contribute in the hippocampus. By extrapolation, the same is probably true of neocortical areas.

The simplest way to interpret this finding is that the areas between cortical areas do not exist during neurogenesis. However, the possibility exists that the boundaries exist without restricting neuronal migration. One might ask what would be the point of boundaries if they did not restrict the movement of cells, yet there are realistic models of corticogenesis that would employ such boundaries. For example, imagine a boundary in the ventricular zone between two cortical areas. Imagine that all the cells on one side of the boundary have a specific marker on their surface (X) by which the cells identify themselves, and that all the cells on the other side of the boundary have a similar but different marker (Y). If cells migrated from the ventricular zone more or less radially but were not constrained by the boundary, then some tangential migration might occur and the sharp border between X and Y would tend to disappear as a boundary zone of mixed cells arises. This is what has been seen to occur in the avian forebrain in chick-quail chimeras (Balaban et al., 1988). Yet all that needs to be proposed to maintain the sharp border is that cells switch fate between X and Y if they find themselves surrounded by cells of the opposite type. Thus any X cell which wanders into the Y region will tend to encounter more Y cells, and hence will switch to Y (and vice versa). So, although we can say that there are no lineage restriction boundaries between cortical fields during neurogenesis, we cannot say that no boundaries of any type exist at this time.

THE STATE OF DETERMINATION OF CORTICAL PRECURSOR CELLS

In this section, I want to consider fate determination and cell autonomy. I have described our data which showed that cortical precursor cells mostly give rise to a single cell type. This seems to suggest that each precursor cell is committed to a restricted fate. Were precursor cells multipotential then a significant proportion of clones should be composed of a mixture of several cell types. This was the result observed by labelling retinal precursor cells, and these cells are consequently thought to be multipotential (Turner & Cepko, 1987; Turner et al., 1990). The result we have observed, the restricted phenotypes, is more difficult to interpret. The fact that most precursor cells only give rise to either neurons or one of the glial cell types suggests that there exist multiple precursor cell types, each committed to one of these fates. Yet other interpretations are possible. It is possible that each cell had a wider potential than it actually exhibited, and that it was limited by circumstance. For example, were gliogenesis and neurogenesis spatially segregated in the ventricular zone as a consequence of factors extrinsic to the cells themselves, then individual cells would lie in either a gliogenetic or a neurogenetic area and behave accordingly. Alternatively, even without such spatial segregation (for which there is no evidence), cell-cell interactions between ventricular zone cells could act to restrict the behaviour of neighbouring cells.

It is difficult to discount categorically interpretations such as these. Traditionally, experimental embryologists have supposed that cells are restricted in their phenotype if they behave as they would in situ when transferred to a different environment. We have performed a similar assay by placing the cells in dissociated cell culture. We discovered that even under these circumstances in which the histogenetic relationships of the ventricular zone cells are disrupted, the same four precursor cell phenotypes are demonstrated: clones are composed of either neurons, astrocytes, oligodendrocytes, or they generate both neurons and oligodendrocytes (Williams et al., 1991). I take this as evidence that precursor cells are indeed restricted to these fates.

THE LINEAGE OF NEURONS AND OLIGODENDROCYTES

In our in vivo studies we found clones made up of both neurons white matter glial cells (Price and Thurlow, 1988). This was the only type of clone that appeared to combine two cell types (although there were a small number of clones, which I have not discussed, that apparently included neurons, gray matter astrocyte, and oligodendrocytes). Again in culture we found one two-cell type clone. These were composed of neurons and oligodendrocytes (Williams et al., 1991). The frequency of occurrence of the mixed clones is very similar in culture and in vivo; we estimate that at E16 between 6 and 9% of all the precursor cells give this mix in vivo, whereas we find 5% of the clones are mixed in cultures from E16 cortex.

These data clearly suggest a link between the neuronal and oligodendrocyte lineages. The question is, what is the nature of that link? An obvious possibility is that the cell that generates both cell types could itself be the precursor of two more restricted precursors, one for neurons and the other for oligodendrocytes. Thus at E16, although most of these neuron-oligodendrocyte (N-O) bipotential cells had already made the transition to either neuronal (N) or oligodendrocyte (O) precursors, some remained bipotential.

Were this hypothesis correct, two predictions would follow. First, as the N-O cell would be the more developmentally primitive cell, earlier in corticogenesis there should be more N-O cells and fewer N and O cells. Second, the proliferative capacity of the N-O cell should tend towards the maximum combined capacity of N cells and O cells. In other words, N-O clones should tend to contain as many neurons as the biggest N clones and as many oligodendrocytes as the biggest O clones. (There are good biological and statistical reasons why this will not be strictly true, but the tendency should be there.) We found that in culture at least, neither of these predictions were fulfilled. First, the mean number of both cell types were similar in N-O clones to the average number of cells in N clones and O clones. Second, in cultures established from earlier cortex, there were fewer N-O clones and more N clones (Williams et al., 1991). These data suggest that the simple relationship between these precursor cells predicted by the hypothesis is incorrect.

A number of models do fit the data, but as yet we cannot distinguish between them. One possibility is that the N-O cell represents an oligodendrocyte-neuronal lineage running parallel to and independently of that provided by the two restricted precursor cells. Thus there would be two different routes by which both cell types could be generated, either via the N-O cell or via the N or O cells. This model would only make sense to me if the two lineages were spatially separate, for example if, say, limbic cortex had the one lineage and neocortex the other. We know this is not the case for this example at least (Grove et al., 1992), but we still cannot exclude some other spatial separation.

More plausible in my opinion is the possibility that the mixed neuron-oligodendrocyte clones do not actually represent a separate precursor cell type. There is no N-O cell, rather some N cells and/or O cells have the propensity to switch between these two phenotypes. So early in corticogenesis, N cells are generated (presumably from an as yet undiscovered multipotential cell); later more O cells and fewer N cells are generated. Most cells then remain in those restricted phenotypes, but some switch. This makes teleological sense; as the need for neurons dwindles, N cells could be pushed into oligodendrocyte production rather than apoptosis or terminal differentiation. This system, therefore, would provide for the maximum utilisation of the generative capacity of the ventricular zone cells. However, there is as yet no data to confirm this hypothesis, although the observation that the N-O phenotype is found with a greater frequency later in corticogenesis rather than earlier is supportive.

At first sight, this last model is superficially similar to the bipotential N-O cell model which I considered first but rejected. Both

46

models propose a period of bipotentiality during which precursors can decide between the two fates. The difference between the models lies in the temporal sequence that is proposed. The first model envisages an earlier bipotential cell giving rise to two later monopotential cells; there is a simple progression from less to more restriction. In the 'switch' model, precursors only display one potential at the time they are generated; they first show the propensity to switch later in corticogenesis. Hence (in one sense) they go from a lesser to a greater developmental potential. It can be argued that this is logically impossible. If cells downstream of a precursor show a potential, then by definition the precursor had at least that potential. The point is that the cells only show the potential later, either because they only acquire it later or because later events are required to trigger it. Whether we call a cell monopotential on the basis of what it is currently capable, or bipotential on the basis of attributes it will later acquire seems to me to be arbitrary. We tend to think of the potential of cells becoming restricted as development proceeds, but what actually happens is that precursors that generate cells required early are replaced by precursors that generate cells required late. It is not at all difficult to envisage circumstances in which a precursor switches from generating one cell type to generating that cell type plus another.

CONCLUSIONS

Using the retroviral lineage-labelling technique we have demonstrated that during the period of neurogenesis, most of the precursor cells of the cortical ventricular zone are restricted in the cell types they can generate. Most give rise to a single cell type, either neurons, astrocytes, or oligodendrocytes. Some precursor cells give rise to both neurons and oligodendrocytes, but we do not yet understand the significance of this apparent link between the lineage of these two cell types. Despite the restriction in terms of the cell types to which precursors contribute, we have been able to discover no restriction in either the lamina, or the cytoarchitectonic area to which precursor cells can contribute. We think this probably means that this aspect of fate is determined after the cells have left, or are leaving, the ventricular zone.

ACKNOWLEDGEMENTS

I would like to acknowledge the help of my colleagues, Dr. Elizabeth Grove and Dr. Brenda Williams, whose work forms the basis of much of what is discussed in this article. I would also like to acknowledge the financial support of the MRC, the EEC, and the Multiple Sclerosis Society of Great Britain and Northern Ireland.

REFERENCES

Balaban, E., Teillet, M-A. and LeDouarin, N. (1988) Application of the quail-chick chimera system to the study of brain development and behavior. Science 241:1339.

Beddington, R.S.P., Morgenstern, J., Land, H., and Hogen, A. (1989) An in situ transgenic enzyme marker for the midgestation mouse embryo and the visualisation of inner mass clones during early organogenesis. Development 106:37.

Berry, M. and Rogers, A.W. (1965) The migration of neuroblasts in the developing cerebral cortex. J. Anat. 99:691.

Fraser, S., Keynes, R., and Lumsden, A. (1990) Segmentation in the chick embryo hindbrain is defined by cell lineage restrictions. Nature 344:431.

Grove, E.A., Kirkwood, T.B.L. and Price, J. (1992) Neuronal precursor cells in the rat hippocampal formation contribute to more than one cytoarchitectonic area. Neuron 8:217.

Luskin, M.B., Pearlman, A.L., Sanes, J.R. (1988) Cell lineage in the cerebral cortex of the mouse studied in vivo and in vitro with a recombinant retrovirus. Neuron 1:635.

Miller, M.W. (1986) Effects of alcohol on the generation and migration of cerebral cortical neurons. Science 233:1308.

Price, J. and Thurlow, L. (1988) Cell lineage in the rat cerebral cortex: a study using retroviral-mediated gene transfer. Development 104:473.

Price, J., Turner, D., and Cepko, C. (1987) Lineage analysis in the vertebrate nervous system by retrovirus-mediated gene transfer. Proc. Natl. Acad. Sci. ULA 84:156.

Price, J., Williams, B. and Grove, E. (1991) Cell lineage in the cerebral cortex. Development Suppl. 2:23.

Rakic, P. (1988) Specification of cerebral cortical areas. Science 241:170.

Sanes, J.R., Rubenstein, J.L.R., Nicolas, J-F. (1986) Use of a recombinant retrovirus to study post-implantation cell lineage in mouse embryos. EMBO J. 5:3133.

Turner, D. and Cepko, C.L. (1987) Cell lineage in the rat retina: A common progenitor for neurons and glia persists late in development. Nature 328:131.

Turner, D.L., Snyder, E.Y. and Cepko, C.L. (1990) Lineage-independent determination of cell type in the embryonic mouse retina. Neuron 4:833.

Walsh, C. and Cepko, C.L. (1988) Clonally related cortical cells show several migration patterns. Science 241:1342.

Williams, B.P., Read, J. and Price, J. (1991) The generation of neurons and oligodendrocytes from a common precursor cell. Neuron 7:685.

HOX GENES AND THE DEVELOPMENT

OF THE BRANCHIAL REGION

Paul Hunt, Edoardo Boncinelli* and Robb Krumlauf

MRC Laboratory of Eukaryotic Molecular Genetics, NIMR
The Ridgeway, Mill Hill, London NW7 1AA, U.K.
*IIGB, Via Marconi 12, 80125 Naples, Italy

One of the key events in early development is positional specification, the process by which initially equivalent parts of a developing structure become different from one another. Once such differences are established the localised production of the substances can occur which eventually causes morphological differences to become apparent in a structure that was originally homogenous. The combination of molecular biology with genetics in the last ten years has begun to indicate how some stages of this process may come about during the early development of the vertebrate central nervous system and the structures associated with it.

INTRODUCTION

Regional Specification in Drosophila

One approach to understanding the events of regional specification is to identify the various genes required. This has been particularly successful in the analysis of the development of the fruit fly *Drosophila*, as large numbers of animals can be screened and it is possible to morphologically identify mutations affecting the very earliest stages of morphogenesis. Three classes of mutants were identified on the basis of their defects in the formation of the segmented body plan (for review see Akam, 1987): the *gap* genes involved in the earliest regional subdivisions of the egg, the *pair-rule* genes in the initial formation of the body segments, and the *segment-polarity* genes in segment maintenance during subsequent development. These groups of genes are hierarchically organised, thus gap gene mutants affect the function of both pair rule and segment polarity genes, while segment polarity genes are not required for the establishment of gap gene activities.

Homeotic Genes

The action of these three classes of genes is to produce a repeating pattern of segments, as mutations in any one of these produce animals with abnormal numbers of metameres. Within this segmental framework a fourth class acts, the *homeotic* genes (Akam, 1987). Their role is to give segments distinct identities, ie they are involved in

Development of the Central Nervous System in Vertebrates
Edited by S.C. Sharma and A.M. Goffinet, Plenum Press, New York, 1992

49

positional specification. Defects in the function of these genes do not alter the number of segments, rather they change the structures that a segment or a group of segments make. One example of such a gene is *Antennapedia*, which is required for the normal development of the thorax. Mutations in this gene which result in expression in parts of the body beyond its normal domains produce thoracic structures in inappropriate parts of the body; for instance ectopic legs form on the head in the place of antennae. The antennal primordium in these mutants is making the same sorts of cells as in normal animals; it is their relative numbers and organisation that have been altered as a result of the mutation, consistent with the idea that the gene is part of a system of supplying positional information to the developing primordia.

Further work has identified a number of homeotic genes in *Drosophila*, some of which, including *Antennapedia*, are involved in specification of regional identity along the A-P axis. The latter, known as *Antennapedia* class homeobox genes, are expressed in particular segment primordia before the appearance of morphological differences between them, consistent with the idea that the particular combination of *Antennapedia* class genes that a segment expresses is part of the system that controls the identity of that segment. The genes are organised into two clusters in which their order along the chromosome reflects both the regions along the A-P axis where they are expressed and the position of segments requiring them for their normal development (Lewis, 1978). When there is overlap between expression domains, posterior genes largely suppress the activity of more anterior genes. Thus expression of a gene in anterior regions of the body where it is not normally expressed results in posterior transformation of anterior segments, while loss of a gene allows more anterior genes to act in posterior parts of the body, resulting in anterior transformations of posterior segments. Isolation and sequencing of individual genes has shown that the proteins they encode contain a DNA binding motif known as the homeobox or homeodomain (Gehring, 1987); thus they are potentially able to act by controlling the expression of other genes.

It has been possible to identify genes in other organisms which share extensive similarities with the genes of the two homeotic gene clusters of *Drosophila*. In the beetle *Tribolium castaneum* a single cluster of genes has been identified, mutations of which cause similar transformations of segment identity along the A-P axis (Beeman, 1987; Beeman et al. 1989). Once again there is collinearity between the position of a gene on the chromosome and its normal segment of action, leading to the suggestion that the ancestral state of insects is for there to be a single cluster of homeotic genes, known as *HOM-C*. This single cluster became split at some stage on the lineage that lead to *Drosophila*.

Vertebrate *Hox* Genes

Vertebrates possess clusters of *Hox* genes with extensive sequence similarity in genomic organisation, sequence and expression domains to the genes of *HOM-C* (Kessel & Gruss, 1990; Simeone et al. 1991), illustrated in figure 1 for the mouse. The vertebrate genes most similar in sequence to a particular *Drosophila* gene also share the same relative anterior limit of expression (Duboule & Dolle, 1989; Graham et al. 1989). The extent of these similarities suggest that the *HOM-C* and *Hox* genes are descended from an ancestral cluster of genes present in the common ancestor of vertebrates and insects, whose primary role of specification along the A-P axis has been conserved (Duboule & Dolle, 1989; Graham et al. 1989). Genes with similar sequence to some components of the three classes of segmentation gene described above have also been isolated in vertebrates, but the evidence to date suggests that while they may have important roles in vertebrate development, they are not involved in the establishment of segments. For instance the vertebrate homologues of the *engrailed* gene, which in

Drosophila and other arthropods is involved in segment maintenance, are not involved in the establishment of rhombomeric segments in the hindbrain or somite formation on the basis of their earliest expression domains (Davis et al. 1991; Hemmati-Brivanlou et al. 1991). Their expression in the midbrain in a number of vertebrates is consistent with a role in specification of that part of the central nervous system, but the time course and sites of expression in other parts of the body suggest roles in the appearance of particular types of cells rather than regional specification.

There are four clusters of *Hox* genes in vertebrates (Simeone et al. 1991), illustrated in figure 1, each containing multiple genes showing similarity to a particular *Drosophila* gene. For example, there are four vertebrate genes, *Hox-1.4*, *Hox-2.6*, *Hox-3.5* and *Hox-4.2* all of which are expressed in anterior parts of the body and show greatest sequence similarity to the *Drosophila* gene *Dfd*, important for the development of the gnathal segments in *Drosophila*. Such groups of vertebrate genes, which show more sequence similarity to each other and to a *Drosophila* gene than they do to the other genes of their cluster are known as members of a *subfamily* or *paralogous group* of genes. The fact that four similar clusters exist suggest that they have arisen by cluster duplication followed by divergence of individual genes from each other.

HOX GENES AND THE DEVELOPMENT OF THE NERVOUS SYSTEM

The expression patterns of *Hox* genes are consistent with axial specification in a number of embryonic contexts. They show overlapping domains along the A-P axes of the limb (Dolle et al. 1989; Izpisua-Belmonte et al. 1991; Nohno et al. 1991), the somitic mesoderm of the trunk (Kessel & Gruss, 1990, 1991), and the central nervous system posterior of the midbrain (Graham et al. 1989; Wilkinson et al. 1989b). This suggests that they have been coopted on different occasions to patterning particular embryonic systems. The early domains of expression in all cases suggest that they are

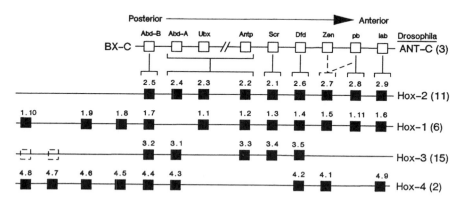

Fig. 1 . Structure of mouse homeobox complexes. Members of a subfamily of genes are aligned vertically with the *Drosophila* gene with which they share most similarity. Note that in the suggested evolutionary relationship between gene complexes indicated at the top by brackets, not all subfamilies of mouse genes have a single equivalent gene in *Drosophila*.

involved in the establishment of regional identity, although as development continues expression becomes restricted to particular cell types within the original A-P expression domain. A particular problem is to understand the different roles of the four clusters of *Hox* genes, as their conservation in all vertebrates suggests important distinct roles which has resulted in their maintenance during evolution. Our work has centred on the development of the branchial region of the head, as there are some indications from experimental embryology as to the mechanism of establishment of antero-posterior specification in this region.

The Development of the Hindbrain and Branchial Region

In the branchial region of the head the neural epithelium plays an important role in patterning (Lumsden, 1990a). At five somites the hindbrain neural plate consists of a series of bulges, the rhombomeres. Their relationships to the first branchial arch are also shown. Lineage analysis with vital dyes has suggested that rhombomeres are compartments (Fraser et al. 1990), and the demonstration that early patterns of neurogenesis also show rhombomeric organisation imply that they represent important units of developmental organisation (Lumsden & Keynes, 1989). Lineage-restricted processes in the hindbrain neural plate may also be controlling aspects of craniofacial skeletogenesis via the neural crest (Noden, 1983; Lumsden, 1990a; Hunt et al. 1991b). The margins of the neural plate produce neural crest which migrates ventrally into the branchial arches, giving rise to the bulk of the connective tissue; crest is also important in the formation of the cranial ganglia (Le Douarin et al. 1986), which show similar spatial relationships to particular arches in all vertebrates (Romer, 1971). The neural crest that gives rise to specific branchial arch structures always arises from particular rhombomeres (Lumsden et al. 1991), suggesting that the developmental processes of the hindbrain and branchial arches are linked (Lumsden, 1990b). The spatial relationships between the hindbrain and the second and third arches are shown in figure 2, based on the studies of Lumsden et al. 1991. There is evidence suggesting that the neural crest is imprinted with its regional identity before migration, which is then transferred to the branchial arches (Noden, 1988). Crest may also be able to direct the development of other tissues within the head, so that they produce structures appropriate to the crest they are in contact with (Noden, 1988). We believe that these properties of head development are reflected in the behaviour of *Antennapedia* class homeobox genes.

In *Drosophila* boundaries of gene expression correlate with specific segments (Akam, 1987), which is also true of the rhombomeric segments of the vertebrate head. In the mouse hindbrain cutoffs of the 5 most 3' *Hox* 2 genes correspond to rhombomeric boundaries, with successive genes showing expression limits separated by 2 rhombomere units as shown in figure 3 (Wilkinson et al. 1989b). A variety of evidence suggests an underlying two segment (rhombomere) periodicity in the structure of the hindbrain (Lumsden & Keynes, 1989; Wilkinson et al. 1989a), which may involve roles for the *Hox* genes in positional specification. Figure 3 illustrates that the branchial arches are each innervated by a cranial motor nerve, whose axons are derived from specific pairs of rhombomeres. Therefore, arch 1 is associated with the r2/r3 pair, arch 2 with r4/r5, and arch 3 with r6/r7. The pattern of expression is such that an arch receives motor innervation from two rhombomeres with differing patterns of gene expression.

Expression of Hox 2 Genes in Migrating Branchial Crest

Previous work has shown that *Hox* genes are expressed in the cranial ganglia, which are derived from neural crest (Holland & Hogan, 1988; Graham et al. 1988; Wilkinson et al. 1989b). In mouse the neural crest begins to leave the margins of the neural plate at 8 days of development (4 somites) in the cranial region, and by the 8½ days (11 somites) , migration is well under way (Verwoerd & van Oostrom, 1979;Nichols, 1981). *Hox-2.8* expression is continuous with the neural plate extending ventrolaterally of it, and can be found in migrating crest as shown in figure 4. Expression in the mesenchyme lateral of the neural plate is not visible at all levels of the neuraxis, which the raises the possibility that some areas of the neural plate do not produce neural crest (Hunt et al. 1991d). Rhombomeres 3 (see fig. 4A) and 5 seem not to have any labelled crest beside

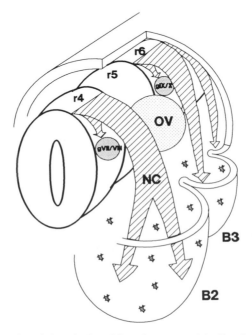

Fig. 2 . Spatial relationships between hindbrain and branchial arches, based on Lumsden et. al., (1991). The arrows indicate routes of crest (nc) migration. The grey shapes within the arches indicate cranial mesenchyme through which the crest cells migrate. ov: otic vesicle.

them. SEM studies of chick and rat embryos at the time of crest emigration suggest the existence of areas of neural tube that are crest free (Anderson & Meier, 1981;Tan & Morriss-Kay, 1985). However, a definitive proof that there are crest-free rhombomeres comes from dye injections at the dorsal midline of chick neural tubes at the start of emigration (Lumsden et al. 1991). This study confirms that rhombomeres 3 and 5 do not produce any neural crest and that rhombomere 4 contributes neural crest to the whole of the second arch in chick and to no other. Thus it seems that in areas where

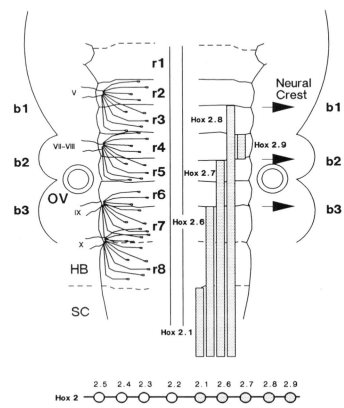

Fig 3. Expression of *Hox-2* genes in the neuroepithelium at 9½ days of mouse development, as described by Wilkinson et al., (1989). The left side of the diagram indicates the pattern of projection of the branchial motor nerves with respect to rhombomere boundaries. Their exit points in rhombomeres 2, 4, 6 and 7 are indicated, as are their relationships with the branchial arches and the otic vesicle. The right hand side of the diagram indicates the anterior expression limits of Hox 2 genes, whose relative positions in the *Hox-2* cluster is shown underneath. Expression domains are overlapping and present throughout the neuroepithelium, such that rhombomere 3 expresses *Hox-2.8* alone and rhombomere 7 a combination of *Hox-2.8*, *Hox-2.7* and *Hox-2.6*.

B1-B3: 1st-3rd branchial arches; V: trigeminal nerve; VII-VIII: facial/acoustic nerve; IX: glossopharangeal nerve; X: Vagus nerve; OV: otic vesicle; r1-r7: rhombomeres 1-7.

crest does arise, it expresses *Hox 2* genes from time of emergence and that the neural crest migrating into the arches has a *Hox 2* label or code. The lack of extensive mixing between different populations of neural crest along the rostro-caudal axis (Lumsden et al. 1991) would mean that crest entering an arch is derived from a restricted number of rhombomeres, and hence pattern of gene expression is maintained. It is interesting to note that these crest-free rhombomeres are the only ones which express *Krox-20* (Wilkinson et al. 1989a).

There is no evidence of *Hox-2.8* expression in the surface ectoderm or in the head mesenchyme through which the crest is migrating.

Expression in the Branchial Region after Migration is Complete

Hox expression persists after crest migration is completed. *Hox-2.8* is expressed at 9 d.p.c. in the VII/VIII cranial ganglion complex (g) that is located opposite rhombomere 4, as shown in Figure 5A. Figure 5C shows a section through the branchial arches of the same embryo hybridised with *Hox-2.8*. It is clear that there is no expression in arch 1, while arch 2 and more posterior regions express *Hox-2.8* in areas colonised by neural crest. The branchial arches are largely derived from neural crest, although there is also contribution from paraxial mesoderm in the core of the branchial arch in chick (Noden, 1988). This paraxial contribution to ventral parts of the arch is small and is confined to the core of the arch, so we believe that the hybridisation seen here is largely due to expression in the neural crest.

When more posteriorly expressed genes of *Hox 2* are examined (Hunt et al. 1991d), they are also found to show a branchial-arch restricted pattern of expression. The expression patterns of the four most anterior *Hox* genes are summarised in figure 6.

The areas of surface ectoderm lateral to the edges of the neural plate are known to produce thickenings or placodes, which generate neural derivatives (D'Amico-Martel & Noden, 1983;Le Douarin et al. 1986). In the light of this and the recent work of Couly and Le Douarin (1990) on the contributions of ectoderm lateral of the neural plate to the head we were interested to see the extent of *Hox 2* expression in the surface ectoderm. In figure 7 expression of *Hox-2.8* is seen in the surface ectoderm (se) of the second branchial arch of a 9½ day embryo, and not in the surface of the first arch (b1). This demonstrates that the surface ectoderm expresses *Hox-2.8* at 9½ days in the same way as the underlying crest mesenchyme. This is in contrast to our observations at 8½ days, when *Hox-2.8* expressing neural crest is seen to be migrating under surface ectoderm that does not express above background levels (figure 4).

Hox genes in developing systems are thought to be one component of the process of assigning different states to otherwise equivalent groups of cells. The maintenance of a state may be manifested by the continued expression of these genes. Each branchial arch has a distinct code of *Hox 2* expression (with arch one not expressing any *Hox* gene), and this arch-specific *Hox 2* pattern is in the neural crest before it has reached the branchial arches. Given that *Antennapedia* class homeobox genes act as positional specifiers (Akam, 1987;Beeman, 1987;Beeman et al. 1989;Kessel et al. 1990), we believe that a specific combination of *Hox 2* expression could provide part of the molecular mechanism for imprinting of cranial neural crest (Hunt et al. 1991b, d).

The Role of Other Subfamilies in the Branchial Region

The hindbrain expression of *Hox 2* genes is characterised by a two rhombomere periodicity, yet each rhombomere has an identity distinct from the rest (Lumsden & Keynes, 1989), thus there are more rhombomeric units than could be individually specified by the genes of a given *Hox* cluster. Therefore we wanted to determine if

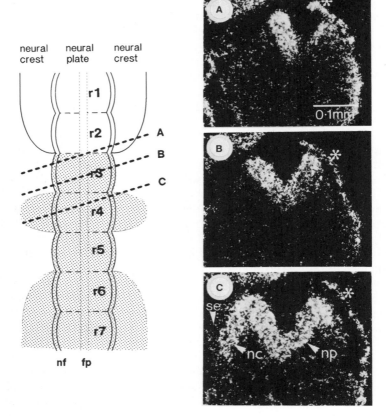

Fig. 4 . Hox 2 expression in migrating and premigratory neural crest; expression
of Hox 2.8 in serial, transverse sections of an 8½ day mouse embryo
hindbrain. The relative position of sections is shown in the diagram on the
left, with A the most anterior section. The sections are slightly oblique,
such that the right hand side of each section is more anterior than the left
hand side. The asterisks indicate extra embryonic membranes that are
expressing Hox 2.8, and serve as a positive control for hybridisation. The
diagram on the left indicates which rhombomeres the sections are passing
through, and the plane of the section. Tissues known to be expressing Hox
2.8 are shaded in grey stipple. The lobes lateral to the neural plate indicate
areas of neural crest that are known to be produced by particular lengths
of neural plate.

nf: neural fold; fp: floorplate; se: surface ectoderm; nc: migrating neural
crest; np : neural plate

genes from all four *Hox* clusters are necessary to generate the full range of rhombomere diversity that is seen. The branchial neural crest is able to give rise to a wide range of cell types (Le Douarin, 1983), so genes of other clusters may be involved in different aspects of crest development as well. For these reasons we have examined the expression of 11 of the 12 *Hox* genes expressed in the hindbrain and branchial arches to define a *Hox* code for this region.

The relationships we have found in the expression of members from a subfamily are exemplified by the genes of the *Zen/pb* group. Expression of two members, *Hox-1.5* and *Hox-2.7*, is shown in Figure 8. *Hox-1.5* is expressed with an anterior limit at the boundary between r5 and r4 in a 9½ day embryo, as shown in Figure 8A-C.

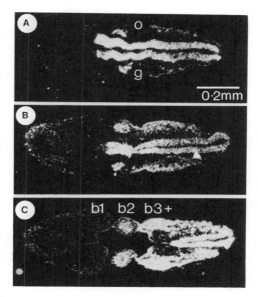

Fig. 5. Hox 2.8 expression in the hindbrain and branchial arches after neural crest migration is complete. A set of serial sections coronal to the hindbrain are shown of a 9 day mouse embryo. Section A is the most dorsal, and shows expression in the hindbrain and the vii\viii ganglion. Section B is ventral to A, and shows expression in the hindbrain and in addition two isolated patches of expression lateral of the neural tube. Section C is more ventral than B, and passes through the branchial arches. The first arch does not express, while the second and more posterior arches express. Expression is seen in those parts of the head known to be colonised by neural crest.

o: otic placode, g: vii\viii ganglion, b1-b3: first-third branchial arches.

The expression pattern of another subfamily member, *Hox-2.7*, is shown in Figure 8D-F. It shows identical anterior expression limits in the rhombomeres (8D), branchial arches (8E), and the surface ectoderm (8F). In addition to identical anterior boundaries of expression, *Hox-1.5* and *Hox-2.7* also show a similar patterns of expression within their rhombomeric domains. There is a high level in r5, and lower levels in more posterior parts of the neural tube. In contrast the third member of the

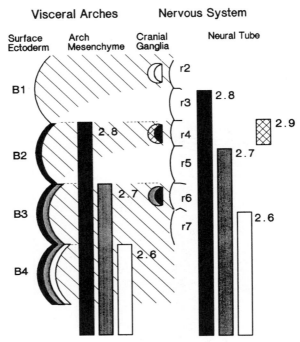

Fig. 6 .Summary of Hox 2 expression found in the hindbrain and branchial arches. The stipple indicates the areas of neural plate where neural crest is produced, and the branchial arch into which it migrates. The ganglion next to rhombomere 2 is the V or trigeminal, that next to rhombomere 4 is the VII/VIII or acoustic-facial complex, and those next to rhombomere 6 are the combined superior ganglia of the IX and X cranial nerves. The shading patterns shown in the cranial ganglia indicate that all the cells in a ganglion express a combination of genes, and do not imply that there is spatial restriction of gene expression within a ganglion. produce crest able to colonise the branchial arches, and so *Hox-1.5* is expressed in the third and more posterior branchial arches, not the second arch (Fig. 8B). There is further support for the idea of an instructive interaction between branchial crest and its overlying ectoderm (Noden, 1988; Hunt et al. 1991d), as Hox 1.5 shows identical expression limits in both tissues as indicated in Fig. 8C.

group, *Hox-4.1*, shows expression at a uniform level up to the r5/6 boundary, then a lower level in r5 (Hunt et al. 1991a). These data show that members of the *Zen/pb* subfamily may differ in levels of expression within their overall domains, but the anterior boundaries and combinations of rhombomeres and branchial arches in which they are expressed are identical. A similar analysis with members of the *Dfd* and *pb* subfamilies shows that each member of a group also has identical boundary of expression in the hindbrain and branchial arches which is characteristic for its subfamily, but there are also regional variations in level (Hunt et al. 1991a). The expression of *Hox* genes expressed in the hindbrain and the levels of expression within these domains are summarised in figure 9.

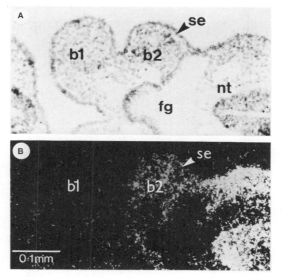

Fig. 7. Expression of Hox 2.8 in surface ectoderm (se) overlying the branchial arches at 9½ days. 4A is a bright field view of 4B. Note lack of expression over first brachial arch (b1), in contrast to the second (b2). Expression is also seen in the wall of the foregut (fg), and the neural tube (nt).

The only exception to this rule of identical patterns among paralogues is in the *labial* group , illustrated in Figure 10. Their expression does not persist into phases of embryogenesis later than 12½ d.p.c. in mouse, and at 9 d.p.c. the three genes exhibit domains of expression distinct from each other. For example *Hox-2.9* is the only gene in the family expressed within the neural tube at 9½ d.p.c., and this domain is restricted to a single rhombomere, r4 (Fig. 10A; Duboule & Dolle, 1989; Murphy et al. 1989; Wilkinson et al. 1989b). In contrast an equivalent section hybridised with *Hox-1.6* shows no expression above background (10B), and *Hox-4.9* expression is confined to the surface ectoderm overlying the hindbrain (10C). *Hox-1.6* is however expressed in non neural tissues elsewhere in the embryo at this stage, as shown in 10D and 10E (Murphy & Hill, 1991). The *labial* group also show differences in behaviour from other subgroups in the way in which their expression patterns develop. At an early stage Hox 1.6 and Hox 2.9 have been shown to have identical expression domains (Murphy & Hill, 1991), but by 8½ d.p.c. expression of Hox 1.6 and part of the Hox 2.9 domain is receding posteriorly. At the same time Hox 2.9 expression is being established in its r4 domain. Even at this stage Hox 4.9 does not show similar expression properties to its two *labial* equivalents in Hox 1 and Hox 2. Figure 10F shows the entirely posteriorly-restricted expression of Hox 4.9 (Hunt et al. 1991a) at a stage at which Hox 2.9 and Hox 1.6 are expressed up to the presumptive r4/r3 boundary (Murphy & Hill, 1991).

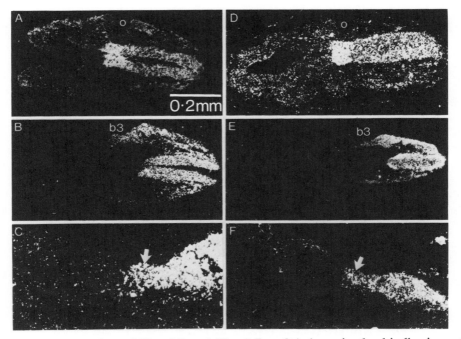

Fig. 8. Expression of Hox-1.5 and Hox-2.7 at 9½ d.p.c. in the hindbrain and branchial region. A-C are hybridised with Hox 1.5, and D-F with Hox-2.7. A and D are coronal sections through the hindbrain, and show expression with an anterior limit at the boundary of r4 and r5. Note highest levels of expression over r5. B and E are coronal sections through the branchial arches, showing expression confined to the third branchial arch and posterior regions. C and F are high magnification views of C and F respectively. The arrows indicate expression in the layer of surface ectoderm that overlies the largely neural crest-derived mesenchyme beneath. G summarises the expression data of the *Zen/pb* family at 9½d.p.c., showing expression up to the third branchial arch and the r4/r5 boundary. Magnification A,B,D,E (×95), C,F(×300).

o: otic vesicle; b3: third branchial arch.

The Hox Code of the Head

Figure 9 is a summary of the patterns of expression of all of the *Hox* genes we have examined at a stage when the rhombomeres have fully formed and neural crest has migrated into the branchial arches. It represents a branchial *Hox* code in which regional differences in expression could be used to specify positional differences in the various tissues.

With the exception of the *labial* subfamily, there do not seem to be any differences in which rhombomeres or branchial arches express members of the same subfamily. In contrast, in the somites the expression limits of members of the same subfamilies can be offset from each other (Gaunt et al. 1989). The presence of areas of reduced crest emigration in rhombomeres 3 and 5 (Kuratani & Kirby, 1991; Lumsden et al. 1991) means that the expression of the *pb* and *zen/pb* groups is one rhombomere out of phase with expression in the hindbrain. Because members of a subfamily apparently have identical patterns of expression it is unlikely that the rhombomeres and the branchial arch structures derived from them are further spatially subdivided at the time of their formation by differential expression of members of a paralogous group. However, expression patterns at the later stages of development when branchial arches are undergoing morphogenesis have not been investigated.

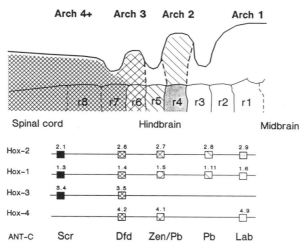

Fig.9. The complete branchial *Hox* code based on gene expression. The diagram indicates the patterns of *Hox* subfamilies expressed in the branchial region after neural crest migration is complete, when distinct rhombomeres are apparent. The shading indicates an overlapping code of *Hox* subfamily expression in the rhombomeres of the hindbrain and the migration of mesenchymal and neurogenic crest from specific rhombomeres, resulting in a transfer of a combinatorial code to the branchial arches. The branchial arch ectoderm subsequently adopts an identical pattern of Hox subfamily expression. Hox 2.9 expression is confined to the ganglionic crest. *Hox* subfamily expression in the hindbrain is out of phase with the branchial arches by one rhombomere as a result of the lack of contribution to branchial arch crest by r3 and r5. This is represented by the absence of crest emanating from r3 and r5. First arch crest that does not have a *Hox* label is also present. The chromosomal relationship of the relevant subfamilies is shown at the bottom of the diagram. This diagram is based on that in Hunt et al 1991a.

61

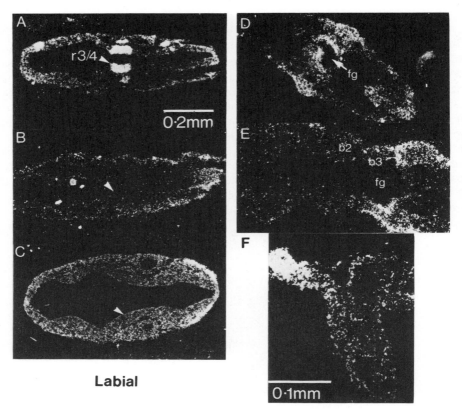

Labial

Fig.10. Expression of the *labial* family of genes in 8 and 9½ day mouse embryos. (A-E) are coronal sections, and (F) is saggital. (A) shows the expression of Hox 2.9 in r4 and the adjacent vii/viii cranial ganglia. An equivalent section with Hox 4.9 (C) shows expression in specific regions of surface ectoderm, but none in the neural tube. (F) shows the expression of Hox 4.9 in the posterior regions of an 8 day embryo. A similar section to (A) and (C) with Hox 1.6 shows no expression in neural tube or cranial ganglia, but more ventral sections of the same embryo show expression in the foregut (fg) and ectoderm and mesenchyme of the posterior branchial arches (D,E). (F) shows the expression of Hox 4.9 in an 8 d.p.c., 1 somite embryo that expressed Hox 2.8 up to the presumptive r2/r3 boundary. At this stage the two other *labial* family genes show r3/r4 boundary restricted expression in the hindbrain.

Based on our findings (Hunt et al. 1991a), we suggest that an early event in the patterning of the head is the establishment of patterns of *Hox* expression in the neural plate that will give rise to the hindbrain. Because the crest that forms the ganglia and branchial arches arises at particular positions along the A-P axis of the neural plate, the arches will have a pattern of *Hox* expression that reflects their level of origin. Rhombomeres 3 and 5 do not contribute crest to the arches which means that the neural crest component in arches 2 and 3 is derived from one rhombomere. The possibility of a link between the development of the hindbrain and the rest of the branmchial region mediated by neural crest has been discussed previously (Lumsden, 1990b).

In the *Hox* code presented in Figure 9 we assume the genes are acting in a simple combinatorial way, in which presence or absence of gene expression is the important property in terms of morphogenesis. However, we have shown that subfamily members can have different levels of expression within the same rhombomeric domains (Hunt et al. 1991a, c). It is possible that expression of subfamily members above a specific threshold may be necessary for morphogenetic function, and that specific subsets of the domains of expression are the only ones involved in combinatorial patterning. These regional variations could also be important for late stage patterning in the neural tube and not implicated in the neural crest specification. The timing of axogenesis, the first morphological criterion of rhombomere identity occurs sufficiently late for this to be a possibility.

Hox Expression in the Developing Spinal Cord

The similarities in early domains of *Hox* subfamily expression in the branchial region do not suggest unique roles for individual genes at this stage of development. However, consideration of the way in which *Hox* expression develops at later stages of development suggests potential roles for different members of the same subfamily of genes (Graham et al. 1991). One indication of a possible reason for conservation of four *Hox* clusters has come from consideration of the change in patterns of *Hox 2* gene expression in the dorsal-ventral axis of the mouse spinal cord during development. At 9 days, expression is homogenous throughout the dorso-ventral extent of the spinal cord. At 10.0 and 11.0 d.p.c. expression is lost from the ventral motor horns, while at the same time there is strong expression in the lateral commissural neurons, which have already performed their final round of cell division. At later stages, 12.0-12.5 d.p.c. RNA distributions are limited to the dorsal sensory regions, without expression in the commissural cells (Graham et al. 1991). Finally, at 14.5 d.p.c. expression reappears in the ventral region. This pattern of expression is the same for all members of the *Hox 2* complex. Thus there is evidence that *Hox 2* expression reflects the birth of particular populations of neurons within the spinal cord and could be used to specify their positional values. Genes of other *Hox* clusters also show dorso-ventral restrictions within the spinal cord (Graham et al. 1991), but they differ from those of the *Hox 2* genes. This raises the possibility that different clusters have distinct roles in particular types of tissues at later stages of development.

DISCUSSION

The development of the vertebrate head is thought to involve a series of interactions between neural plate, neural crest, mesoderm, surface ectoderm and pharyngeal endoderm. Despite this complexity, it is possible to define a sequence of events by which some components of this system are spatially specified. The developmental and spatial relationships between neural tube and branchial arches suggest that primary patterning events in the neural plate could be transmitted to other parts of the head by migrating neural crest (Lumsden, 1990b). We believe that the vertebrate *Hox* genes are a component of the process that achieves this spatial specification. The similarity of expression domains between members of a subfamily suggests that there is redundancy in the earliest aspects of the specification of morphological units in the branchial region by *Hox* genes. It is better to think in terms of a subfamily of *Hox* genes together specifying a pair of rhombomeres and a branchial arch. The specification of pairs of rhombomeres would be consistent with the two segment patterns of both branchial and somatic motor nerve development observed in the hindbrain (Lumsden & Keynes, 1989). There are sufficient subfamilies to uniquely specify each branchial arch, and system that was able to distinguish odd from even rhombomeres would be able to uniquely specify each rhombomere in combination with a subfamily of *Hox* genes. *Krox-20* could provide the information necessary to distinguish all but r1 and r7, so perhaps other genes in concert with *Krox-20* may be responsible for this. There is evidence from rhombomere grafting experiments that odd and even rhombomeres differ in their cellular properties, as the apposition of part of an odd rhombomere with part of an even one results in the formation of a new rhombomere boundary, while the other possibilities result in the formation of a large, compound rhombomeres (Guthrie & Lumsden, 1991). The specific roles for which particular subfamily members are required occur after primary specification of rhombomeres and branchial arches (Hunt et al. 1991c).

Phenotypes of Mice Lacking Particular *Hox* Genes

These ideas of the way in which the *Hox* code of the head acts to specify morphological units is supported by the phenotype of mice lacking normal *Hox-1.5* (Chisaka & Capecchi, 1991) and *Hox-1.6* protein (Lufkin et al. 1991). The rhombomere morphologies of *Hox-1.5* and *-1.6* deleted mice appear normal, supporting the idea that Hox genes are involved in spatial specification of units rather than their initial establishment. The *Hox-1.5* mice have normal cranial ganglia and defects in tissues dependent upon mesenchymal neural crest for their development such as the heart outflow tract and the glands of the neck (Kirby, 1989; Chisaka & Capecchi, 1991), some of which correspond to the normal domain of *Hox-1.5* expression. The fact that normal ganglia are formed suggest that there is sufficient information to spatially specify them in the absence of *Hox-1.5*, supporting the idea of redundancy in the early role of Hox genes, spatial specification of the neural epithelium. The defects could mean that *Hox-1.5* is required to maintain spatial specification in mesenchymal crest derivatives, or that *Hox-1.5* has a specific role in some other aspect of development of mesenchymal crest. In contrast the *Hox-1.6* mice show normal mesenchymal structures, but disrupted nuclei of branchial nerves VII, VIII, IX and X, and their associated ganglia (Lufkin et al. 1991). The fact that two members of the same *Hox* complex produce defects in different ranges of tissues argues against a simple model where a particular cluster of Hox genes is solely responsible for spatial specification and/or differentiation in a particular group of tissues.

It is interesting that cranial ganglia which do not normally express the gene are disrupted in *Hox-1.6* mutant mice, although the neural plate from which both the ganglia and the rhombomeres derive did at 8 d.p.c. (Murphy & Hill, 1991). It may be that in the absence of *Hox-1.6* it is not possible to establish or maintain normal patterns of expression of other genes, which may result in defects later in development in tissues that do not normally express *Hox-1.6*. It is not clear how the other 3' *Hox* genes are expressed in the branchial region of mice lacking *Hox* genes. In *Drosophila* posterior genes are known to repress the expression of genes expressed in more anterior domains (Akam, 1987), thus it is possible that interactions between vertebrate *Hox* genes are necessary to maintain appropriate patterns of gene expression. It is also known that the transcription patterns within vertebrate *Hox* complexes are complex (Simeone et al. 1988; M-H. Sham, in preparation), and that transcripts for one gene may originate within another. It may be that deletion of one gene may alter expression patterns of other genes, perhaps by disturbing the genetic circuitry necessary to establish and maintain gene expression by removing one of its components. Alternatively the large genomic insertions used to disrupt a genes may destroy transcription start sites of other genes, and hence alter their patterns of expression. This is a general problem in the interpretation of the phenotype of mice lacking a specific *Hox* gene; until the effects of the loss of specific gene on the expression of the other members of the cranial *Hox* gene network are known it is not possible to interpret phenotypes in terms of alterations in the cranial *Hox* code. Homologous disruption of a Hox gene could also perturb the expression of other genes important for head development.

The *Hox-1.5* gene is normally expressed in an identical way to its homologue *Hox-2.7* in the crest at early stages (figure 8), which populates the third and posterior branchial arches. There are skeletal abnormalities in neural crest derivatives which do not normally express *Hox-1.5*, such as the first branchial arch derived mandibles and maxillae, and absence of the lesser wing of the hyoid bone, a second arch derivative (Chisaka & Capecchi, 1991). However, the greater wing of the hyoid bone, derived from the *Hox-1.5* expressing third arch, appears more normal. The defects seen with *Hox-1.6* lie within a smaller region, but also show evidence of perturbations of structures which never express *Hox-1.6* (Lufkin et al. 1991; Murphy & Hill, 1991). These are mainly associated with the bony parts of the ear, some of which are derived from the otocyst, a structure which is produced by an induction from the underlying hindbrain. There is much evidence of the importance of interactions between different tissues in the head for normal morphogenesis (Moody & Heaton, 1983a, b; Hall, 1987; Thorogood, 1988; Ruiz-i-Altaba, 1990), and the role of *Hox* genes in the endoderm and head paraxial mesoderm are not clear. The defects in more anterior arches beyond the normal regions of *Hox-1.5* and *Hox-1.6* gene expression may be due to interactions between structures of different arches necessary to produce normal development.

The Requirement for Four *Hox* Clusters in Vertebrates

One possibility is that each gene in a subfamily has a distinct role at the earliest stage of structure specification, with a different range of structures specified by each member, for example cranial ganglia, rhombomeres or branchial cartilages. Thus members of a subfamily would act in parallel and independently to specify regional identity in the different derivatives of the hindbrain neural plate, hence coincident expression domains. The apparent similarities in expression domains could reflect the lack of cellular resolution in the radioactive *in situ* hybridisation technique and its inability to demonstrate the presence of active protein product; a technique with higher resolution may reveal differences between subpopulations of cells.

The lineage relationships between cells of the cephalic neural plate are not as clear as in the trunk, where evidence suggests that there is multipotency in cells while within the neural plate, in that descendants of a single cell can contribute to the neural tube, dorsal root ganglia, the adrenal medulla and pigment cells (Bronner-Fraser & Fraser, 1988). In the head also there is some preliminary *in vivo* data (Bronner-Fraser & Fraser, 1988) and *in vitro* data that suggests that both mesenchymal and neurogenic derivatives can derive from a single crest cell precursor (Baroffio et al. 1991). Given this apparent level of plasticity in crest differentiative potential, it is hard to imagine how cells belonging to subpopulations of crest lineages can be defined before crest emigration occurs. Thus if *Hox* subfamily members are supplying information in parallel to different lineages of crest from the same axial level they must be doing so after the crest precursors have left the neural tube and have made the decisions as to which lineage they will represent.

There cannot be a simple relationship between the genes of a particular *Hox* complex and spatial specification of particular crest lineages. Crest cells contributing to the first four branchial arches are able to give rise to the same range of cell types, yet there are no Hox genes expressed in the first arch, no *Hox 3* or *Hox 4* members in the second arch, and no *Hox 3* member expressed in the third arch. This suggests that Hox genes are not a requirement for the establishment of early crest lineages, unless there are great differences in how particular crest lineages arise at different axial levels. For the same reason it is hard to imagine why the different components of more posterior branchial arches require independent complexes of *Hox* genes for their early spatial patterning while more anterior arches employ fewer genes to perform apparently the same task, if a cluster of *Hox* genes is required to generate particular lineages.

Subgroup members probably have important distinct roles in the head later on in development as part of the mechanism causing cells to follow particular differentiation pathways, hence the specific problems in particular crest derivatives. It is probable that there is functional redundancy in the early morphogenetic developmental events with unique functions arising later in development, which would explain our findings, the specificity of defects seen in mutant mice and the later-arising differences of expression in specific structures (Gaunt et al. 1989). Detailed comparisons of somite domains reveal that subgroup members differ in which somites they are expressed (Gaunt et al. 1989, 1990; reviewed in Kessel & Gruss, 1991), leading to the suggestion that each somite is uniquely specified by a particular combination of gene expression or *Hox* code. There are more somites than could be individually specified by an overlapping code of *Hox* genes from any one cluster. Members of the more posteriorly expressed subfamilies such as the *Abd-B* group also show differences in A-P expression limits in the nervous system and somites (Izpisua-Belmonte et al. 1990). Therefore part of the reason for the conservation of four *Hox* clusters in vertebrates may be to individually specify parts of the trunk nervous system and paraxial mesoderm.

The Development of the Anterior Head

The parts of the head anterior of the hindbrain do not express *Antennapedia* class *Hox* genes, so some other mechanisms must be involved in their specification. In *Drosophila* the anterior head is also beyond the domains of expression of the *HOM-C* genes, and seem to be specified by an independent patterning system (Cohen & Jurgens, 1990; Finkelstein & Perrimon, 1990). In vertebrates there is emerging molecular evidence for groups of genes distinct from the four clusters of *Antennapedia* class *Hox* genes involved in the specification of head development. The murine homologue of the cell signalling molecule, *Wnt-1* is expressed in the mesencephalon (Wilkinson et al. 1987), which is deleted in homologous recombinant mice lacking the gene function (McMahon & Bradley, 1990). The expression patterns of other genes suggests an involvement in the patterning of brain and neural crest. In more anterior parts of the mouse neuroepithelium there is evidence for a gene related to the *Distal-less* gene of *Drosophila* showing spatially-restricted domains of expression consistent with regional patterning (Price et al. 1991). Striking differences in gene expression in specific branchial arches is also apparent with retinoic acid receptor ß (Dolle et al. 1990; Rowe et al. 1991) and the cytoplasmic retinoic acid binding protein (Dencker et al. 1990;

Vaessen et al. 1990; Maden et al. 1991), suggesting a role in anterior crest specification. That these molecules show spatially-restricted distributions is particularly interesting in the light of evidence for differential sensitivity of facial primordia to retinoic acid (Morriss & Thorogood, 1978; Sulik et al. 1988; Durston et al. 1989). Other genes may play a role in specification of the anterior neural plate such as *BMP-4* and *Vgr-1* (Jones et al. 1991). Some of the genes mentioned here may be involved in the actual establishment of pattern in the head anterior of the hindbrain, others may be early markers of regionally-restricted differentiation events. A more detailed comparison of the onset of expression of such genes coupled with the emerging technology of directed mutagenesis in mice will elucidate the relative positions of such genes in the developmental hierarchy of the head.

There is also evidence for head patterning strategies that do not involve genetic specification of the neural plate followed by transfer of patterning information to other parts of the head by imprinted neural crest. Evidence suggests that crest prespecification may be less important in more anterior parts of the head (McKee & Ferguson, 1984; Noden, 1988). The distribution of type II collagen suggests that aspects of craniofacial morphogenesis may be controlled by the distribution of molecules on cranial epithelia that arrest crest migration and induce chondrogenesis at specific sites (Thorogood et al. 1986; Wood et al. 1991). In this "flypaper" model patterning information resides in the neural plate but also in other head epithelia such as the primordia of the paired sense organs (Thorogood, 1988), while there is little intrinsic information in the crest. These epigenetic mechanisms are likely to be the more important in craniofacial morphogenesis, as the bulk of cranial and facial structures are derived from this region.

Thus the vertebrate body axis appears to be show three zones of *Hox* expression; the anterior head, without any expression by *Antennapedia* class genes, the branchial region, with an overlapping code of rhombomere and branchial arch specification, and the trunk, where offsets in subfamily expression mark particular somites and parts of the spinal cord.

Future Directions

There seems little doubt that the *Hox* family is an important part of the system specifying regional identity. The descriptive studies suggested that they played an important role in the head, which has been directly demonstrated by the phenotypes observed in mice bearing mutated *Hox* genes. It will now be essential to identify their primary and secondary roles, and to determine how the signals for establishing the patterns are established. In this regard the identification of transcriptional control regions which are required to produce a particular aspect of the expression pattern will be useful to test the *Hox* code by dominant overexpression in transgenic mice and to identify potential upstream factors able to regulate the expression of the genes themselves.

ACKNOWLEDGEMENTS

We thank Drs. Andrew Lumsden, Drew Noden, Peter Thorogood and David Wilkinson for valuable discussions. This work was funded by the UK MRC, and Paul Hunt is in receipt of an MRC studentship.

Figure is adapted from Hunt and Krumlauf (1991), Cell 66, pp 1075-1078. Figures 3 and 7 are adapted from Hunt et al. (1991b), 4, 5 and 6 from Hunt et al. (1991d) and 8 and 10 from Hunt et al. (1991c).

REFERENCES

AKAM, M. (1987). The molecular basis for metameric pattern in the *Drosophila* embryo. *Development* **101**, 1-22.

ANDERSON, C. & MEIER, S. (1981). The influence of the metameric pattern in the mesoderm on migration of cranial neural crest cells in the chick embryo. *Devl Biol.* **85**, 385-402.

BAROFFIO, A., DUPIN, E. & LE DOUARIN, N. (1991). Common precursors for neural and mesenchymal derivatives in the cephalic neural crest. *Development* **112**, 301-305.

BEEMAN, R. (1987). A homeotic gene cluster in the red flour beetle. *Nature* **327**, 247-249.

BEEMAN, R., STUART, J., HAAS, M. & DENELL, R. (1989). Genetic analysis of the homeotic gene complex (HOM-C) in the beetle *Tribolium castaneum*. *Devl Biol.* **133**, 196-209.

BRONNER-FRASER, M. & FRASER, S. (1988). Cell lineage analysis reveals multipotency of some avian neural crest cells. *Nature* **335**, 161-164.

CHISAKA, O. & CAPECCHI, M. (1991). Regionally restricted developmental defects resulting from targetted disruption of the mouse homeobox gene *hox1.5*. *Nature* **350**, 473-479.

COHEN, S. & JURGENS, G. (1990). Mediation of *Drosophila* head development by gap-like segmentation genes. *Nature* **346**, 482-485.

D'AMICO-MARTEL, A. & NODEN, D. (1983). Contributions of placodal and neural crest cells to avian cranial peripheral ganglia. *Am. J. Anat.* **166**, 445-468.

DAVIS, C., HOLMYARD, D., MILLEN, K. & JOYNER, A. (1991). Examining pattern formation in mouse,chicken and frog embryos with an *En*-specific antiserum. *Development* **111**, 287-298.

DENCKER, L., ANNERWALL, E., BUSCH, C. & ERIKSSON, U. (1990). Localization of specific retinoid-binding sites and expression of cellular retinoic-acid-binding protein (CRABP) in the early mouse embryo. *Development* **110**, 343-352.

DOLLE, P., IZPISUA-BELMONTE, J. C., FALKENSTEIN, H., RENUCCI, A. & DUBOULE, D. (1989). Coordinate expression of the murine Hox-5 complex homoeobox-containing genes during limb pattern formation. *Nature* **342**, 767-772.

DOLLE, P., RUBERTE, E., LEROY, P., MORRISS-KAY, G. & CHAMBON, P. (1990). Retinoic acid receptors and cellular retinoid binding proteins. I. A systematic study of their differential pattern of transcription during mouse organogenesis. *Development* **110**, 1133-1151.

DUBOULE, D. & DOLLE, P. (1989). The structural and functinal organization of the murine HOX gene family resembles that of Drosophila homeotic genes. *EMBO* **8**, 1497-1505.

DURSTON, A., TIMMERMANS, J., HAGE, W., HENDRIKS, H., DE VRIES, N., HEIDEVELD, M. & NIEUWKOOP, P. (1989). Retinoic acid causes an anteroposterior transformation in the developing central nervous system. *Nature* **340**, 140-144.

FINKELSTEIN, R. & PERRIMON, N. (1990). The orthodenticle gene is regulated by *bicoid* and *torso* and specifies *Drosophila* head development. *Nature* **346**, 485-488.

FRASER, S., KEYNES, R. & LUMSDEN, A. (1990). Segmentation in the chick embryo hindbrain is defined by cell lineage restrictions. *Nature* **344**, 431-435.

GAUNT, S. J., KRUMLAUF, R. & DUBOULE, D. (1989). Mouse homeo-genes within a subfamily, Hox-1.4, -2.6 and -5.1, display similar anteroposterior domains of expression in the embryo, but show stage- and tissue-dependent differences in their regulation. *Development.* **107**, 131-141.

GAUNT, S. J., COLETTA, P. L., PRAVTCHEVA, D. & SHARPE, P. T. (1990). Mouse Hox-3.4: homeobox sequence and embryonic expression patterns compared with other members of the Hox gene network. *Development* **109**, 329-339.

GEHRING, W. (1987). Homeoboxes in the study of development. *Science* **236**, 1245-1252.

GRAHAM, A., PAPALOPULU, N., LORIMER, J., MCVEY, J., TUDDENHAM, E. & KRUMLAUF, R. (1988). Characterization of a murine homeo box gene, *Hox 2.6*, related to the drosophila deformed gene. *Genes Dev.* **2**, 1424-1438.

GRAHAM, A., PAPALOPULU, N. & KRUMLAUF, R. (1989). The murine and *Drosophila* homeobox clusters have common features of organisation and expression. *Cell* **57**, 367-378.

GRAHAM, A., MADEN, M. & KRUMLAUF, R. (1991). The murine Hox-2 genes display dynamic dorsoventral patterns of expression during central nervous system development. *Development* **112**, 255-264.

GUTHRIE, S. & LUMSDEN, A. (1991). Formation and regeneration of rhombomere boundaries in the developing chick hindbrain. *Development* **112**, 221-229.

HALL, B. (1987). Tissue Interactions in Head Development and Evolution. In *Developmental and Evolutionary Aspects of the Neural Crest* (ed. P. F. A. Maderson), pp. 215-259. New York: John Wiley.

HEMMATI-BRIVANLOU, A., DE LA TORRE, J., HOLT, C. & HARLAND, R. (1991). Cephalic expression and molecular characterisation of *Xenopus En-2*. *Development* **111**, 715-724.

HOLLAND, P. & HOGAN, B. (1988). Expression of homeo box genes during mouse development: a review. *Genes Dev.* **2**, 773-782.

HUNT, P., GULISANO, M., COOK, M., SHAM, M., FAIELLA, A., WILKINSON, D., BONCINELLI, E. & KRUMLAUF, R. (1991a). A distinct *Hox* code for the branchial region of the head. *Nature* **353**, 861-864.

HUNT, P., WHITING, J., MUCHAMORE, I., MARSHALL, H. & KRUMLAUF, R. (1991b). Homeobox genes and models for patterning the hindbrain and branchial arches. *Development* **112 (Supplement: Molecular and cellular basis of pattern formation)**, 187-196.

HUNT, P., WHITING, J., NONCHEV, S., SHAM, M., MARSHALL, H., GRAHAM, A., ALLEMANN, R., RIGBY, P., GULISANO, M., FAIELLA, A., BONCINELLI, E. & KRUMLAUF, R. (1991c). The branchial *Hox* code and its implications for gene regulation, patterning of the nervous system and head evolution. *Development* **113 (Supplement, Developmental Nerve Cell Biology)**, In press.

HUNT, P., WILKINSON, D. & KRUMLAUF, R. (1991d). Patterning the vertebrate head: murine Hox 2 genes mark distinct subpopulations of premigratory and migrating neural crest. *Development* **112**, 43-51.

IZPISUA-BELMONTE, J.-C., DOLLE, P., RENUCCI, A., ZAPPAVIGNA, V., FALKENSTEIN, H. & DUBOULE, D. (1990). Primary structure and embryonic expression pattern of the mouse *Hox-4.3* homeobox gene. *Development* **110**, 733-745.

IZPISUA-BELMONTE, J.-C., TICKLE, C., DOLLE, P., WOLPERT, L. & DUBOULE, D. (1991). Expression of homeobox *Hox-4* genes and the specification of position in chick wing development. *Nature* **350**, 585-589.

JONES, C. M., LYONS, K. & HOGAN, B. (1991). Involvement of *Bone Morphogenetic Protein-4 (BMP-4)* and *Vgr-1* in morphogenesis and neurogenesis in the mouse. *Development* **111**, 531-542.

KESSEL, M. & GRUSS, P. (1990). Murine developmental control genes. *Science* **249**, 374-379.

KESSEL, M. & GRUSS, P. (1991). Homeotic transformations of murine prevertebrae and concommitant alteration of Hox codes induced by retinoic acid. *Cell* **In press**.

KESSEL, M., BALLING, R. & GRUSS, P. (1990). Variations of cervical vertebrae after expression of a *Hox 1.1* transgene in mice. *Cell* **61**, 301-308.

KIRBY, M. (1989). Plasticity and predetermination of the mesencephalic and trunk neural crest transplanted into the region of cardiac neural crest. *Devl Biol.* **134**, 402-412.

KURATANI, S. & KIRBY, M. (1991). Initial Migration and distribution of the cardiac neural crest in the avian embryo: An introduction to the concept of the circumpharyngeal crest. *Am. J. Anat.* **191**, 215-227.

LE DOUARIN, N. (1983). *The Neural Crest.* Cambridge: Cambridge University Press.

LE DOUARIN, N., FONTAINE-PERUS, J. & COULY, G. (1986). Cephalic ectodermal placodes and neurogenesis. *TINS* **9**, 175-180.

LEWIS, E. (1978). A gene complex controlling segmentation in *Drosophila*. *Nature* **276**, 565-570.

LUFKIN, T., DIERICH, A., LEMEUR, M., MARK, M. & CHAMBON, P. (1991). Disruption of the Hox-1.6 homeobox gene results in defects in a region corresponding to its rostral domain of expression. *Cell* **66**, 1105-1119.

LUMSDEN, A. (1990a). The cellular basis of segmentation in the developing hindbrain. *TINS* **13**, 329-335.

LUMSDEN, A. (1990b). The Development and Significance of Hindbrain Segmentation. In *Seminars in Developmental Biology: The Evolution of Segmental Patterns*, vol. 1, issue 2 (ed. C. Stern), pp. 117-125. Philadelphia: W.B. Saunders.

LUMSDEN, A. & KEYNES, R. (1989). Segmental patterns of neuronal development in the chick hindbrain. *Nature* **337**, 424-428.

LUMSDEN, A., SPRAWSON, N. & GRAHAM, A. (1991). Segmental origin and migration of neural crest cells in the hindbrain region of the chick embryo. *Development* **113**, In press.

MADEN, M., HUNT, P. N., ERIKSSON, U., KUROIWA, A., KRUMLAUF, R. & SUMMERBELL, D. (1991). Retinoic acid-binding protein and homeobox expression in the rhombomeres of the chick embryo. *Development* **111**, 35-44.

MCKEE, G. & FERGUSON, M. (1984). The effects of mesencephalic neural crest cell extirpation on the development of chicken embryos. *J. Anat.* **139**, 491-512.

MCMAHON, A. & BRADLEY, A. (1990). The *Wnt*-1 (*int*-1) proto-oncogene is required for development of a large region of mouse brain. *Cell* **62**, 1073-1085.

MOODY, S. & HEATON, M. (1983a). Developmental relationships between trigeminal ganglia and trigeminal motorneurons in chick embryos. I. ganglion development is necessary for motorneuron migration. *J. Comp. Neurol.* **213**, 327-343.

MOODY, S. & HEATON, M. (1983b). Developmental relationships between trigeminal ganglia and trigeminal motorneurons in chick embryos. II. ganglion axon ingrowth guides motorneuron migration. *J. Comp. Neurol.* **213**, 344-349.

MORRISS, G. M. & THOROGOOD, P. V. (1978). An Approach to Cranial Neural Crest Migration and Differentiation in Mammalian Embryos. In *Development in Mammals*, vol. 3 (ed. M. H. Johnson), pp. 363-411. Amsterdam: Elsevier North-Holland.

MURPHY, P. & HILL, R. (1991). Expression of mouse *labial*-like homeobox-containing genes, *Hox 2.9* and *Hox 1.6*, during segmentation of the hindbrain. *Development* **111**, 61-74.

MURPHY, P., DAVIDSON, D. & HILL, R. (1989). Segment-specific expression of a homeobox-containing gene in the mouse hindbrain. *Nature* **341**, 156-159.

NICHOLS, D. (1981). Neural crest formation in the head of the mouse embryo as observed using a new histological technique. *JEEM* **64**, 105-120.

NODEN, D. (1983). The role of the neural crest in patterning of avian cranial skeletal, connective, and muscle tissues. *Devl Biol.* **96**, 144-165.

NODEN, D. (1988). Interactions and fates of avian craniofacial mesenchyme. *Development* **103**(Supplement; Craniofacial Development), 121-140.

NOHNO, T., NOJI, S., KOYAMA, E., OHYAMA, K., MYOKAI, F., KUROIWA, A., SAITO, T. & TANAGUCHI, S. (1991). Involvement of the Chox-4 chicken homeobox genes in determination of anteroposterior axial polarity during limb development. *Cell* **64**, 1197-1205.

PRICE, M., LEMAISTRE, M., PISCHETOLA, M., DI LAURO, R. & DUBOULE, D. (1991). A mouse gene related to *Distal-less* shows a restricted expression in the developing forebrain. *Nature* **351**, 748-751.

ROMER, A. (1971). *The Vertebrate Body, Shorter Version*, Fourth edn. Philadelphia: W. B. Saunders Company. (pp 163-167)

ROWE, A., RICHMAN, J. & BRICKELL, P. (1991). Retinoic acid treatment alters the distribution of retinoic acid receptor beta transcripts in the embryonic chick face. *Development* **111**, 1007-1016.

RUIZ-I-ALTABA, A. (1990). Neural expression of the Xenopus homeobox gene Xhox3: evidence for a patterning neural signal that spreads through the ectoderm. *Development.* **108**, 595-604.

SIMEONE, A., PANNESE, M., ACAMPORA, D., D'ESPOSITO, M. & BONCINELLI, E. (1988). At least three human homeoboxes on chromosome 12 belong to the same transcription unit. *N.A.R.* **16**, 5379-5390.

SIMEONE, A., ACAMPORA, D., NIGRO, V., FAIELLA, A., D'ESPOSITO, M., STORNAIUOLO, A., MAVILIO, F. & BONCINELLI, E. (1991). Differential regulation by retinoic acid of the homeobox genes of the four HOX loci in human embryonal carcinoma cells. *Mechanisms of Development* **33**, 215-227.

SULIK, K., COOK, C. & WEBSTER, W. (1988). Teratogens and craniofacial malformations: relationships to cell death. *Development* **103**, 213-232.

TAN, S. S. & MORRISS-KAY, G. (1985). The development and distribution of the cranial neural crest in the rat embryo. *Cell Tissue Res.* **240**, 403-416.

THOROGOOD, P. (1988). The developmental specification of the vertebrate skull. *Development* **103**, 141-153.

THOROGOOD, P., BEE, J. & VON DER MARK, K. (1986). Transient expression of collagen type II at epitheliomesenchymal interfaces during morphogenesis of the cartilaginous neurocranium. *Devl Biol.* **116**, 497-509.

VAESSEN, M.-J., MEIJERS, J., BOOTSMA, D. & VAN KESSEL, A. (1990). The cellular retinoic-acid-binding protein is expressed in tissues associated with retinoic-acid-induced malformations. *Development* **110**, 371-378.

VERWOERD, C. & VAN OOSTROM, C. (1979). *Advances in Anatomy, Embryology and Cell Biology*, 58: *Cephalic Neural Crest and Placodes*. Berlin: Springer-Verlag.

WILKINSON, D., BAILES, J. & MCMAHON, A. (1987). Expression of the proto-oncogene *int*-1 is restricted to specific neural cells in the developing mouse embryo. *Cell* **50**, 79-88.

WILKINSON, D., BHATT, S., CHAVRIER, P., BRAVO, R. & CHARNAY, P. (1989a). Segment-specific expression of a zinc finger gene in the developing nervous system of the mouse. *Nature* **337**, 461-464.

WILKINSON, D., BHATT, S., COOK, M., BONCINELLI, E. & KRUMLAUF, R. (1989b). Segmental expression of hox 2 homeobox-containing genes in the developing mouse hindbrain. *Nature* **341**, 405-409.

WOOD, A., ASHHURST, D., CORBETT, A. & THOROGOOD, P. (1991). The transient expression of type II collagen at tissue interfaces during mammalian craniofacial development. *Development* **111**, 955-968.

DISTRIBUTION OF THE HOMEOBOX *ENGRAILED* GENE EXPRESSION DURING THE

EMBRYONIC DEVELOPMENT OF THE TROUT CNS

Elena Vecino

Department of Cell Biology and Pathology
University of Salamanca
Salamanca 37007, Spain

One of the main interests in neurobiology is to understand the cellular and molecular mechanisms that regulate the organization of the nervous system during development. Recent studies have suggested some genes as responsible for controlling critical developmental events such as neuronal diversification and neural crest cell fate. Strong candidates are several gene families of the development-regulating genes from *Drosophila,* e.g. the homeobox genes. The description of mutant phenotypes have shown that some of the *Drosophila* homeobox genes play a very different role, i.e. to control position-specific characteristics in the early embryio and in the CNS (Doe and Scott, 1988). In vertebrates, a number of genes have been isolated by virtue of their homology with the conserved homeobox sequence of *Drosophila* pattern formation genes (Carrasco et al., 1984; Levine et al., 1984; Mc Ginnis et al., 1984).

The *engrailed (en)* is a homeobox gene that has been suggested to play an important role during development to control position-specific characteristics in the early embryo and in the CNS (Holland, 1989; Martinez et al., 1990; Martinez et al., 1991). *En* has been identified in a wide range of metazoans, including vertebrates (for review: Patel et al., 1989). There appears to be a strong sequence conservation between fish and mammalian *engrailed*-containing genes. Thus, zebrafish have two *engrailed*-like sequences that are conserved as much as those found in mouse and Drosophila (Fjöse et al., 1988).

In mouse CNS, the expression of this *en* gene has been shown to be limited to one band of the neural tube that includes portions of posterior mesencephalon and anterior metencephalon. Similar patterns of *en* distribution have been found in chicken, frog and zebrafish (Patel et al., 1989). In mammals, the *en* expression increases in its spatial complexity as the animal develops while there is a reduction in the extent of expression (Davis et al., 1988).

More primitive vertebrates where embryos can be easily accessed at all developmental stages, should be amenable for investigation of homeobox-containing genes. Thus, fish are well suited.

The description of gene sequence, organization and expression is prerequisite for the formulation of an hypothesis regarding the function of the vertebrate homeobox genes. In the present paper, the spatial

Development of the Central Nervous System in Vertebrates
Edited by S.C. Sharma and A.M. Goffinet, Plenum Press, New York, 1992

expression pattern of the *en* in trout *(Salmo fario)* CNS is analyzed and compared to the mammalian *en* distribution. To this end, the monoclonal antibody Mab 4D9 that specifically recognize engrailed proteins (Davis et al., 1988) was used for immunohistochemistry according to the peroxidase-antiperoxidase (PAP) method (Stermberger, 1970).

Twenty trout embryos of five different developmental stages (146°C, 154°C, 227°C, 280°C, and 440°C) and four alevins (one day old) were used in the present study. These developmental stages are expressed in day-degrees, i.e. the water temperature times the number of days until hatching, expressed in ^{0}C. In these units, eclosion takes place at 440°C.

The embryos and alevins were fixed by immersion in 4% paraformaldehyde in phosphate buffer (0.1 M, pH 7.2) for 4 hours. The neural tubes were dissected from ten embryos, washed three times in phosphate-buffered saline (PBS), and then processed *in toto* for immunohistochemistry with the Mab 4D9 antibody (Patel et al., 1989). The other fixed embryos and the fixed alevin brains were rinsed in PBS, and then placed in 30% sucrose until they sank. Transverse and sagittal sections were cut in a cryostat, collected on slides subbed with chrome alum-gelatin, and allowed to dry at room temperature. These slides were processed for immunohistochemistry with the Mab 4D9 according to the indirect PAP method (Stermberger et al., 1970), using diaminobenzidine for visualization of the immunoreaction.

Stages 146°C and 154°C

Trout embryos express the *engrailed* protein from the earliest developmental stage analyzed (146°C, when the optic vesicles appear). At these stages, *en* was expressed in the presumptive posterior mesencephalon and anterior metencephalon. A caudo-rostrally decreasing gradient of immunoreactivity was observable in *in toto* preparations (Fig. 1A).

Stages 227°C and 280°C

Embryos at these stages were analyzed *in toto* and *in sections*. At these stages, the mesencephalic optic tectum was clearly defined, while the cerebellum was represented by a sheet of pseudostratified epithelium consisting of proliferating cells, the matrix layer (Powels, 1978). In *in toto* preparations, the caudorostrally decreasing gradient now extended across the indentation between the optic tectum and the cerebellar matrix layer (Fig. 1B). The distribution of the *en* expression could be observed in detail in sections where, besides the immunoreactive cells located in the periventricular matrix layers L and M of the cerebellum (Powels, 1978), immunoreactive cells were also found within hypothalamic areas and in the caudal optic tectum.

Stages 440°C and 440°C + 1 day

In 440°C embryos (just before hatching) and in alevins one day after hatching, *en* expression was found in the hypothalamus (Fig. 2A), in cells located in the mesencephalic tegmentum (Fig. 2B, C), periventricular matrix layers L and M of the cerebellum, caudal optic tectum and within the boundaries of the trigeminal motor nucleus (Fig. 3).

Not all the cell nuclei where the *en* was expressed showed the same stain intensity (Fig. 2C). Thus, weakly stained cell nuclei were found in the hypothalamic areas (Fig. 2A), trigeminal motor nucleus (Fig. 3C), and rostral proliferating matrix layer of the cerebellum; contrasting with the strong stain found in the caudal proliferating matrix layer of the cerebellum, cells located in the part of the mesencephalic tegmentum that

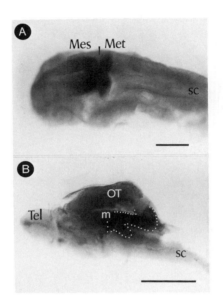

Fig. 1. Mab 4D9 immunoreactivity in the toto preparation (rostral is to
the left) of: A) 154° embryo. *Engrailed* is expressed in the posterior
mesencephalon (Mes) and anterior metencephalon (Met) in a caudorostrally
decreasing gradient. B) 280° embryo, the *engrailed* caudo-rostrally
decreasing gradient now extended across the identation between the optic
tectum (OT) and the cerebellar matrix layer (m) area marked with dots.
(Tel) telencephalon, (sc) spinal cord. Bars=100 μm.

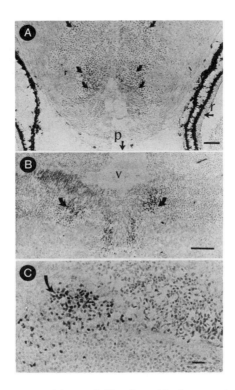

Fig. 2. A) Transverse section of the hypothalamus at the level of the pituitary (P) of a embryo 440°. Mab 4D9 immunoreactive cells are pointed by arrows. (r) retina. B) Mab 4D9 immunoreactive cells expressing the *engrailed* protein with different intensity. The picture was taken at approximately the same level of Fig. 3B (frame). C) Cells from the mesencephalic tegmentum of a embryo 440°C showing different intensity of *engrailed* expression. Bar=50 μm.

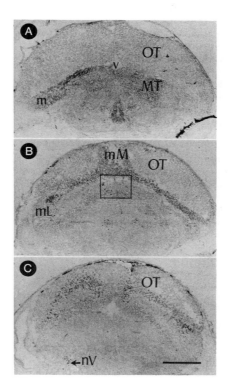

Fig. 3. Transverse rostro-caudal sections (A to C) of a 440° embryo. Mab
4D9 immunoreactive cells located: A in the matrix layer (m) ventral to
the third ventricle (V) and in the mesencephalic tegmentum (MT). B) in
the stratum periventiculare (SPV) of the optic tectum (OT), matrix zone M
(mM) and L (mL) of the cerebellum and isolated intense labelled cells
located close to the midline of the mesencephalic tegmentum (arrows) C) in
the OT and in the boundaries of the trigeminal motor nucleus (nV).
Bar=100 μm.

is immediately ventral to the matrix layer of the cerebellum and in the caudal optic tectum.

The *en* protein is located in the cell nucleus, supporting the notion that the *engrailed* protein is a regulatory factor. In the present study, we have found that not all immunoreactive nuclei stain equally with the Mab 4D9 antisera. Similar observations have also been make in *Drosophila* (Di Nardo et al., 1985) which, similar to zebrafish and mouse, has two different *en* genes (*en-1* and *en-2*) (Fjöse et al., 1988). Both *en* genes are found in the developing brain and, at least in some cases, in the same cells, and the activity of these genes is controlled according to cell position as well as cell type (Davidson et al., 1988). It is possible that the trout also possesses two *en* genes. In this case, the products of these two genes could have been recognized with different intensity by the Mab 4D9 antisera used in the present study. However, recent studies have shown that in *Xenopus* the Mab 4D9 antibody only recognizes the homeobox-containing protein *en-2* (Hemmati-Brivanlou et al., 1990).

The results of this study show that the expression of *en* in the fish neural tube first appeared when the somites were already delineated. This is in agreement with the *en* patterns found in other chordates (Patel et al., 1989), indicating that *en* is not involved in the process of segmentation in chordates.

One of the most interesting features of the *en* expression during embryogenesis is, however, the transition from uniform *en* expression in the early stages of the development to a more complex pattern seen in the later embryonic stages. The pattern of expression of *en* in the late embryonic developmental stages opens the possibility that *en* may be involved in specification of different cell populations in the brain (Davis et al., 1988).

The pattern found in the present study resembles the *en* expression patterns described in mouse (Davis et al., 1988) and in chick (Gardner et al., 1988) where, besides the immunoreactive cells found in the developing cerebellum and optic tectum a faint *en* stain was also found in hypothalamic areas and trigeminal nucleus. The spatial pattern of *en* gene expression has been conserved in at least these three vertebrate classes.

In fish embryos, the presence of serotonin (Ekstrom et al., 1985) and substance P (Vecino and Sharma, 1990) has been described in the same hypothalamic areas where we have found *en* expression. The meaning of the possible colocalization of en, serotonin or substance P in hypothalamic areas is unknown. However, the three substances are known to appear early during development, and are thus available at a time suitable to play a role in the differentiation of the CNS (Senba et al., 1982; Ekstrom et al., 1985; Du et al., 1987).

I thank Dr. Alvarado-Mallart for the lab-facilities, advice during the Work and helpful comments on the manuscript. To Dr. Patel for the gift of the antibody. The study was supported by grants from the Spanish Ministery of Education.

REFERENCES

Carrasco, A.E., Mc Ginnis, W., Gehring, W.J. and De Robertis, E.M. (1984) Cloning of an *X. laevis* gene expressed during early embryiogenesis coding for a peptide region homologous to *Drosophila* homeotic genes. Cell 37:409-414.

Davidson, D., Graham, E., Sime, C. and Hill, R. (1988) A gene with
    sequence similarity to Drosophila engrailed is expressed during the
    development o the neural tube and vertebrae in the mouse. Development
    104:305-316.
Davis, A.C., Noble-Tophan, S.E., Rossant, J. and Joyner, A.L. (1988)
    Expression of the homeo boxcontaining gene En-2 delineates a specific
    region of the developing brain. Genes Dev. 2:361-371.
Di Nardo, S., Kuner, J.M., Theis, T. and O'Farrell, P.H. (1985)
    Development of embryonic pattern in D. melanogaster as revealed by
    accumulation of the nuclear engrailed protein. Cell 43:59-69.
Doe, C.Q. and Scott, M.P. (1988) Segmentation and homeotic gene function
    in the developing nervous system of Drosophila. Trends Neurosci.
    11:101-106.
Du, F., Chamay, Y. and Dubois, P. (1987) Development and distribution of
    substance P in the spinal cord and ganglia of embryonic and newly
    hatched chick: An immunofluorescence study. J. Comp. Neurol.
    263:436-454.
Ekström, P.,Nyberg, L. and van Veen, T. (1985) Ontogenetic development of
    serotoninergic neurons in the brain of a teleost, the three-spined
    stickeleback. An immunocytochemical analysis. Dev. Brain Res.
    17:209-224.
Fjöse, A., Eiken, H.G., Njblstad, P.R., Molven, A. and Hordvik, I. (1988)
    A zebrafish engrailed-like homeobox sequence expressed during
    embryogenesis. FEB Lett. 231:355-360.
Gardner, C.A., Darnell, D.K., Poole, S.J., Ordahl, C.P. and Barald, K.F.
    (1988) Expression of an engrailed-like gene during development of the
    early embryonic chick nervous system. J. Neurosci. Res. 21:426-437.
Hemmati-Brivanlou, A., Stewart, R.M. and Harland, R.M. (1990) Region-
    specific neural induction of an engrailed protein by anterion
    notochord in Xenopus. Science 250:800-802.
Holland, P.W.H. (1989) Pursing the functions of vertebrate homeobox
    genes: progress and prospects. Trends Neurosci. 12:206-209.
Levine, M., Rubin, G.M. and Tjian, R. (1984) Human DNA sequences
    homologous to a protein coding region conserved between homeotic genes
    of Drosophila. Cell 38:667-673.
Martinez, S., Alvarado-Mallart, R.M. (1990) Expression of the homeobox
    Chick-en gene in chick/quail chimeras with inverted mes-metencephalic
    gaits. Dev. Biol. 139:432-436.
Martinez, S., Wassef, M., Alvarado-Mallart, R.M. (1991) Induction of a
    mesencephalic phenotype in the 2-day-old chick posencephalon is
    preceded by the early expression of the homeobox gene en. Neuron
    6:971-981.
McGinnis, W., Hart, C.P., Gehring, W.J. and Ruddle, F.H. (1984) Molecular
    cloning and chromosome mapping of a mouse DNA sequence homologous to
    homeotic genes of Drosophila. Cell 38:675-680.
Patel, N.H., Martin-Blanco, E., Coleman, K.G., Poole, S.J., Ellis, M.C.,
    Komberg, T.B. and Goodman, C.S. (1989) Expression of engrailed
    proteins in arthropods, annelids, and chordates. Cell 58:955-968.
Powels, E. (1978) On the development of the cerebellum of the trout,
    Salmo gairdneri. Anat. Embryol. 152:291-308.
Senba, E., Shiosaka, S., Hara, Y., Inagaka, S., Sakanaka, M., Takatsuki,
    K., Kawai, Y. and Tohyama, M. (1982) Ontogeny of the peptidergic
    system in the rat spinal cord: Immunohistochemical analysis. J.
    Comp. Neurol. 208:54-66.
Stemberger, L.A., Hardy, P.H. Jr., Cuculis, J.J. and Meyer, H.G. (1970)
    The unlabeled antibody method of immunohistochemistry. Preparation
    and properties of soluble antigen complex and its use in
    identification of spirochetes. J. Histochem. Cytochem. 18:315-333.
Vecino, E. and Sharma, S.C. (1990) Localization of substance P-like
    immunoreactivity in the developing goldfish. Eur. J. Neurosci. Suppl.
    4187:278.

A GENERAL MODEL OF CORTICAL HISTOGENESIS: STUDIES IN THE DEVELOPING CEREBRAL WALL OF THE MOUSE

V.S. Caviness, Jr. and T. Takahashi

Massachusetts General Hospital
Boston, MA   02114   USA

The cerebral neocortex is formed of large populations of neurons, divisible into multiple classes in terms of their shapes and their patterns of connectivity and interaction with other neurons (Jones, 1984a). Neocortical neurons are arrayed in a series of five lamina, VI - II, deep to the overlying molecular layer I. Each of these is dominated by a principal class of neurons: polymorphic neurons in layer VI, large pyramidal neurons in layer V, granular neurons in layer IV and medium and small pyramidal neurons in layers III and II, respectively. The patterns of distribution of neuronal somata and axons within these laminae vary regionally throughout the entire neocortex (Jones, 1984a,b). These variations in pattern have served as criteria for multiple architectonic subdivisions or parcellations of the neocortex. Certain of these systems of parcellation, in particular that of Brodmann (1909) for which there is close homology across mammalian species, is reliably correlated with the underlying functional organization of the cerebrum (Zilles, 1990).

The neurons of the neocortex arise in a generative epithelium, referred to as the ventricular zone (VZ), because it forms the lining of the cerebral ventricles in the depths of the developing cerebral wall (His, 1904; Boulder Committee, 1970; Rakic, 1988). There is a systematic relationship between the sequence in which young neurons undergo their terminal divisions in the VZ and the depth at which they ultimately come to lie in the cortex. Thus, the earliest formed neurons are the polymorphic neurons of layer VI followed by the large pyramidal neurons of layer V. The granular neurons and medium and small pyramidal neurons of the successively overlying layers are formed at progressively later dates (Sidman and Rakic, 1973; Caviness et al., 1981).

Neurons find their way from the VZ to the developing cortex by migrating as freely motile elements. It has been recognized that the young neurons are guided in their migrations by following the surfaces of radial glial cells, a bipolar cell form of astroglial lineage (Rakic, 1972, 1978). The soma of the radial glial cells lies in or near the VZ. The soma gives rise to a descending process with which the cell is attached at the ventricular surface. An ascending process extends outward through the intermediate or migratory zone.

Rakic has drawn attention to the observation that both the developing VZ and cortex have a radially striated appearance (Rakic,

Development of the Central Nervous System in Vertebrates
Edited by S.C. Sharma and A.M. Goffinet, Plenum Press, New York, 1992

83

1988). He has suggested that both are formed of columnar groupings of subpopulations of cells. This hypothesis has been the starting point for a uniquely comprehensive general hypothetical formulation interrelating the full sweep of histogenetic events of the cerebral cortex. The columns within the VZ he designated "proliferative units" while those of the neocortex were referred to as "ontogenetic columns". In the general formulation proliferative units and ontogenetic columns were interrelated by subsets of hypotheses which proceed from the most fundamental cytogenetic events in the VZ to the ontogeny of the organizational map of the fully developed neocortex (Rakic, 1988).

The general neocortical histogenetic model of Rakic has two principle tenets. The first is the proposition that the proliferative units are mapping units which collectively constitute a protomap of the neocortex still within the VZ. The second is a model of the VZ neuronal production fundamental to neocortical histogenesis. The formulation with respect to a VZ protomap holds that the neocortical ontogenetic columns are mapped units which collectively make up the architectonic parcellation system and the basis of the functional organization of the neocortex. The mapping and mapped units are proposed to relate to each other spatially in an orderly one-to-one topologic fashion. That is, the cellular progeny coming from a specified proliferative unit is delivered exclusively to its corresponding ontogenetic column within the cortex.

The orderly translation of proliferative units upon ontogenetic columns is assured by the organization of the overall radial glial fiber system. More specifically, it is proposed that the radial fibers all have a full transcerebral span and that this cell configuration is stable throughout the migratory epoch of neocortical histogenesis (Rakic, 1988). One glial fiber, or perhaps a fascicle of fibers, arises from each of the mapping units and extends fully to the corresponding mapped unit.

The second tenet of the general formulation of Rakic provides what is, to our knowledge, the first model for the proliferative output behavior of the cerebral VZ. Thus, it is postulated that the generative epithelium initially goes through a phase of exponential growth during which polyclonal populations of the proliferative units become established. During this initial phase, both daughter cells arising from mitotic division in the VZ return to the proliferative pool of cells. The onset of neuronal cytogenesis is associated with a shift to steady state growth. During this phase the daughter cells arising from a division will have different fates. Whereas one will return to the proliferative pool of cells in the respective proliferative unit, the other will become post-mitotic and initiate its migration toward the cortex. At the end of the cytogenetic epoch each proliferative cell will undergo a terminal division. At this point both daughter cells will become postmitotic and migrate to the cortex.

The formulation of Rakic directs our attention in a comprehensive way to the successive cellular events upon which cortical histogenesis is dependent. The formulation is strong analytically in that it provides specific hypotheses relating to events and mechanisms of histogenesis which may be actively examined experimentally. Now, a half decade since it was set forth, we will revisit the principle tenets of the Rakic formulation. The perspective of this reconsideration derives largely from a series of experimental studies, certain of them still in progress, which are based upon the developing murine cerebrum.

We will consider two distinct sets of studies. The first, based upon investigations now completed, is concerned with the organization and ontogeny of the radial glial fiber system and patterns of neuron migration through the fiber system. The observations to be reviewed are pertinent to the plausibility of the protomap hypothesis. The second block of investigations to be reviewed, currently ongoing, are concerned with the cytokinetic behavior and cell output of the VZ. These experiments address directly the mode of cell division which underlies the Rakic formulation. They go considerably further, however, in that they will arrive at a histogenetic model which includes both quantitative estimates of cell production in the cerebral VZ and estimates of cortical growth during the early developmental phases.

THE RADIAL FIBER SYSTEM AND NEURONAL MIGRATION

Ontogeny and Structure of the Radial Glial Fiber System

The image of the radial glial cell, upon which the Rakic protomap hypothesis is based, was derived from the appearance of the cell in Golgi impregnations and by study with electron microscopy (Rakic, 1972, 1978; Rakic et al., 1974). These methods presented the radial glial cell in its simplest configuration and provided an incomplete picture of the organization the radial fiber system as a whole. Studies based upon subsequently developed monoclonal antibodies, RC1 and RC2, each with high selectivity and sensitivity for cells of astroglial lineage within the developing nervous system including the radial glial cell, have substantially enlarged upon the earlier perspective (Misson et al., 1988a,b; Edwards et al., 1990; Takahashi et al., 1990a). It has become clear that the radial glial cellpopulation becomes differentiated within the neural tube at least as early as the ninth embryonic day (E9) in the mouse, a developmental stage within hours of neurulation (Misson et al., 1988a,b; Edwards et al., 1990).

Even at this earliest phase of CNS histogenesis in the mouse, the organization in the radial glial fiber system is already complex with fibers gathered together in fascicles which span the full width of the neural tube (Fig. 1A; Gadisseux et al., 1988, 1989; Misson, et al., 1988a,b; Edwards et al., 1990). Several days later by E12 - E13, at the outset of cerebral development in the mouse, the general fasciculated pattern of the fiber system is conspicuous within the cerebral vesicle (Mission et al, 1988a,b; Edwards et al., 1990). Initially the fascicles of glial fibers ascend across the cerebral wall in a radially symmetric fashion. Through E14 - E15 there is no apparent difference in the density of the fibers in their span across the full thickness of the cerebral wall.

By E16 - E17, however, a fundamental change has occurred in the pattern of fiber span (Fig 1B). Specifically there appear to be step-like decreases in the density of the fibers with ascent across the cerebral wall (Gadisseux et al., 1989; Misson et al., 1991a). These stepwise gradients, visible to the eye in suitably stained material, have been quantified by counts of fibers crossing successive tangential planes through the full thickness of the cerebral wall (Gadisseux et al., 1992). The quantitative studies establish that at E17, there is a step drop of nearly 50% in the density of fibers, corrected for tissue expansion, in ascent from the intermediate zone through the subplate to the upper layers of the cortical plate (Gadisseux et al., 1992). This gradient is iniated at a level corresponding to the external sagittal stratum. This stratum is a fiber plane which carries the thalamocortical and cortical thalamic fibers and lies at the future inferior border of the neocortex (Crandall and Caviness, 1984). It becomes apparent as early as E14 - E15, soon after the developmental stratification pattern of the cerebral wall becomes established.

The gradients of radial fiber density with ascent across the cerebral wall are a reflection of dynamic properties of the radial glial cells themselves. The radial glial cell population is actively proliferative (Misson et al., 1988a,b). Cells, found by staining with RC1 or RC2 to have all the characteristic morphological features of radial glial cells, may be demonstrated to be replicating DNA by the incorporation of tritiated thymidine (^{3}H-TdR).

During G2 phase, the ascending and descending processes of such cells, marked autoradiographically with ^{3}H-TdR, appear to retain their characteristic bipolar forms. The ascending process appears not to be present as the cell goes through M-phase but must be subsequently re-elaborated by daughter cells. During the period of neuronal migration, growth cone tipped ascending processes of these cells, forming part of the transcerebral fascicles, are encountered at high density throughout the upper intermediate zone (Takahashi et al., 1990a). There is a step drop in growth cone density at the level of the external sagittal stratum and subplate at E17 (Fig 1B). Then, in the final few days before birth, E18 - P0, there is a surge of entry of growth cone-tipped radial glial fibers into the subplate and lower cortical plate (Fig. 1C).

We have previously suggested that this late surge of radial fibers supports principally the terminal segment of migration of supragranular neurons (Gadisseux et al., 1989, 1992; Takahashi et al., 1990a). This view is consistent with the observation that there are small columns of supragranular pyramidal cells intercalated in the cortex between other larger columns formed of pyramidal cell somata and apical dendrites which extend through all five cellular layers (Escobar et al., 1986).

The dramatic change in the gradient of density of radial glial fibers, occurring in the external sagittal stratum and continuing into the cortical plate, is associated with an equally dramatic change in the pattern of migration of neurons through the radial fiber system. Specifically, neurons traversing the intermediate zone migrate between fascicles of fibers (interfascicular mode of migration) whereas they appear to penetrate into the fascicles (intrafascicular mode of migration) as they ascend beyond the external sagittal stratum (Gadisseux et al., 1988).

Certain cerebral malformations encountered in man may reflect a differential vulnerability of the migration process to the interfascicular compared to the intrafascicular modes of cell migration (Caviness et al., 1988). Thus, pachygyria (also referred to as the "double cortex" malformation), lissencephaly and the Zellweger malformation are associated with arrest of neuron migration at and superficial to the external sagittal stratum, that is over the migratory path that would have been intrafascicular. Other less common malformations have been associated with a more central arrest of migration between the VZ and the external sagittal stratum, that is over the interfascicular segment of migration.

Neuronal Migration through the Radial Fiber System

The migratory path and the ultimate distributions of neuronal progeny of VZ clones are traceable by retroviral intra-genomic insertion of the gene for histochemically detectable enzyme beta-galactosidase when the clonal progenitor is proliferating (Cepko, 1988; Luskin et al., 1988). The apparent clonally related progeny of VZ progenitors, identified in this way, are distributed according to patterns which suggest that neurons arising at the same point (proliferative unit) do not follow an orderly path to a common point (ontogenetic column) in the cortex (Walsh and Cepko, 1988). The apparent degree of divergence in the rodent brain has been estimated by this method to be on the order of hundreds of microns.

The observations of Austin and Cepko (1990) indicate that degree of divergence is systematically different in the rostral-caudal as compared to the medial-lateral dimensions of the cortex. Thus, the progeny are relatively closely grouped within a narrow range of distances with regard to the rostral-caudal dimension, though the separation of neurons of common clonal origin within the cortex is still as much as several hundreds of microns. In comparison, the range of divergence in the medial-lateral dimension is very much greater than in the rostral-caudal dimension. Statistically considered, neurons arising in the dorsomedial regions of the cerebral VZ also tend to migrate to positions within several hundred microns of each other with a degree of divergence similar to that seen generally in the rostrocaudal dimension. With increasingly lateral point of origin in the VZ, however, the degree of spread is very much greater than for those arising dorsomedially. Further, the degree of divergence is very much greater among clones of cells labeled with the enzyme at progressively later stages of cerebral histogenesis.

This pattern of divergence observed with the retroviral gene insertion-based experiments is strongly predicted by the patterns of deployment of radial glial fibers and the observed patterns of neuronal migration through the fiber system (Fig. 2; Misson et al., 1991b). The fibers ascend in only slightly divergent fashion in the medial and dorsomedial cortical regions, the zone of the cerebral wall where clonal divergence is least. At increasingly lateral positions, however, fibers ascending from the VZ become increasingly deflected laterally, converging to form a massive radial fiber fascicle which continues laterally in a plane parallel to the pial surface. Ultimately the radial fiber fascicle intersects the external sagittal stratum where the fibers again become separated so as to ascend radially with equal spacing across the cortex. The fibers of this system do not, however, mingle with the more inferiorly and laterally placed radial fibers which take origin from the infraventricular striatal region (Edwards et al., 1990).

Radial glial fibers may be stained with RC2 in the same histological sections in which migrating cells are marked with beta-galactosidase by viral insertion (Misson et al., 1991b). In such double labeled preparations it is observed that the migrating cells follow closely the alignment of radial glial fibers, whether their alignment is divergent or convergent. As predicted by the studies of Austin and Cepko (1990), those in medial and dorsomedial cortical regions ascend in a pattern which is approximately "truly radial". Those directed more laterally, on the other hand, enter the tangentially aligned fiber fascicle with the consequence that cells arising from widely distant points in the VZ initially converge toward each other as they cross the intermediate zone. Then in their approach to the cortex, they diverge widely from each other as they follow the divergent pattern of alignment of fibers of the fascicle. In their migrations, the more laterally directed progeny of a given clone of neurons appear to move in an unsystematic way through the convergent fiber bundle. They ultimately appear to leave the fascicle in widely separated points for their final and radial ascent through the external sagittal stratum and lower levels of the developing cortex (Misson et al., 1991b).

The set of studies reviewed thus far do not support the hypothesis that points within the generative epithelium map in a one to one fashion upon points in the cerebral cortex. The radial glial fiber system develops and is deployed in such a way that it would not be expected to provide such an orderly and fine-grain translation of one surface upon the other. The pattern of movement through the fiber system is clearly not a systematically constrained point to point movement. To the extent that these observations, which are drawn entirely from experiments in rodents, apply generally to the mammalian cerebrum, they argue against the existence of a fine-grained protomap within the VZ as an antecedent to the columnar and architectonically parcellated map of the fully developed neocortex.

The determinants of the neocortical map remain to be identified. Conceivably broad regional attributes of the final map may prove to be anticipated by regional variations within the generative epithelium. The sharper boundary conditions of the neocortical map, on the other hand, might then reflect the patterns of conjunction of reciprocal connections which register nuclei of the thalamus with the cortical mantle at the earliest phases of deployment of these two projection systems. Experiments with the analytic power needed to test this hypothesis have not as yet been devised.

A MODEL OF CYTOGENESIS AND CORTICAL GROWTH

The second principal tenet of the histogenic formulation of Rakic is a model of neuronal production by the VZ. It is proposed specifically that the VZ is initially in an exponential growth mode as the proliferative units are built up. Then, with the onset of neuronal production, when young neurons become definitively postmitotic, the VZ shifts to a steady state mode of growth. With this shift in growth mode, each division will yield both a postmitotic neuron and a cell with continuing proliferative activity. The overall cycle of cell production would be concluded by a final division within each lineage in which both daughter cells would become postmitotic neurons.

We consider here a program of experiments designed to examine the mode of neuronal production directly. The analysis requires preliminary measurements of cytokinetic parameters. The fully developed methodology will allow an even more elaborated histogenetic model than that provided by Rakic in that it will predict the growth relations between the cortical neuronal number and volume and the size of the VZ proliferative pool of origin.

The set of studies, at present only partially completed, are being undertaken in the murine brain. The analysis is being conducted in a dorsomedial sector of the cerebral wall where radial glial fiber alignment is only slightly divergent and the pattern of neuronal migration appears to be approximately radial (Gadisseux et al., 1989). Thus neurons within the cortical segment of this cerebral sector will have arisen from the segment of the VZ which forms the base of the cerebral wall sector.

The most complete set of analyses thus far have been conducted on embryos of E14. On this embryonic date in the mouse brain the full architectonic stratification pattern becomes established (Takahashi et al., 1992c). At the outset of E14, the cerebral wall is constituted of the proliferative zone at the margin of the ventricular system with the narrow overlying zone including both the earliest postmitotic cells and fibers. This overlying area was originally referred to as the primordial plexiform zone by Marin-Padilla (1971).

Near the midpoint of E14, intermediate zone, subplate, cortical plate and molecular layer become sublaminated within the primordial plexiform zone. Within several hours, there is abrupt expansion in the thickness of the intermediate zone, corresponding presumably to a massive influx of thalamocortical and cortical thalamic fibers. The expansion of outer strata of the cerebral wall is not matched by a similar change in the thickness of the generative epithelium which remains relatively constant at 70-80 microns throughout E14.

Cytokinetic Parameters

The generative epithelium, as viewed in general cell stains, has relatively few differentiated features. Mitoses are concentrated at the ventricular surface. A much smaller complement of mitoses which belongs to a second proliferative population is distributed through the ventricular, subventricular and intermediate zones (Boulder Committee, 1970).

The proliferative population of the VZ itself has been recognized to be a pseudostratified eptihelium with S-phase occuring in the abventricular region of the epithelium (S-phase zone) and M-phase at the ventricular surface (His, 1909; Sauer, 1935; Sauer and Walker, 1959; Sidman et al., 1959). Such a to-and-fro cycling pattern does not occur, apparently, among the proliferative cells of the secondary proliferative population.

The cells of the proliferative zone may be assumed to include, variably through the full histogenetic epoch, both proliferating and non-proliferating cells. The proliferative populations are referred to as the growth fraction (Nowakowski et al., 1989). It may also be assumed that the proliferative population is constituted of multiple cellular lineages. Thus, as noted earlier, from early in neocortical histogenesis, an astroglial population marked by RC1 or RC2 may be distinguished from the remainder of cells which do not stain with the antibody. It is to be considered that the diverse lineages may have different cytokinetic parameters.

The strategy of study of the cytokinetic cycle is predicated upon the assumption that neuronal progenitors of the proliferative zone divide asynchronously. That is, the nuclei of the proliferative zone will be distributed through the separate phases of the cell cycle in proportion to the length of that stage in relation to the overall cell cycle. The method entails cumulative labeling of all cell nuclei of a given cycle as these nuclei progress through S-phase. This requires that the S-phase marker be injected at intervals which are less than the length of S-phase. The series of injections must be continued through an interval which is longer than the complete cell cycle (Tc) minus the duration of S-phase (Ts) (Fig. 3; Nowakowski et al., 1989).

The dependent experimental variable is the labeling index (LI: the proportion of labeled with respect to the total cell population) as this changes through time. The LI may be expected to increase with cumulative S-phase labeling to a maximum value which will correspond to the growth fraction (Fig. 3; Nowakowski et al., 1989). The growth fraction will be completely labeled at a time which corresponds to Tc-Ts. The LI at time of the initial injection at the outset of the cumulative labeling schedule will correspond to Ts/Tc. The two equations expressing this relationship may be solved simultaneously to provide a values for Tc and Ts. The length of G2 phase may be estimated as the interval between the initial injection of BUdR and the time that the first cell in M-phase is labeled at the ventricular surface. The length of M-phase may then be estimated as the additional time required to label 100% of cells observed in M-phase at the ventricular surface.

The set of observations available for this discussion is based upon the use of thymidine analog, bromodeoxyuridine (BUdR), as the S-phase marker, administered according to cumulative labeling protochols at 50 ug/g per body weight per injection (Fig. 3; Miller and Nowakowski, 1988; Nowakowski, et al, 1989). It has been demonstrated by other investigators that this dose of the tracer is not associated with an augmentation of cell death among the proliferative cells and their progeny (Al-Ghoul and Miller, 1989; Nowakowski et al., 1989). Nuclei in S-phase are concentrated in the outer half of the VZ (S-phase zone). Preliminary studies establish that a dose of 50 ug/g BUdR provides effective labeling of 100% of the nuclei in S-phase ("saturation labeling") through a period extending from 15 minutes to greater than 2 hours following a single injection (Takahashi et al., 1992a).

At survival times greater than 2 hours following a single injection of 50 ug/g, a small portion of nuclei in S-phase are not labeled. These unlabeled S-phase nuclei are distributed preferentially to the outer aspect of the S-phase zone. This observation suggests that DNA replication is initiated with the nucleus of the cell in the outer aspect of the S-phase zone. The descending process evidently shortens progressively as the nucleus continues from the outset to the end of S-phase (Takahashi et al., 1992a).

When sequential injections beginning at 9:00 am on E14 are given every 3.0 hours through a period of 12 hours, with animal sacrifice 30 minutes after the last injection, all nuclei of the VZ become labeled (Takahashi, 1992b). The first mitotic figures are labeled within 1 hour while 100% of mitotic figures at the ventricular surface are labeled within 2 hours. The slope of ascent of the LI is linear with the interval T_cT_s corresponding to 11.3 hours and the LI at the initiation of injections corresponding to $T_s/T_c = 0.25$ (Fig. 3). T_c is calculated to be 15.1 and T_s 3.8 hours (Takahashi et al., 1992). The growth fraction of the E14 murine cerebral VZ is 100% (i.e., maximum LI = 1.0). The linearity of the slope of ascent of LI suggests that there is only a single proliferative population in the murine VZ at E14 by the criterion of length of T_c.

Similar experiments undertaken on each of the embryonic days, E12 through E16, indicate that T_c increases from approximately 10 to 20 hours while T_s as a proportion of T_c declines from nearly 50% to 20%. The growth fraction holds constant at 1.0 (Caviness et al., 1991).

Cell Production and Migration

A somewhat different S-phase labeling strategy (Takahashi et al., 1991) allows computation of the fractions of daughter cells produced by a given cell cycle which will either leave the cycle and migrate to the cortex (the Q fraction; Fig. 4) or re-enter S-phase and continue to proliferate (the P fraction). If an initial injection of ^{3}H-TdR is given at the start of the experiment and this is followed in two hours by a cumulative labeling sequence with BUdR, there will come to be three subsets of labeled cells within the VZ. These are a "2 hour" cohort of cells labeled only with ^{3}H-TdR (T cells), a cohort of cells labeled both with [3]HTdR and BUdR (T + B cells), and finally, a population of cells labeled only with BUdR (B cells; Fig. 5).

The T cells are allowed to progress through M-phase to some time before their daughter cells, also T cells, would re-enter into S-phase. These daughter cells will represent a fraction of the total population of daughter cells of the cell cycle at that time (Fig. 6). A portion of the daughter T cells will ultimateĺy re-enter S-phase. This fraction of the daughter T cells, referred to as the P fraction (P = proliferative and persisting in the cycle) will become labeled with BudR. The remainder of the T daughter cells will leave the proliferative pool and begin their migrations (the Q or quiescent fraction of the T cells). It is assumed here that none of the T cells is eliminated by cell death. The proportion of daughter cells that will leave the cell cycle (q = quits the cycle) is then represented as

$$Q = Nq/Nq + Np)$$

where Nq is the number of T cells that quit and Np the number of T cells that remain in the proliferative cycle.

The value for q must ascend from 0, prior to the onset of cytogenesis, to 1.0 as cytogenesis is terminated. The Rakic hypothesis, based upon a simple linear growth model, implies that the value for q will step up immediately with the onset of cytogenesis to 0.5 where it will remain until a terminal sharp upward step to 1.0. Our preliminary determinations indicate that the value of q is substantially less than .4 in the early E14 murine brain (Takahashi et al., 1991). This date, near the middle point of the cytogenetic epoch (Caviness, 1982), corresponds to the time of birth of neurons of the infragranular layers. This observation implies that at E14 more than 60% of daughter cells will return to the proliferative population while less than 40% will leave it.

This value for the output fraction at E14 clearly does not support the hypothesis of steady state growth. The value is more consistent with the hypothesis that q will ascend relatively slowly from its initial value of 0. The full course of ascent of q to reach 1.0 at the conclusion of cytogenesis may inscribe an "S-shaped" curve. A satisfactory test of this hypothesis must await a more complete set of values for q sampled throughout the cytogenetic epoch.

Cell Migration

The T cells that represent the Q fraction may be tracked through their migrations and into their final positions within the postnatal cortex. The patterns of disposition of this cohort may be used to estimate the statistics of distribution within the cortex of the output of the cell cycle initiated at 9:00 am on E14. A preliminary set of experiments of this type indicates that there are at least two delays in the ascent of cells across the cerebral wall. An initial delay appears to occur with the emergence of the cells from the VZ itself. The second delay appears to occur as the T cohort of cells reaches and attempts to ascend beyond the external sagittal stratum. Additional data will be required to allow estimates of rates of migration and statistics of dispersion.

Growth

The number of T cells in the Q fraction for an integral cell cycle on any given day from E12 - 17, multiplied by the respective Tc/2 hr (i.e., the Q fraction is a "2 hr cohort"), will provide an estimate of the total cell output for the respective integral cell cycle. The calculation assumes a constant value for Q throughout each cycle. Experiments in progress will determine the value for the total cell output for each integral cycle.

At the same time the final distributions of the T cells arising with each cycle will be mapped within the cortex. These T cell distributions, by interpolation, will provide estimates for the ultimate intracortical distributions of the full output of each integral cycle. This data will allow computations of the growth relationships between the number of progenitor cells and (1) the size of the VZ that they occupy and (2) the volume of cortex that will ultimately come to contain this cell population.

GENERAL IMPLICATIONS

The overall experimental program will define quantitatively, in terms of both magnitude and rates, the progression of the complex sequence of cellular events through which the murine neocortex is assembled. This comprehensive and quantitative vision may be expected to provide additional levels of understanding of the points of action of regulatory controls which govern the operation of the histogenetic program.

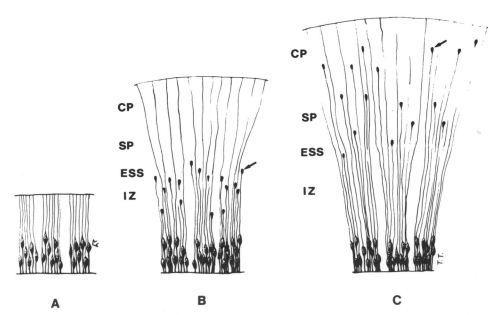

Fig. 1. Schematic representation of the organization of the radial glial fiber system of the dorsomedial murine neocortex at early (A), intermediate (B) and late (C) stages of histogenesis. A. Fibers are grouped in fascicles, and there is uniform fiber density across the full thickness of the cerebral wall. The open arrow indicates a soma of a radial glial cell. B. There is a step drop in fiber density at the level of the external sagittal stratum (ESS). Large numbers of growth cone-tipped fibers (arrow) are observed at the ESS and in the subjacent intermediate zone (IZ). C. Growth cones at the tips of radial fibers (arrow) are more uniformly distributed through ESS, subplate (SP) and lower cortical plate (CP).

Subsequent experiments may then be concerned with the molecular regulation of these processes. Studies in a wide variety of species establish, for example, that a complex of genetically regulated proteins serves to gate the movement of cells into S-phase and beyond into M-phase (Murray and Kirschner, 1991). Conceivably, histologically applicable probes for the expression of the genes encoding these proteins will allow visualization of these critical regulatory processes within the VZ.

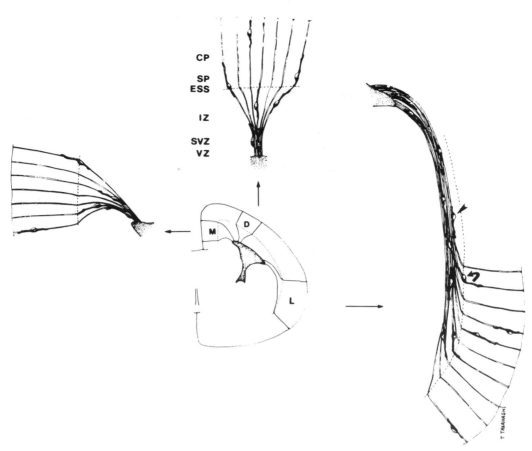

CP
SP
ESS

IZ

SVZ
VZ

M   D

L

Fig. 2. Schematic representation of neuron migration with respect to the
differential patterns of radial glial fiber organization in medial (M) ,
dorsomedial (D) and lateral (L) regions of the late embryonic murine
neocortex. Fibers arising in the medial and dorsomedial regions of the
ventricular zone (VZ) and subventricular zone (SVZ) diverge slightly in
their transcerebral span. Neurons undergoing their terminal divisions in
these regions of the VZ follow the diverging course of the fibers into the
cortex. There is relatively little dispersion of postmigratory neurons in
these cortical regions (M and D), the tangential dimensions of the cortex
considered. Fibers arising laterally (L) converge initially to form a
compact fiber fascicle which extends across the intermediate zone (IZ).
This fascicle courses approximately in parallel to the cerebral surface.
At the level of the external sagittal stratum (ESS) and subplate (SP),
fibers of this fascicle diverge again prior to ascending in parallel
fashion across the cortical plate (CP). (The interface between ESS and SP
is indicated by a broken line.) Neurons arising from widely separated
points in the lateral ventricular zone become substantially intermixed in
their ascent through this fascicle. In comparison to neurons arising
medially (M) and dorsomedially (D) within the VZ, those arising laterally
(L) become more widely dispersed within the cortex. An arrowhead
indicates a neuron migrating by interfascicular mode; a curved arrow
indicates a neuron migrating by intrafascicular mode. (Modified from
Misson et al., 1991b.)

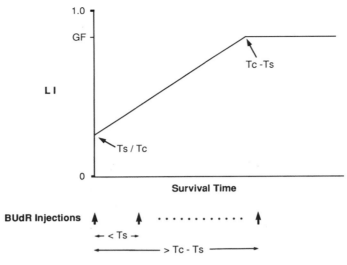

Fig. 3. Graphic representation of the change in the labeling index (LI) in the ventricular zone throughout a period of cumulative S-phase labeling with BUdR. The period of labeling is of greater duration than the length of the cell cycle minus the length of S-phase (i.e., > Tc - Ts). Each BUdR injection is indicated by an arrow along the abscissa. The interinjection interval in the cumulate labeling schedule is less than the length of S-phase (i.e., < Ts). The LI is observed here to ascend linearly from its value at the Y intercept, corresponding to (Ts/Tc)*GF. It reaches a maximum value, less than 1.0 in this hypothetical case, when the total pool of proliferating cells has been labeled. The labeling index when the total proliferating pool is labeled corresponds to the growth fraction (GF). The time required to label the growth fraction is Tc - Ts.

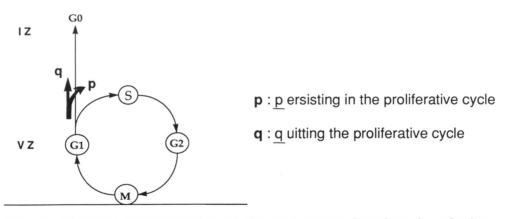

p : p ersisting in the proliferative cycle

q : q uitting the proliferative cycle

Fig. 4. Schematic representation of the cell ouptut fractions in relation to the cell division cycle of the cerebral ventricular zone (VZ). S-phase (S) occurs with the cell nucleus in the outer zone of the VZ while mitosis or M-phase (M) occurs only after the nucleus has approximated the ventricular surface. Nuclei in G2-phase (G2) and G1-phase (G1) are found at an intermediate depth of the VZ. Following M-phase a fraction of daughter cells, referred to as the P fraction (p), will re-enter S-phase. The remaining fraction of daughter cells, referred to as the (q) fraction will become permanently postmitotic and quit the proliferative pool to migrate across the intermediate zone (IZ) toward the cortex.

Double Labeling Sequence : The Three Cohorts

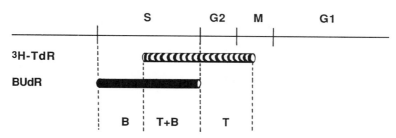

Fig. 5. Schematic representation of the three cohorts of cells that may be distinguished by a staggered ^{3}H-TdR - BUdR double labeling schedule. The schedule is initiated with a single injection of ^{3}H-TdR which labels all nuclei in S-phase (striped cylinder). The ^{3}H-TdR injection is followed in 2 hr by a cumulative BUdR labeling schedule which will label all cells which are in S-phase when the marker is injected or which will enter S-phase subsequently as repeated injections of the marker are given (filled cylinder). A cohort of cells whose nuclei will be labeled only with ^{3}H-TdR (T cells) will have moved into G2-phase and M-phase in the 2 hr following the ^{3}H-TdR injection but before the first BUdR injection. Because S-phase is longer than the 2 hr interval between the ^{3}H-TdR and initial BUdR injections, a second cohort will be labeled with both markers (T + B cells). Finally, a third cohort of cells which enters S-phase after the ^{3}H-TdR has been cleared from the VZ cell environment will be labeled only with BUdR (B cells).

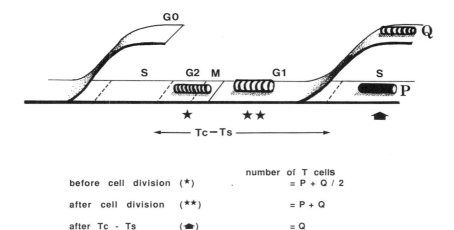

	number of T cells
before cell division (*)	= P + Q / 2
after cell division (**)	= P + Q
after Tc - Ts (⬆)	= Q

Fig. 6. Schematic representation of the separate paths of Q and P fractions following cell division. A T cell cohort (*) is defined as illustrated in Fig. 5. In the course of cell division, the size of this cohort will double (**). After an interval equal to the length of the cell cycle minus the length of S-phase (i.e., > Tc - Ts, arrow) a portion of the T cells will re-enter S-phase (P) and the complementary portion will become post-mitotic and quit the proliferative cycle in the VA (Q) to begin their migrations. The fraction of the output of the cell cycle (q) which will quit the proliferative pool (q) corresponds to $Nq/(Nq+Np)$ where Np+Nq and Nq are the numbers of T cells after cell division and before Tc-Ts and the numbers of T cells after cell division but before Tc - Ts, respectively.

REFERENCES

Al-Ghoul, W.M. and Miller, M.W. (1989) Transient expression of Alz-50 immunoreactivity in developing rat neocortex: a marker for naturally occurring neuronal death. Brain Res. 481:361.

Austin, C.P. and Cepko, C.L. (1990) Cellular migration patterns in the developing mouse cerebral cortex. Development 110:713.

Boulder Committee (1970) Embryonic vertebrate nervous system: revised terminology. Anat. Rec. 166:257.

Brodmann, K. (1909) "Vergleichende Lokalisationslehre der Grosshirnrinde," Leipzig, Barth.

Caviness, V.S., Jr. (1982) Neocortical histogenesis in normal and reeler mice: a developmental study based upon [3H]thymidine autoradiography. Dev. Brain Res. 4:293.

Caviness, V.S., Jr., Pinto-Lord, M.C. and Evrard, P. (1981) The development of laminated pattern in the mammalian neocortex. In: "Morphogenesis and Pattern Formation," L.L. Brinkley, B.M. Carlson, and I.G. Connolly, eds., Raven Press, New York.

Caviness, V.S., Jr., Misson, J.-P. and Gadisseux, J.-F. (1988) Abnormal neuronal patterns and disorders of neocortical development. In: "From Reading to Neurons," A. Galaburda, ed., MIT Press, Boston.

Caviness, V.S., Jr., Takahashi, T., Jacobson, M. and Nowakowski, R.S. (1991) Cytokinetic parameters of the ventricular zone in developing mouse neocortex. Soc. Neurosci. Abst. 17:29.

Cepko, C.L. (1988) Retrovirus vectors and their applications in neurobiology. Neuron 1:345.

Crandall, J.E. and Caviness, V.S., Jr. (1984) Axon strata of the cerebral wall in embryonic mice. Dev. Brain Res. 14:185.

Edwards, M.A., Yamamoto, M. and Caviness, V.S., Jr. (1990) Organization of radial glial and related cells in the developing murine CNS: Analysis based upon a new monoclonal antibody marker. Neuroscience 36:121.

Escobar, M.I., Pimienta, H., Caviness, V.S., Jr., Jacobson, M., Crandall, J.E. and Kosik, K.S. (1986) Architecture of apical dendrites in the murine neocortex: dual apical dendritic systems. Neuroscience 17:975.

Gadisseux, J.-F., Kadhim, H., Van DeBosch de Aguilar, J.P., Caviness, V.S., Jr. and Evrard, P. (1988) Neuron migration within the radial glial fiber system of the developing murine cerebrum. An electron microscopic autoradiographic analysis. Dev. Brain Res. 52:39.

Gadisseux, J.-F., Evrard, P., Misson, J.-P. and Caviness, V.S., Jr. (1989) Dynamic structure of the radial glial fiber system of the developing murine cerebral wall. An immunocytochemical analysis. Dev. Brain Res. 50:56.

Gadisseux, J.-F., Evrard, P., Misson, J.-P. and Caviness, V.S., Jr. (1992) Dynamic changes in the density of radial glial fibers of the developing cerebral wall: a quantitative immunohistological analysis. J. Comp. Neurol., in press.

His, W. (1904) "Die Entwicklung des Menschlichen Gehirns wahrend der ersten Monate," Hirzel, Leipzig.

Jones, E.G. (1984a) History of cortical cytology. In: "Cerebral Cortex: Cellular Components of the Cerebral Cortex," A. Peters and E.G. Jones, eds., Plenum Press, New York.

Jones, E.G. (1984b) Laminar distribution of cortical efferent cells. In: "Cerebral Cortex: Cellular Components of the Cerebral Cortex," A. Peters and E.G. Jones, eds., Plenum Press, New York.

Luskin, M.B., Pearlman, A.L. and Sanes, J.R. (1988) Cell lineage in the cerebral cortex of the mouse studied in vivo and in vitro with a recombinant retrovirus. Neuron 1:635.

Marin-Padilla, M. (1971) Early prenatal ontogenesis of the cerebral cortex (neocortex) of the cat (Felis domestics). A Golgi study. I. The primordial neocortical organization. Z. Anat. Entwickl. Gesch. 134:117.

Miller, M.W. and Nowakowski, R.S. (1988) Use of bromo-deoxyuridine-immunohistochemistry to examine the proliferation, migration and time of origin of cells in the central nervous system. Brain Res. 457:44.

Misson, J.-P. Edwards, M.A., Yamamoto, M. and Caviness, V.S., Jr. (1988a) Mitotic cycling of radial glial cells of the fetal murine cerebral wall: A combined autoradiographic and immunohistochemical study. Dev. Brain Res. 38:183.

Misson, J.-P., Edwards, M.A., Yamamoto, M. and Caviness, V.S., Jr. (1988b) Identification of radial glial cells within the developing murine central nervous system: studies based upon a new immunohistochemical marker. Dev. Brain Res. 44:95.

Misson, J.-P., Takahashi, T. and Caviness, V.S., Jr. (1991a) Ontogeny of radial and other astroglial cells in murine cerebral cortex. Glia 4:138.

Misson, J.-P., Austin, C.P., Takahashi, T., Cepko, C.L. and Caviness, V.S., Jr. (1991b) The alignment of migrating neural cells in relation to the murine neopallial radial glial fiber system. Cereb. Cort., 1: 221.

Murray, A.W. and Kirschner, M.W. (1991) What controls the cell cycle. Sci. Am. 264:56.

Nowakowski, R.S., Lewin, S.B. and Miller, M.W. (1989) Bromodeoxyuridine immunohistochemical determination of the lengths of the cell cycle and the DNA-synthetic phase for an anatomically defined population. J. Neurocytol. 18:311.

Rakic, P. (1972) Mode of cell migration to the superficial layers of fetal monkey neocortex. J. Comp. Neurol. 145:61.

Rakic, P. (1978) Neuronal migration and contact guidance in the primate telencephalon. Postgrad. Med. J. 54:25.

Rakic, P. (1988) Specification of cerebral cortical areas. Science 241:170.

Rakic, P., Stensaas, L.J., Sayer, E.P. and Sidman, R.L. (1974) Computer aided three-dimensional reconstruction and quantitative analysis of cells from serial electron microscopic montage of foetal monkey brain. Nature 250:31.

Sauer, F.C. (1935) Mitosis in the neural tube. J. Comp. Neurol. 62:377.

Sauer, M.E. and Walker, B.E. (1959) Radioautoradiographic study of interkinetic nuclear migration in the neural tube. Proc. Soc. Exlp. Biol. and Med. 101:557.

Sidman, R.L., Miale, I.L. and Feder, N. (1959) Cell proliferation and migration in the primitive ependymal zone: an autoradiographic study of histogenesis in the nervous system. Exp. Neurol. 1:322.

Sidman, R.L. and Rakic, P. (1973) Neuronal migration, with special reference to developing human brain: a review. Brain Res. 62:1.

Takahashi, T., Misson, J.-P. and Caviness, V.S., Jr. (1990a) Glial process elongation and branching in the developing murine neocortex: a qualitative and quantitative immunohistochemical analysis. J. Comp. Neurol. 302:15.

Takahashi, T., Jacobson, M., Nowakowski, R.S. and Caviness, V.S., Jr. (1990b) Cell cycle kinetics of the E14 murine cerebral ventricular zone: estimates based upon S-phase labeling with BUdR. Soc. Neurosci. Abst. 16:1147.

Takahashi, T., Nowakowski, R.S., Jacobson, M. and Caviness, V.S., Jr. (1991) Cell output of the ventricular zone of the E14 mouse neocortex. Soc. Neurosci. Abst. 17:29.

Takahashi, T., Nowakowski, R.S. and Caviness, V.S., Jr. (1992a) BUdR as an S-phase marker for quantitative studies of cytokinetic behavior in the murine cerebral ventricular zone.

Takahashi, T., Nowakowski, R.S. and Caviness, V.S., Jr. (1992b) Cytogenesis in the secondary proliferative population of the murine cerebral wall. Soc. Neurosci. Abst., in press.

Takahashi, T., Nowakowski, R.S. and Caviness, V.S., Jr. (1992c) Cell cycle
    parameters and patterns of nuclear movement in the neorcortical
    proliferative zone of the fetal mouse. J. Neurosci., in press.
Walsh, C. and Cepko, C.L. (1988) Clonally related cortical cells show
    several migration patterns. Science 241:1342.
Zilles, K. (1990) Cortex. In: "The Human Nervous System", G. Paxinos,
    ed., San Diego, Academic Press.

THE USE OF EXPERIMENTAL GENETICS TO STUDY PATTERN FORMATION IN THE

MAMMALIAN CNS

Karl Herrup

Division of Developmental Neurobiology
E.K. Shriver Center
200 Trapelo Road
Waltham, MA 02254

The mammalian cerebellum has long intrigued neurobiologists as an attractive model system in which to approach the study of pattern formation because of its simple, highly repetitive cytoarchitecture. Overlaid on the apparent homogeneity, however, is a large scale pattern of sagittally organized bands and clusters that is seen at all levels, from the molecular constituents of the cells to the network properties of the region. It is rapidly becoming recognized that this pattern reflects a fundamental organizing principle of the cerebellum.

History. Jansen and Brodal (1940) were the first to notice this organization in their study of rabbit cerebellar cortico-nuclear connections. Subsequently, the theme of a longitudinal banding pattern has recurred in many different studies. Voogd (1967), used retrograde methods to show that the projections of the inferior olive to the cortex of each hemicerebellum are organized into approximately half a dozen sagittal bands. He further demonstrated that the olive cell collaterals (sent to the neurons of the deep cerebellar nuclei) contact nuclear cells in the same region to which the Purkinje cells innervated by the cortical branch of these olivary fibers project (Groenewegen and Voogd, 1977, Voogd, 1967). Voogd has also suggested that the mossy fiber afferents to the cerebellar cortex respect the same landmarks and the same sagittal organization. This is strong evidence that the pattern defined by the projections is one that is recognized by many different cell types. Additional confirmation of the fundamental basis of the pattern can be found in studies from many species on the anatomical (Chambers and Sprague, 1955, Chan-Palay et al., 1977, Courville, 1975, Scheibel, 1977) and physiological (Armstrong, 1974, Oscarson, 1969) organization of the olivary projections. In addition, a variety of histochemical (Chan-Palay et al., 1982, Marani and Voogd, 1977, Scott, 1963, Scott, 1964) immunological (Chan-Palay et al., 1981, Gravel et al., 1987, Hawkes et al., 1985, Hawkes and Leclerc, 1987, Leclerc et al., 1990, Wassef and Sotelo, 1984), and, significantly, genetic (Greenberg et al., 1990, Wassef et al., 1987) heterogeneities have been discovered. These data emphasize that a fundamental longitudinal pattern exists and that it affects the cells in all layers of cerebellar cortex. Researchers including Voogd (Voogd, 1969), Komeliussen (Korneliussen, 1969), and Wassef et al. (Wassef and Sotelo, 1984) have stressed the developmental importance of the sagittal organization. Others have suggested that the bands might have originated in evolution from two initially separate populations of cells

Development of the Central Nervous System in Vertebrates
Edited by S.C. Sharma and A.M. Goffinet, Plenum Press, New York, 1992

99

(Brochu et al., 1990, Lannoo et al., 1991). Even in the malformed
cerebellar environment of several of the mouse neurological mutants, a
recognizable semblance of the sagittal pattern is retained (Blatt and
Eisenman, 1988, Blatt and Eisenman, 1989, Goffinet, 1984). This
underlines the strong, possibly intrinsic, nature of the pattern - if a
cerebellum can form at all it will have aspects of a longitudinal
organization associated with it.

The Zebrin sagittal bands. As their name suggests, Zebrins are a
series of antibodies against antigens that define a pattern of sagittal
bands, visible as prominent stripes in either horizontal or coronal
sections. MabQ113, against the Zebrin-1 antigen, and the newly
characterized Zebrin-2 antibody are the best known of these. The antigens
form a bilaterally symmetric pattern of seven to eight bands in each half
cerebellum. Zebrin-1 is a 120 kd intracellular antigen located throughout
Purkinje cells from dendritic spine to axon tip. Zebrin-2 migrates as a
36 kd species (Doré et al., 1990) and has an identical cell localization
to Zebrin-1 (Brochu et al., 1990, Lannoo et al., 1991). Leclerc and
Hawkes have shown that the banded staining pattern arises postnatally
(Leclerc et al., 1988).

Many features of CNS development are dependent on cell:cell
interactions for their expression, and the development of heterogeneous,
Zebrin[+] and Zebrin[-], Purkinje cells would seem at first to be a likely
candidate for such a feature. The appearance of the pattern begins at P6
with the development of antigenicity in all Purkinje cells. By P12,
antigen expression is fully developed and the banding pattern begins to
emerge through the loss of staining from the cells that will constitute
the Zebrin[-] band. At birth, the climbing fiber system is already
sagittally organized (Sotelo et al., 1984), and while the Zebrin staining
transition is coincident with the maturation of the climbing fibers, the
Zebrin stripes are unaffected by deafferentation. In the adult,
pedunculotomy has no effect on the maintenance of the banding pattern and
a similar operation in the neonate (before staining develops) is likewise
ineffective in preventing the development of the stripes (Leclerc et al.,
1987). Perhaps the most dramatic demonstration of the resistance of
Zebrin staining to manipulation is that transplantation of embryonic
cerebellar anlagen, either to the anterior chamber of the eye, to a
cavity in cerebral cortex (Wassef et al., 1990), or to kainate depleted
adult cerebellar cortex (Rouse and Sotelo, 1990) has no effect on the
development of Purkinje cells that are both Zebrin[+] and Zebrin[-]. While a
role for cell:cell interactions among Purkinje cells is not eliminated by
these findings, the results strongly suggest that the Zebrin[+/-] phenotype
is a cell autonomous property of the developing Purkinje cells. If the
Zebrin-positive or negative character of a given Purkinje cell is
intrinsically determined, then where does the spatially regulated staining
pattern come from?

Since Zebrin banding is one of only several methods that reveals the
sagittal organization of cerebellum, one question that arises is to what
extent do the various banding patterns recognize common boundaries in the
brain. The data of Gravel et al. (1987) demonstrate that the afferent
bands of olivary climbing fibers do largely respect the boundaries defined
by Zebrin. Other authors have demonstrated that this is true for AChE
(Boegman et al., 1988), 5'-nucleotidase (Eisenman and Hawkes, 1989) as
well as cytochrome oxidase (Leclerc et al., 1990) - though in this case
whether the Zebrin[+] cells correlate with a CO[+] or a CO[-] band varies from
species to species. Underlying all of these questions, however, is more
fundamental one. If the pattern of sagittal banding is intrinsic to
proper cerebellar development and if, in particular, the Zebrin staining
of cerebellar Purkinje cells is cell autonomous, then is this pattern

specified in a genetically more rigid way? Preliminary evidence from my laboratory supports the hypothesis that, in the cerebellum, the sagittal banding pattern that demarcates the Zebrin staining is the same pattern respected by polyclones of adult Purkinje cell lineages (see below). This finding suggests that to fully understand the adult pattern it may be necessary to look at early times (before the mitosis of precursors is complete).

Zebrin bands may represent developmental "compartments"

As discussed, the Zebrin antibodies define a series of sagittal bands whose boundaries are coincident with the functional architecture of the cerebellum. Sotelo and colleagues were among the first to draw the analogy between the bands in cerebellum and the concept of a developmental genetic "compartment" in *Drosophila* (Wassef et al., 1985). The importance of this analogy is emphasized by a newly described monoclonal antibody, P-path, developed by Dr. Miyuki Yamamoto (Edwards et al., 1989). P-path recognizes one major, and 3 minor, 9-0-acetylated gangliosides expressed on the plasma membrane of many embryonic brain cells. Based on its chromatographic mobility (Chou et al., 1990), the major P-path inununoreactive species is likely to be an acetylated derivative of disialolactoneotetrosylceramide. One of the minor bands chromatographs with the 9-0-acetyl-GD3 standard.

Immunocytochemistry of the adult mouse cerebellum shows that P-path staining is primarily associated with the cell surface of Purkinje cells. The pattern of immunoreactivity is such that the immunopositive Purkinje cells are organized into distinct parasagittal bands separated by negative ones. Zebrin II immunopositive Purkinje cells are also distributed in bands - 6 symmetrical parasagittal compartments, 3 per side, with two additional bands defining the boundaries between the hemisphere and vermis (Brochu et al., 1990, Doré et al., 1990). The bands of Zebrin II-positive Purkinje cells imply the existence of 6 additional bands made up of the Zebrin II-negative cells. Definition of a group by the absence of a substance is not totally satisfying, however, since subdivisions of the negative group can go undetected. Double staining with anti-Zebrin II and P-path antibodies eliminates this uncertainty - all Purkinje cells that are Zebrin II-negative are P-path-positive. A complete reconstruction of the staining patterns of the vermis reveals the existence of a third class of Purkinje cell. Throughout the vermis, the $P3^+$ compartment is both zebrin II-positive and P-path-positive. We were unable to identify Purkinje cells in any region of the mouse cerebellum that were unstained by both antigens. Therefore, the fourth compartment - Zebrin II^- negative/P-path-negative - does not exist.

The implication of the complementarity between the P-path and Zebrin bands is that the antibodies define subsets of Purkinje cells each of which comprises a fundamental unit of cerebellum. At it is unlikely that the presence of one of these compounds is directly responsible for the presence or absence of the other, there are likely to be many qualities that characterize (and differ between) these Purkinje cell types - Zebrin and P-path are only part of the description. The conclusion that there are deep developmental genetic distinctions among the three types of Purkinje cells supports the analogy between the Zebrin bands and *Drosophila* compartments. In *Drosophila*, after the establishment of compartment boundaries, the cells are intrinsically set to display certain phenotypic characteristics as they mature. The hypothesis that this arrangement might apply to cerebellum was put forth several years ago by Wassef and Sotelo (1984) and strengthened by the recent observation of Rouse and Sotelo (1990) that grafts of dissociated Purkinje cells precursors, transplanted into adult cerebellum depleted of Purkinje cells by kainate, develop an organized banding pattern as revealed by staining with anti-zebrin I.

If the Zebrin bands represent "compartments" of the cerebellar Purkinje cell population, established early in the development of the CNS then the bands (as compartments) would be defined before cell division is complete. In this case, evidence for this event might be apparent in the different lineages of cells. Unlike the fly, several decades of examination of mouse mosaics has clearly established that significant amounts of cell mixing occur during the developmental process (e.g., Dewey et al., 1976, Herrup, 1987, Mullen, 1977) - see also below). Nonetheless, recent evidence from lineage studies in cerebellum and cerebral cortex suggest that restrictions to mixing do occur and are visible in the pattern of neuronal cell lineages of the brain (Crandall and Herrup, 1990, Herrup et al., 1991).

The relationship of the Zebrin "compartments" to Purkinje cell lineages

In many ways cell lineage relationships represent an interface between development and genetics. Cells essentially acquire the information needed to attain their adult characteristics from two sources: intrinsic and extrinsic. Cell lineage provides a vehicle for translating the intrinsic information from a progenitor cell, in whom the information was acquired, to the descendant, in whom the information must be used. Given this, it seems nearly self evident that knowledge of the mitotic ancestry of a cell will be one essential part in the understanding of the developmental genetic machinery that guides ontogeny.

One of the strongest motivations for studying neuronal cell lineage is that the observed clonal relationships may help to explain the logic of basic features of CNS organization and function. To suggest that a particular lineage distribution pattern has significance for the development of an area, it is necessary to demonstrate that regions defined by such lineage patterns are coextensive with other significant features of the structure such as anatomy, physiology or biochemistry. We are pursuing this goal in cerebellum by comparing the distribution of Purkinje cell lineages to the structure/function boundaries delineated by the Zebrin bands. Our preliminary data suggest, as predicted above, that the basic sagittal banding plan of cerebellar architecture is laid down early in neural development.

If the Zebrin bands are used to define the boundaries of a cell lineage grouping in a $Gus^h/Gus^h \leftrightarrow Gus^b/Gus^b$ chimera, then, according to a χ^2 test, the spatial distribution of the Gus^h/Gus^h to Gus^b/Gus^b ratio of Purkinje cells is significantly non-random ($p < 0.05$) with respect to the bands (and interbands). If these same boundaries are shifted out of alignment with the actual Zebrin bands, the χ^2 test of the distribution is no longer significant ($p < 0.22$). These data support the conclusion that the progenitors of the Purkinje cells in the different bands are not identical. The fact that this lineage segregation is apparent only when the boundaries used for the χ^2 are aligned with the actual Zebrin bands means that it is not simply due to a general sagittal organization of the cerebellar lineages (Hallonet et al., 1990).

These findings of significant inhomogeneities in the Purkinje cell lineage map coupled with their close registration with the functional architecture indicates that important mixing restrictions are likely to be established before neurogenesis is completed in the ventricular zone of the fourth ventricle. The lineage maps that we have reconstructed from adult chimeras represent the end of a process involving differentiation, mitosis, migration and cortical expansion. Thus the factors involved in establishing each Purkinje cell's final location will evade simple explanation. Our current hypothesis is that specific boundaries to cell mixing are established in the ventricular zone and are maintained through subsequent developmental events. The process of compartmentation in *Drosophila* offers one analogy for this scheme (Crick and Lawrence, 1975, Lawrence, 1981), and recent work in chick suggests that some aspects of this model may well apply to the vertebrate CNS (Avarado-Mallart et al., 1990, Fraser et al., 1990, Martinez et al., 1991). Until more data are accumulated, however, we propose a less rigid modification of this model. If one begins with the Purkinje cell progenitors as they are selected in the early neuroepithelium (Herrup, 1986, Herrup and Sunter, 1986, Wetts and Herrup, 1982) our hypothesis is that at some stage before the proliferation of this population is complete, an independent process sets up restrictions to mixing that bounds off small cohorts of cells. If these restrictions are roughly maintained during the translocation of cells from the ventricular zone to the cerebellar cortical plate, then variations in the ratios of the founder populations will be retained and produce the non-random distributions that we observe in the adult cerebellar Purkinje cell layer. Presumably the specific paths of cell migration and pattern of formation of the Purkinje cell monolayer will affect the final form of the lineage maps. Our early examination of the cell lineages in the ventricular zone itself (see below) suggests that while these post-mitotic processes may degrade the crispness of ventricular mosaic somewhat, the pattern in the adult bears striking similarities to that found in the embryo.

Transgenes as novel cell markers for CNS lineage studies

Advancements in techniques of both molecular biology and experimental embryology have made it possible to custom design cell markers of considerable value for developmental neurobiologists. The production of transgenic mice is done by introducing a specifically designed DNA fragment, via microinjection, into one of the two prenuclei of a fertilized embryo. The transgene integrates into the host genome and is thus heritable, passing to the offspring of the original transgenote as a simple Mendelian element. Any piece of DNA can be used as a transgene. Thus a cloned construct carrying an appropriate promoter and an easily detectable "marker" gene can be introduced. If designed properly, this element will be expressed as protein product in some or all cells of the body. This expression is likely to be cell autonomous; therefore, a chimera can be made between a transgenic embryo and any other embryo and it will appear mosaic for the expression of the transgene.

Together with Dr. Kevin Kelley a novel construct was made using the 5' regulatory elements of Thy-1.2 (a cell surface protein expressed at high levels on most CNS neurons and Tlymphocytes) and the structural gene for the bacterial ß-galactosidase gene (easily distinguished histologically from mammalian ß-galactosidase by its pH optimum). This construct was used to make fifteen different DNA positive mice. Three of these were found to express the bacterial transgene off the mouse promoter in one or more tissues. The pattern of expression confirms much about the molecular anatomy of the Thy-1 gene. The Thy-1 promoter/enhancer correctly directs expression to the CNS. Northern analysis of 11 different tissues reveals that expression of the transgene is restricted to "brain". The fact that thymus is negative for mRNA expression is evidence that the immunological enhancer (responsible for the expression of Thy-1 on the surface of mature thymocytes) is contained either within the structural sequences of the gene or (less likely) in the 3'region. Histological analysis of transgene activity (bacterial ß-galactosidase activity as determined with Xgal staining) confirms that expression is restricted to nervous tissue. There was substantial variation among various neuronal regions in the level of expression. The neurons of the cerebellar cortex were particularly low while cells in area CA1 of hippocampus and neurons in the septal nucleus were particularly high. The large neurons of the brain stem nuclei were also high in ß-galactosidase activity. Neural crest derivatives were uniformly negative in the adult; this included cells of the mesencephalic nucleus of the trigeminal nerve which are of crest origin, but located in the CNS. Within this general scheme, the pattern of transgene expression matched, almost precisely, the pattern of expression of the nominal Thy-1 gene.

Surprisingly little is known about the expression of endogenous Thy-1 in the embryo. Most authors (Morris, 1985) speak of its appearance on neurons concomitant with the growth of the neurites of the cell. In our own efforts to determine the age of onset of LacZ staining, embryos from the TBG/1 line were found to exhibit ß-galactosidase activity as early as embryonic day 10 (E10 - Kelley et al., 1989)). By E13, the neuroepithelial cells lining the ventricular zone are heavily labeled, and this staining persists through later stages (Appendix - Fig 4A & B). In addition to the neuroepithelial expression, neural crest derivatives such as the dorsal root ganglia are labeled in the embryo. This staining diminishes by E15 and is never seen in the adult. The relationship of this staining pattern to the endogenous Thy-1 gene is under investigation.

Cell lineage in the ventricular zone

The above model, describing the behavior of cells in the ventricular zone prior to migration, is based on observations made in adult chimeric animals. The specific predictions of the model are, first, that the lineages of cells must mix extensively within the plane of the ventricular zone during the early stages of neurogenesis. This cellular behavior is needed to explain the observed spatial dispersion of the descendents of the 8 to 12 Purkinje cell founders (proposed on the basis of adult *lurcher* chimera cell counts (Herrup, 1987, Vogel et al., 1991, and Wetts and Herrup, 1982)). Yet the highly non-random spatial distributions of cell lineages in the adult cerebellar Purkinje cell layer (Herrup et al., 1991, Herrup and Sunter, 1986) and the cerebral cortex (Crandall and Herrup, 1990) require two additional predictions. First, during the final cell divisions there must be a reduction in cell mixing (to account for the observed establishment of real or virtual boundaries), and second the resulting mosaic of clustered cell families must be retained, at least in rough representation, during the migration from the ventricular zone cells to the final position in the cortical plate. One of the prime motivations behind the development of a new generation of transgenic cell markers has been to approach these questions directly in the embryo itself. With the ventricular zone expression of the *tbg-1* transgene, the first glimpse of the organizations of cell lineage within the ventricular zone has now been achieved. Aggegation chimeras were made with one embryo derived from a *tbg-1/tbg-1* by +/+ mating and one embryo from a separate mating of two non-transgenic parents. The resulting *tbg-1/+* ⟷ +/+ chimeras were removed by Caesarian section on the 12th and 13th day of gestation. After fixation, the embryo was whole mount stained for ß-galactosidase activity and subsequently bisected on the midline.

In spinal cord, a very fine gained mosaicism of cells is observed. Based on analyses of *tbg-1/tbg-1* embryos of this age, the cells observed

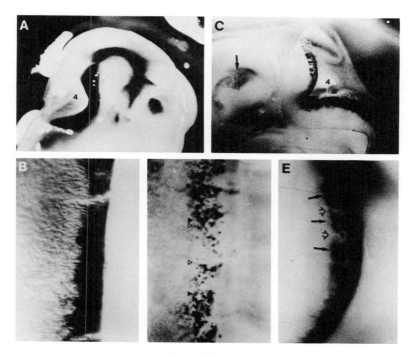

FIGURE 1

A: The ventricular zone of a *Thy-1:lacZ* transgenic mouse on embryonic day
12. The embryo has been whole mount stained for Xgal activity and
bissected on the midline to reveal the pattern of staining.

B: A cryostat 12μm section through the ventricular zone of the hindbrain
of an embyro such as the one shown in A. Note that every single cell in
the neurogenic region is positive for the Xgal product.

C: The ventricular zone of a chimera made from one Thy-1:*lacZ* embryo and
one wild-type. The mosaicism of the cell lineages in the ventricular zone
in obvious (compare with A). Note the more thorough mixing in the more
caudal regions of the CNS as contrasted with the "patch" like arrangement
of clones in the roof of the fourth ventricle (4).

D: A higher magnification of the spinal cord of a transgenic wild-type
chimera. Note that although the lineages are well mixed there is an order
apparent as the ratio of the genotypes (density of transgenic, stained,
cells) changes over very short anatomical distances. The open triangles
border a region of low transgenic cell density; the filled triangles
border a region of higher density.

E: Higher magnification of the roof of the fourth ventricle in the embryo
shown in C. Note the transverse, near segmental organization to the
lineages appearent in this view. The filled arrows indication regions of
higher transgenic cell density while the open arrows highlight regions of
lower transgenic cell density.

are predominantly post-migratory neurons of the spinal grey matter. The arrangement of the lineages in lumbar regions is least ordered in spatial terms. By contrast, in cervical and thoracic cord, areas with high densities of +/tbg-1 cells have clear anterior/posterior boundaries with areas where the ratio of +/tbg-1 to +/+ cells noticeably changes (Figure 1D). Although precise registration with the overall segmentation pattern of the embryo is difficult, examination of several such transitions in animals of different ages was highly suggestive of a correlation with the segmentation of the cord as marked by the cartilage of the vertebrae. Leber et al. (1990) used recombinant retrovirus infections of early chick embryos to suggest that the descendent clones of any one spinal cord progenitor cell were scattered in the transverse plane, but were restricted in their anterior/posterior mobility. Our analysis of +/tbg-1↔ +/+ chimeras suggests that the observed anterior/posterior restriction applies not only to single clones, but to the spinal population as a whole. The well defined anterior/posterior regions of cord with noticeably different ratios of +/tbg-1 to +/+ cells suggests that the progenitor cells for adjacent "regions" cannot be the same. The implication is that each "region" represents a polyclone of a relatively small number of progenitor cells, and that the descendents of these progenitors do not freely intermix.

In the the fourth ventricle, lineages of cells in the final stages of neurogenesis and early migration show a different arrangement. Most, though not all, areas show small clusters of cells of like genotype interspersed with cells of the opposite genotype. In some areas the clusters can be quite distinct (solid/open arrows Figure 1C, E) while in other regions the lineages are more finely interspersed. In the former regions, it is noteworthy that, while the clusters are readily apparent, no one cluster is monolithic in genotype. Each has at least a few cells of the opposite lineage in evidence. There is a strong tendency for clusters to be elongated mediolaterally and stacked in the anterior/posterior direction. At a coarser scale, the ventricular zone of the myelencephalon and metencephalon may be organized in transverse stacks of cells that are similar to those seen in the spinal cord. It has been suggested previously (West, 1977) that neurogenesis in the mammal proceeds through a period of near random interspersion of cell lineages followed by a final period of coherent clonal growth. A similar conclusion was reached by Gray et al. (Gray et al., 1988, Gray and Sanes, 1991) in their analysis of recombinant retroviral infection of chicken embryos. In the adult cerebellum, Oster-Granite and Gearhart (1981) have provided evidence that the Purkinje cells of one lineage exist in non-random clusters of from four to eight cells. Together with the results from the tbg-1 chimeras, these findings suggest that the lineage "patches" of Purkinje cells, described above for adult cerebellar cortex, represent the descendants of these distinct ventricular zone patches. The appearance of the ventricular zone of these animals is a gratifying confirmation of many of the predictions that we had made based on the analysis of adult mosaics, but, as our experiments have only just begun, many questions remain to be answered.

Conclusions

For decades, the study of the genetic control pattern formation has been the province of the invertebrate biologist. While much important data has been gained from the study of vertebrate limb development, the stunning advances in our understanding of the process of segmentation in the fly have far exceeded even the most optimistic projections of only ten years ago. Coupled with the advances in Drosophila biology, however, has come the discovery that the networks of genes involved in specifying invertebrate development bear strong molecular homology to similar genes in organisms from frog to chick to man. The time is ripe for strong model systems to be developed in the mouse - systems that will apply the lessons learned in *Drosophila* to the developing systems of the mammal. It is hoped that the data presented in this chapter reinforce the contention that the developing mouse cerebellum may well be such a system.

ACKNOWLEDGEMENTS

The author wishes to thank his colleagues and collaborators, Dr. Kevin Kelley, Dr. Nicole Leclerc, Dr. Richard Hawkes, and Mr. Andy Ahn, whose work is liberally cited here. Further thanks go to Drs. Sharma and Goffinet for the time and effort spent in organizing a stimulating course, the results of which are represented in this volume. Finally, no acknowledgement section would be complete without thanks to the organizations who foot the bill for this work, specifically, The March of Dimes Birth Defects Foundation (#1-1175) and the NIH (NS # 18381 and NS # 20591).

REFERENCES

Armstrong, D.M. (1974) Topographical localization in the olivo-cerebellar projection: an electrophysiological study in the cat. <u>J. Comp. Neurol.</u> 154:287-302.

Avarado-Mallart, R.-M., Martinez, S. and Lance-Jones, C. (1990) Pluripotentiality of the 2 day old avian genninative neuroepithelium. <u>Devel. Biol.</u> 139:75-88.

Blatt, G. and Eisenman, L. (1988) Topographic and zonal organization of the olivocerebellar projection in the reeler mutant mouse. <u>J. Comp. Neurol.</u> 267:603-615.

Blatt, G.J. and Eisenman, L.M. (1989) Regional and topographic organization of the olivocerebellar projection in homozygous staggerer *(sg/sg)* mutant mice: an anterograde and retrograde tracing study. <u>Neurosci.</u> 30:703-715.

Boegman, R., Parent, A. and Hawkes, R. (1988) Zonation in the rat cerebellar cortex: patches of high acetylcholinesterase activity in the ganular layer are congruent with Purkinje cell compartments. <u>Brain Res.</u> 448:237-251.

Brochu, G., Maler, L. and Hawkes, R. (1990) Zebrin II: A polypeptide antigen expressed selectively by Purkinje cells reveals compartments in rat and fish cerebellum. <u>J. Comp. Neurol.</u> 291:538-552.

Chambers, W.W. and Sprague, J.M. (1955) A functional localization in the cerebellum: I. Organization in longitudinal cortico-nuclear zones and their contribution to the control of posture, both extrapyramidal and pyramidal. <u>J. Comp. Neurol.</u> 130:105-130.

Chan-Palay, V., Nilaver, G., Palay, S.L., Beinfeld, M.C., Zimmerman, E.A., Wu, J.U. and O'Donohue, T.L. (1981) Chemical heterogeneity in cerebellar Purkinje cells: existence and coexistence of glutamic acid decarboxylase-like and motilin-like immunoreactivities. <u>Proc. Nat. Acad. Sci.</u> 78:7787-7791.

Chan-Palay, V., Palay, S.L., Brown, J.L. and Van Itallie, C. (1977) Sagittal organization of olivocerebellar and reticulocerebellar projections: autoradiogaphic studies with ^{35}S-methionine. <u>Exp. Brain Res.</u> 30:561-576.

Chan-Palay, V., Palay, S.L., Brown, J.L. and Van Itallie, C. (1982) Sagittal cerebellar microbands of taurine neurons: immunocytochemical demonstration by using antibodies against the taurine synthesizing enzyme sulfinic acid decarboxylase. <u>Proc. Nat. Acad. Sci. U.S.A.</u> 79:4221-4225.

Chou, D., Flores, S. and Jungalwala, F. (1990) Identification of disialosyl paragloboside and 9-acetyl-disialosyl paragloboside in cerebellum and embryonic cerebrum. J. Neurochem. 54:1598-1607.

Courville, J. (1975) Distribution of climbing fibers demonstrated by a radioautogaphic tracing method. Brain Res. 95:253-263.

Crandall, J. and Herrup, K. (1990) Patterns of cell lineage in the cerebral cortex reveal evidence for developmental boundaries. Exp. Neurol. 109:131-139.

Crick, F.H.C. and Lawrence, P.A. 1975. Compartments and polyclones in insect development. Science 189:340-347.

Dewey, M.J., Gervais, A.G. and Mintz, B. (1976) Brain and ganglion development from two genotype classes of cells in allophenic mice. Devel. Biol. 50:68-81.

Doré, L., Jacobson, C. and Hawkes, R. (1990) Organization and postnatal development of Zebrin II antigenic compartmentation in the cerebellar vermis of the grey opossum, Monodelphis domestica. J. Comp. Neurol. 291:431-449.

Edwards, M., Schwarting, G. and Yamamoto, M. (1989) Expression of the disialoganglioside GD3 in developing axon tracts of the fetal mouse brain. Neurosci. Abst. 15:959.

Eisenman, L. and Hawkes, R. (1989) 5'-nucleotidase and the mabQ113 antigen share a common distribution in the cerebellar cortex of the mouse. Neurosci. 31:231-235.

Fraser, S., Keynes, R. and Lumsden, A. (1990) Segmentation in the chick embryo hindbrain is defined by cell lineage restrictions. Nature 344:431-435.

Goffinet, A.M. (1984) Events governing organization of postmigratory neurons: studies on brain development in normal and reeler mice. Brain Res. Rev. 7:261-296.

Gravel, C., Eisenman, L.M., Sasseville, R. and Hawkes, R. (1987) Parasagittal organization of the rat cerebellar cortex: direct correlation between antigenic Purkinje cell bands revealed by mabQ113 and the organization of the olivocerebellar projection. J. Comp. Neurol. 265:294-310.

Gray, G., Glover, J., Majors, J. and Sanes, J. (1988) Radial arrangement of clonally related cells in the chicken optic tectum: lineage analysis with a recombinant retrovirus. Proc. Nat. Acad. Sci. 85:7356-7360.

Gray, G. and Sanes, J. (1991) Migratory paths and phenotypic choices of clonally related cells in the avian optic tectum. Neuron 6:211-225.

Greenberg, J., Boehm, T., Sofroniew, M., Keynes, R., Barton, S., Norris, N., Surani, M., Spillantini, M.-G. and Rabbitts, T. (1990) Segmental and developmental regulation of a presumptive T-cell oncogene in the central nervous system. Nature 344:158-160.

Groenewegen, H.J. and Voogd, J. (1977) The parasagittal zonation within the olivocerebellar projection I. Climbing fiber distribution in the vermis of cat cerebellum. J. Comp. Neurol. 174:417-488.

Hallonet, M., Teillet, M.-A. and Le Douarin, N. (1990). A new approach to the development of the cerebellum provided by the quail-chick marker system. Development 108:19-31.

Hawkes, R., Colonnier, M. and Leclerc, N. (1985) Monoclonal antibodies reveal sagittal banding in the rodent cerebellar cortex. Brain Res. 333:359-365.

Hawkes, R. and Leclerc, N. (1987) Antigenic map of rat cerebellar cortex: the distribution of parasagittal bands as revealed by monoclonal anti-Purkinje cell antibody mabQ113. J. Comp. Neurol. 256:29-41.

Herrup, K. (1986) Cell lineage relationships in the development of the mammalian CNS. III. Role of cell lineage in regulation of Purkinje cell number. Devel. Biol. 115:148-154.

Herrup, K. (1987) Roles of cell lineage in the developing mammalian brain. In: Neural Development, Hunt, R.K., ed. Academic Press, New York, pp. 65-97.

Herrup, K., Carman, G. and Bower, J. (1991) Spatial distribution of Purkinje cell lineages in cerebellar cortex suggests early developmental restrictions to neuroblast mixing. J. Neurosci. (submitted).

Herrup, K., Letsou, A. and Diglio, T.J. (1984) Cell lineage relationships in the development of the mammalian CNS: The facial nerve nucleus. Dev. Biol. 103:329-36.

Herrup, K. and Sunter, K. (1986) Lineage dependent and independent control of Purkinje cell number in the cerebellar cortex of lurcher chimeric mice. Devel. Biol. 117:417-427.

Herrup, K., Wetts, R. and Diglio, T.J. (1984) Cell lineage relationships in the development of the mammalian CNS. II. Bilateral independence of CNS clones. J. Neurogenet. 1:275-88.

Jansen, J. and Brodal, A. (1940) Experimental studies on the intrinsic fibers of the cerebellum. II. The cortico-nuclear projection. J. Comp. Neurol. 73:267-321.

Kelley, K.A., Manjunath, G.S. and Herrup, K. (1989) Neuroepithelial expression of a Thy-1.2/lacZ fusion gene in the developing CNS of transgenic mice. Neurosci. Abst. 15:957.

Korneliussen, H.K. (1969) Cerebellar organization in light of cerebellar nuclear morphology and cerebellar corticogenesis. In: Neurobiology of Cerebellar Evolution and Development. Llinas, R., ed. Amer. Med. Assoc., Chicago, pp. 515-523.

Lannoo, M., Brochu, G., Maler, L. and Hawkes, R. (1991) Zebrin II immunoreactivity in the rat and in the weakly electric teleost Eigeninannia (Gymnotiformes) reveals three modes of Purkinje cell development. J. Comp. Neurol. 310:215-233.

Lawrence, P.A. (1981) The cellular basis of segmentation in insects. Cell 26:3-10.

Leber, S., Breedlove, S. and Sanes, J. (1990) Lineage, arrangement, and death of clonally related motoneurons in chick spinal cord. J. Neurosci. 10:2451-2462.

Leclerc, N., Doré, L., Parent, A. and Hawkes, R. (1990) The compartmentalization of the monkey and rat cerebellar cortex: Zebrin I and cytochrome oxidase. Brain Res. 506:70-78.

Leclerc, N., Gravel, C. and Hawkes, R. (1987) Parasagittal zonation in the cerebellar cortex develops independently of afferent input. Neurosci. Abst. 13:118.

Leclerc, N., Gravel, C. and Hawkes, R. (1988) The development of parasagittal zonation in the rat cerebellar cortex: MabQ113 andgenic bands are created postnatally by the suppression of antigen expression in a subset of Purkinje cells. J. Comp. Neurol. 273:399-420.

Levitt, P., Cooper, M. and Rakic, P. (1981) Coexistence of neuronal and glial precursor cells in the cerebral ventricular zone of the fetal monkey: an ultrastructural immunoperoxidase study. J. Neurosci. 1:27-39.

Luskin, M., Pearlman, A. and Sanes, J. (1988) Cell lineage in the cerebral cortex of the mouse studied in vivo and in vitro with a recombinant retrovirus. Neuron 1:635-647.

Marani, E. and Voogd, J. (1977) An acetylcholinesterase band-pattern in the molecular layer of the cat cerebellum. J. Anat. 124:335-345.

Martinez, S., Wassef, M. and Alvarado-Mallart, R.-M. (1991) Induction of a mesencephalic phenotype in the 2-day-old chick prosencephalon is preceded by the early expression of the homeobox gene. en Neuron 6:1-20.

Morris, R. (1985). Thy-1 in developing nervous tissue. Dev. Neurosci. 7:133-160.

Mullen, R.J. (1977) Site of pcd gene action and Purkinje cell mosaicism in cerebella of chimeric mice. Nature 270:245-247.

Mullen, R.J. (1978) Mosaicism in the central nervous system of mouse
    chimeras. In: The Clonal Basis of Development - 36th Symposium of
    the Society for Developmental Biology. Subtelney, S. and Sussex,
    I.M., ed. Academic Press, New York, pp. 83-101.

Mullen, R.J. and Herrup, K. (1979). Chimeric analysis of mouse cerebellar
    mutants. In: Neurogenetics: A Genetic Approach to the Central
    Nervous System. Breakefield, X.O., ed. Elsevier-North Holland, New
    York, pp. 271-297.

Oscarson, O. (1969) The sagittal organization of the cerebellar anterior
    lobe as revealed by the projection patterns of the climbing fiber
    system. In: Neurobiology of Cerebellar Organization and
    Development. Llinas, R., ed. Amer. Med. Assoc., Chicago, pp. 525-
    532.

Oster-Granite, M.L. and Gearhart, J. (1981) Cell lineage analysis of
    cerebellar Purkinje cells in mouse chimeras. Devel. Biol. 85:199-
    208.

Price, J. and Thurlow, L. (1988) Cell lineage in the rat cerebral cortex:
    a study using retroviral-mediated gene transfer. Development
    104:473-482.

Price, J., Tumer, D. and Cepko, C. (1987) Lineage analysis in the
    vertebrate nervous system by retrovirus-mediated gene transfer.
    Proc. Nat. Acad. Sci. 84:156-160.

Rouse, R. and Sotelo, C. (1990) Grafts of dissociated cerebellar cells
    containing Purkinje cell precursors organize into Zebrin I defined
    compartments. Exp. Brain Res. 82:401-407.

Sanes, J. (1989). Analysing cell lineage with a recombinant retrovirus.
    Trends Neurosci 12:21-28.

Scheibel, A. (1977) Sagittal organisation of mossy fiber terminal systems
    in the cerebellum of the rat: a Golgi study. Exp. Neurol. 57:1067-
    1070.

Scott, T.G. (1963) A unique pattern of localization in the cerebellum.
    Nature 200:793.

Scott, T.G. (1964) A unique pattern of localization within the cerebellum
    of the mouse. J. Comp. Neurol. 122:1-8.

Sotelo, C., Bourrat, F. and Triller, A. (1984) Postnatal development of
    the inferior olivary complex in the rat. II. Topographic
    organization of the immature olivocerebellar projection. J. Comp.
    Neurol. 222:177-199.

Tumer, D. and Cepko, C. (1987) Cell lineage in the rat retina: a common
    progenitor for neurons and glia persists late in development.
    Nature 328:131-136.

Vogel, M., Mclnnes, M. and Herrup, K. (1991) A theoretical and
    experimental examination of cell lineage relationships among
    cerebellar Purkinje cells in the mouse. Neuron (submitted).

Voogd, J. (1967) Comparative aspects of the structure and fibre
    connexions of the mammalian cerebellum. Prog. Brain Res. 25:94-135.

Voogd, J. 1969. The importance of fibre connections in the comparative
    anatomy of the mammalian cerebellum. In: Neurobiology of
    Cerebellar Evolution and Development. Llinas, R., ed. Amer. Med.
    Assoc., Chicago, pp. 493-514.

Walsh, C. and Cepko, C. (1988) Clonally related cortical cells show
    several migration patterns. Science 241:1342-1345.

Wassef, M. and Sotelo, C. (1984) Asynchrony in the expression of
    guanosine 3':5' phosphate dependent protein kinase by clusters of
    Purkinje cells during the perinatal development of rat cerebellum.
    Neuroscience 13:1217-1241.

Wassef, M., Sotelo, C., Cholley, B., Brehier, A. and Thomasset, M. (1987)
    Cerebellar mutations affecting the postnatal survival of Purkinje
    cells in the mouse disclose a longitudinal pattern of differentially
    sensitive cells. Devel. Biol. 124:379-389.

Wassef, M., Sotelo, C., Thomasset, M., Granholm, A.-C., Leclerc, N.,
    Rafrafi, J. and Hawkes, R. (1990) Expression of compartmentation
    antigens in cerebellar transplants. J. Comp. Neurol. 294:223-234.
Wassef, M., Zanetta, J., Brehier, A. and Sotelo, C. (1985) Transient
    biochemical compartmentalization of Purkinje cells during early
    cerebellar development. Devel. Biol. 111:129-137.
West, J. (1977) Analysis of clonal growth using chimaeras and mosaics.
    In: Development in Mammals. Johnson, M.H., ed. Elsevier-North
    Holland, New York, pp. 413-460.
Wetts, R. and Herrup, K. (1982) Cerebellar Purkinje cells are descended
    from a small number of progenitors conunitted during early
    development: quantitative analysis of lurcher chimeric mice. J.
    Neurosci. 2:1494-1498.

DEVELOPMENT AND FATE OF CAJAL-RETZIUS CELLS *IN VIVO* AND *IN VITRO*

P. Derer and M. Derer

Lab. de Neurobiologie du Développement
Institut des Neurosciences, Université P. et M. Curie
9, quai Saint Bernard, 75005 Paris France

INTRODUCTION

Tangentially oriented neurons in the first layer of the developing mammalian cerebral cortex, were first described by Cajal (1891) and by Retzius (1893) independently. These neurons have been called Cajal-Retzius cells (CRc). Using ^{3}H thymidine and autoradiography, it has been established in different mammalian species that CRc were the earliest generated neurons of the cerebral cortex and were cogenerated with cells located under the cortical plate which are known as the subplate neurons (Raedler and Sievers 1975, 1976, Konig et al., 1977, Raedler and Raedler 1978, Shoukimas and Hinds 1978, Raedler et al., 1980, Caviness 1982, Luskin and Shatz 1985, Chun and Shatz 1989, Jackson et al., 1989).

In the adult, the first layer is largely a neuropil and therefore contains only sparse neurons, thus the fate of CR neurons has often puzzled neurobiologists and has been the object of continuous debate among them. For some authors, these cells persist until adulthood, and are only diluted in the expanding neuropil of the first layer (Fox and Inman 1966, Baron and Gallego 1971, Rickman et al., 1977, Shoukimas and Hinds 1978, Marin-Padilla 1978, 1988, Larroche 1981), while others have suggested that the CRc are transient and disappear once corticogenesis is finished. The mode of this disappearance could be either a transformation into another neuronal type, hence the disappearance could be only apparent (Marin-Padilla 1971, 1972, Edmund and Parnavelas 1982, Parnavelas and Edmund 1983, Meyer and Ferres-Torres 1984), or disappearance by neuronal death and subsequent elimination by transient brain macrophages, (Purpura et al., 1960, Noback and Purpura 1961, Duckett and Pearse 1968, Sas and Sanides 1970, Bradford et al., 1977, Luskin and Shatz 1985, Ferrer et al., 1990).

Thus the aim of this study was to search for data which support one of these hypotheses. For this purpose, three approaches have been used:
1) To find out if morphological changes of the CRc occur during ontogenesis, a new staining method using the Dil was carried out,
2) The quantitative analysis of the amount of CRc during development using a specific visualization of the CRc with acetylcholinesterase cytochemistry,
3) The environment of these cells has been modified by explanting the CRc, to test *in vitro* the influences of intrinsic versus extrinsic factors upon CRc's fate.

Development of the Central Nervous System in Vertebrates
Edited by S.C. Sharma and A.M. Goffinet, Plenum Press, New York, 1992

MATERIAL AND METHODS

Material came from normal and reeler (rl^{Orl}) mice fetuses, new born, and young pups up to 15 days of age. All were of the BAlb/C strain. These animals were processed in different ways:

1) For Global viewing of the CRc

The cells were stained with a lipophilic dye of the carbocyanine family, recently introduced by Honig and Hume (1986, 1989). The dye is 1,1'dioctadecyl-3-3-3'3'tetramethyl indocarbocyanine perchlorate known as DiI, (Molecular Probe, Eugene, Oregon). The stain was performed on brains fixed with 4% paraformaldehyde (Godement et al., 1987). The method is described in detail elsewhere (Derer and Derer 1991). It consisted mainly of applying tiny crystals of DiI over the cortex and allowing the subsequent migration of the dye in the phospholipidic part of the cell plasmalemma. Within two weeks up to twelve months we obtained global revelation of the CRc, whose shape was best observed from superficial thich sections parallel to the meningeal surface.

2) Quantitative evaluation of CRc

The density of CRc was estimated on tangential sections of the cortex after histochemical staining of acetylcholinesterase activity by the Koelle method, which is specific of the CRc. The method is described elsewhere (Derer 1985). Cell density estimates were obtained by direct counting on the microscope using a square reticule in the ocular lens. At 4OX magnification, 10.000μm^2 were viewed at the same time. According to the age of the animals, about 150 to 500 fields per brain were counted randomly.

The total number of CRc per hemisphere was calculated as the product of the density at each stage by the surface of the cortex of the same age. To estimate the total surface of the cortex at each stage, the hemispheres were sliced coronally into 500μm thick serial sections for newborn and young pups and 200μm thick sections for prenatal animals. The surface of the cortical rim of each slice can be assimilated to a trapezium whose height is the thickness of the section and whose lengths of the two parallel sides are the length of the cortical borders of each section. These lengths were measured with a curvimeter on successive camera lucida drawings. The limits of the cortex were put at the edge of the cingulate cortex medially and rhinal fissure laterally. All partial areas were summed up to give the total cortical area.

3) Culture technique

To establish the cultures of CRc, we took advantage of the reeler mutation in whose inverted cortex, the CRc lie close to the surface, in direct apposition to the basal lamina (Derer 1979, 1985). Brains were dissected from new-born animals, cortical meninges were carefully removed and a tangential cortical section was made and sticked by its internal face to a millipore filter; then the section was applied by its external face onto a coverslip coated with collagen. After withdrawal of the section an almost monolayered "cortical print" containing a large number of CRc remained on the coverslip. Medium consisting of L15 + 10% fetal calf serum + 10% horse serum + penicillin 100 U/ml + streptomycine 100 mg/ml + 0.6% glucose, was added and cultures were incubated in humid air atmosphere at 36°C for a time ranging from a few hours to 40 days. At given time intervals, the cultures were fixed and processed either for acetylcholinesterase activity or for immunocytochemistry of GFAP (antiserum from Bio Makor) and GABA (antiserum from Seguela et al., 1984). Cultures were also examined with electron microscope after Koelle reaction to identify CRc.

RESULTS

1) Developmental Aspect of the CRc as Revealed with Dil

Dil appeared to demonstrate CRc very efficiently especially on tangential sections. In mice, CRc appeared as early as E13 with their bipolar shape and were tangentially oriented (fig. 1a). A dendrite proximal swelling was coming off an oblong pericaryon and was prolonged by a short dendrite which ended by a large and flat growth cone like terminal (fig. 1 b). Opposite to the dendrite was a very thin and smooth axonal process (under 0.5μm in diameter) which wandered in the tangential plane. From E14 onward, the CRc shape remained bipolar, only the processes lengthened (fig. 1 c-d-e). The dendrite grew from an average of 50μm at E13 until it reached at least 300μm around birth. After birth, the dendrite did not increased very much, nevertheless at all stages a growing

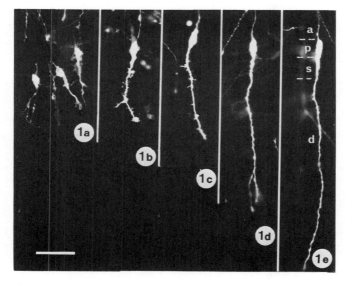

Fig. 1. All figures come from superficial tangential sections of cerebral hemispheres. Dil staining. Figures (a) to (e) display CRc dendritic elongation as a function of time. a) E13, b) E14, the dendrite terminates with a large growth cone. c) E15. d) E18, the rectilinear dendrite continue to grow in a plane strictly parallel to the meningeal surface. e) P2, even after birth, the CRc remain a monodendritic neuron. p: pericaryon; s: dendrite proximal swelling; d: dendrite; a: axon. Scale bar: 50μm

cone was present at the end of this process. The length of the dendrite increased mainly before birth.

An important feature was that all the CRc processes grew along a precise plane of orientation which was parallel to the cortical surface. After birth, numerous vertically oriented thin appendages appeared which joined the soma and all the processes of the CRc to the surface. There, these appendages bended and spread under the cortical basal lamina along several hundred of micrometers. In the tangential plane, in the most superficial layer of sections, only the horizontal parts of these appendages were observed, making a loose network (fig. 2a) above the plane containing the soma and the main processes of the CRc of origin that were lying 20 to 30μm under the meningeal surface (fig. 2b).

As seen before with HRP (Derer and Derer 1990), DiI staining showed likely contacts between the apex of young pyramidal cells and CRc axons, especially at early stages (not illustrated).

2) Electron microscopic studies

With EM, it is usually soma and the dendrite proximal swelling that were best viewed. The most remarkable feature was the presence of Nissl bodies made of parallely stacked RER cisterns filled with fibrillar material. Usually the Golgi complex was encased in a sleeve of RER inside the dendrite proximal swelling (fig. 3). In the axonal pole, similarly stacked cisterns were present. These features gave the CRc an aspect of advanced neuronal maturation, which was reached well before birth. By contrast, most of the cortical plate neurons had few organelles even at birth indicating an immature state of development. Few type II synapses with en passant axons of unknown origin, were found on the CRc somata and proximal swellings (fig. 4).

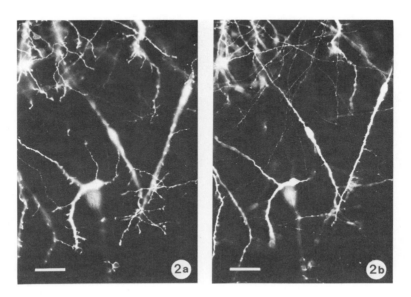

Fig. 2. Two day old pup. Tangential section. DiI staining. Focusing on two planes of the same field which are 20μm apart. a) CRc thin appendages are in focus, they make a loose network under the meninges. b) CRc of origin of the above appendages. Note a rare CRc with a bifurcate dendrite. Scale bar: 50μm.

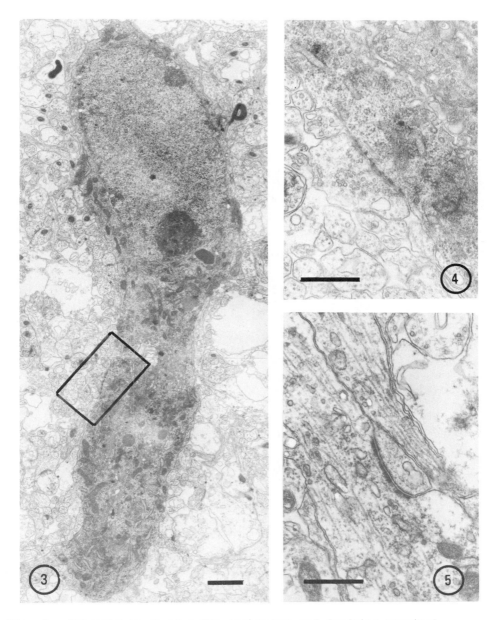

Fig. 3. Ultrastructure of a CRc pericaryon and dendrite proximal swelling. Newborn, Coronal section. Only one synapse was seen on the process (rectangle). The Golgi complex is encased in the RER. Scale bar: 1μm.

Fig. 4. Detail of the synaptic ending seen on the preceeding CRc. Scale bar: 0.5μm.

Fig. 5. New-born. Tangential section. Desmosome-like junction occurring only on CRc process with an unidentified orthogonally oriented process. Extensive symmetrical thickenings were prominent. Scale bar: 0.5μm.

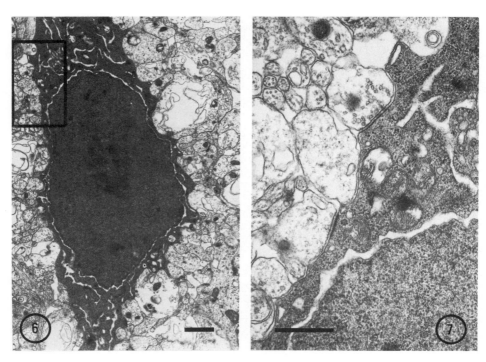

Fig. 6. P7. Tangential section. This CRc was in the process of death.
It exhibits overall darkening which contrasts with surrounding neuropil.
Golgi complex and RER cisterns appear empty. Scale bar: 1μm.

Fig. 7. Enlargement of the rectangle of figure 6, showing the dying CRc in
synaptic contact with two normal looking afferent endings. These synapses
are of Gray type II. CRc nucleoplasm and cytoplasm are homogeneously dark
and granular. Scale bar: 0.5μm.

In addition, desmosome-like junctions were observed between proximal swellings and perpendicularly oriented processes which could be radial glia or the apical dendrites of pyramidal cells (fig. 5). In the first cortical layer, the CRc appeared to be the only neurons engaged in such non synaptic interactions. Soon after birth, aspects of CRc degeneration were observed beginning at P4. Degeneration appeared as overall cytoplasmic darkening with swelling of Golgi complexes, followed by the RER whose dilated cisterns became empty. The nucleus also became uniformly darkened, masking the prominent nucleolus (fig. 6). Such aspects of neuronal degeneration resembled cell necrosis according to Oppenheim's classification (1991) and is definitely different from apoptosis characterized by a breakdown occurring at first in cell nucleus. During the process of breakdown, CRc were usually seen in contact with few but normally looking afferent axonal endings (fig. 7).

3) Fate of CRc Population during Corticogenesis

a) Qualitative aspect

As described elsewhere (Duckett and Pearse 1968, Kristt 1979, Derer 1985), Koelle reaction gave a specific product only in CRc during development. The reaction product was only observed in the soma, the axonal pole, and the dendrite proximal swelling, i.e. the parts of the cell where the RER cisterns were present (fig. 8). The whole CRc population observed from tangential sections formed a network of spindle shaped neurons. The CRc density diminished drastically as a function of time (fig. 9,10,11,12). Since the chemical reagents used for Koelle reaction reach uniformly all cortical cells, the method can be used quantitatively.

b) Quantitative data

The data are given in table 1. At each stage, the density was estimated as the mean of the number of CRc per $10.000\mu m^2$ field. From E16 onward, this density decreased continuously with a break occurring at P2. Between P2 and P5, the decrease was speeding up, and slowed down afterwards. During the same period of time, the cortical surface increased linearly. So estimate of the total amount of CRc per hemisphere could be calculated for each stage. This indicate that a stable number of CRc was reached between E18 and P2: around 20000 CRc per hemisphere. A steep drop in the number of CRc took place after P2 which made that about 50% of them were already gone by P5. The decrease of these neurons slowed down until P10 where only 25% of CRc were left (table 1).

Counts were difficult to perform after P10 since the CRc became very sparse in the first layer. Moreover, the few remaining CRc presented a shrunken dendrite proximal swelling .

Thus this part of the work along with EM observations argue very strongly in the disappearance of the CRc. The process of CRc removal began early after birth and appeared as a fairly rapid phenomenon since in one week most of the CRc had been withdrawn from the first cortical layer.

4) Fate of CRc *in vitro*

Having shown that the CRc disappear rapidly from the developing mammalian cortex *in vivo,* this prompted us to put the CRc *in vitro* to test if the viability of CRc changed in a different environment. We made a "print" of the new-born reeler cortical surface which usually appeared as a monolayered explant as seen on figure 13 taken one hour after explantation. In phase contrast, most of the cells that stuck to the

Table 1. Variations of CRc density, cortex area, and total CRc number as a function of age.

age	number of CRc per $10^{-2}mm^2$	cortex area in mm^2	total number of CRc
E16	20.78 ± 4.93 (n=157)	8.5	17 671
E19	15.20 ± 3.67 (n=259)	12.6	19 010
PO	13.49 ± 3.71 (n=380)	13.8	18 666
P2	11.32 ± 2.86 (n=175)	16.7	18 972
P4	7.04 ± 2.88 (n=506)	19.5	13 660
P5	4.50 ± 2.01 (n=290)	20.9	9 367
P8	2.82 ± 1.69 (n=454)	25	7 036
P1O	1.85 ± 1.41 (n=221)	27.8	5 132

n=number of unit area ($10,000\mu m^2$) examined at each stage.
After P2, CRc number diminishes drastically and only 25% are left at P10

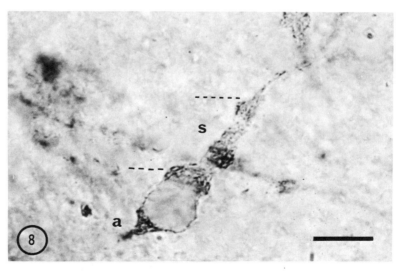

Fig. 8. E16 fetus. Tangential section. Early CRc stained with Koelle method. The acetylcholinesterase enzyme activity, specific of CRc, yield a coarse granular reaction product which outlines only the dendrite proximal swelling (s) and the axonal pole (a). The dendrite, nucleus and axon are devoid of the enzyme activity. Scale bar: $25\mu m$.

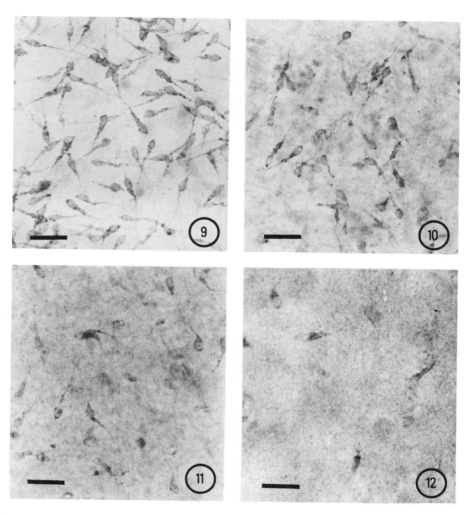

Fig. 9 to 12. Tangential sections. Koelle reaction. These four figures show that: 1) CRc population forms a network in one plane of the first cortical layer only; 2) CRc density diminish strikingly as corticogenesis goes on. Fig. 9: E19; Fig. 10: P4; Fig. 11: P8: Fig. 12; P10. Scale bar: 50μm.

collagen surface were spindle shaped and their pattern in the fresh explant was very similar to CRc observed *in situ* (fig. 13). Two to three days after explantation, flat cells began to spread and reached confluence some days later (fig. 14). These cells were strongly immunoreactive with anti GFAP (data not shown) and had the aspect of type I astrocytes, according to the classification of Raff et al. (1983). These astrocytes did not extend further than the area occupied by the piece of basal lamina that was picked up with the cortical print. Above that glial carpet, two kind of neurons survived:

 - multipolar neurons which gave rise to an extensive axonal network consisting of many varicose collaterals which sometimes ran parallel to one another making concentric arrays. These cells presented a strong reaction with an antibody against GABA (fig. 15).

- The second type of neurons were the CRc since they were spindle shaped (fig. 16) and presented a positive reaction for AchE activity (fig. 17). These neurons were non immunoreactive for GABA. Many of them persisted as long as forty days *in vitro*, which is well beyond their lifespan *in vivo*. During all this time period the CRc retained the same characteristic shape and AchE activity.

At the ultrastructural level, somata displaying the Koelle reaction were seen in synaptic contact with many axon terminals. These contacts were of Gray type II, having symmetric thickenings and clear vesicles (fig. 18) and thus were likely inhibitory.

DISCUSSION

1) CRc do disappear

a) In a previous work, some aspects of CRc degeneration were observed at the ultrastructural level, beginning at P4 (Derer and Derer 1990). This observation is in agreement with the drop of the total number of CRc observed here with another technique.

The morphological aspect of CRc degeneration seems to account for cell necrosis (Oppenheim 1991) or cytoplasmic type of cell death according to Cunningham (1982). We had mentioned that degeneration begins first as a cytoplasmic alteration, by swelling in the Golgi complex followed by that of the RER cisterns. This type of cytoplasmic cell death occurring naturally was also reported in different models of peripheral (Pilar and Landmesser 1976) and central nervous system (Chu-Wang and Oppenheim 1978, Giordano et al., 1980, Valverde and Facal-Valverde 1987, 1988). This primary alteration of the cell's synthetic apparatus may explain why CRc undergoing cell death could not express AchE activity anymore, instead of the alternate interpretation of a down regulation of the enzyme activity.

b) The morphology of the CRc seemed to be conserved throughout their development, even in the course of degenerescence. As observed previously (Derer and Derer 1990), CRc can always be distinguished from the few multipolar cells remaining in the adult first layer (Cajal 1891, Bradford et al., 1977, Parnavelas and Edmunds 1983).

c) From culture experiments, we have shown that even after 40 days *in vitro* CRc were still present, and continued to express their AchE activity. Thus, as long as the CRc are alive *in vitro*, the enzyme activity is not down regulated and allows the demonstration of these cells.

All these arguments converge in favour of a CRc disappearance "in situ" by an actual cell death resulting of the destruction of the cellular integrity. The alternate hypothesis of a change in the cellular metabolism which should make the cell's marker disappear, seems difficult to maintain.

2) Hypothesis on the cause of CRc death *in vivo*

What could account for the disappearance of CRc so early in the life of the animal? Since no experimental data are yet available on this subject, only speculations can be put forward.

The reported aspect of CRc degeneration accounts for cell necrosis

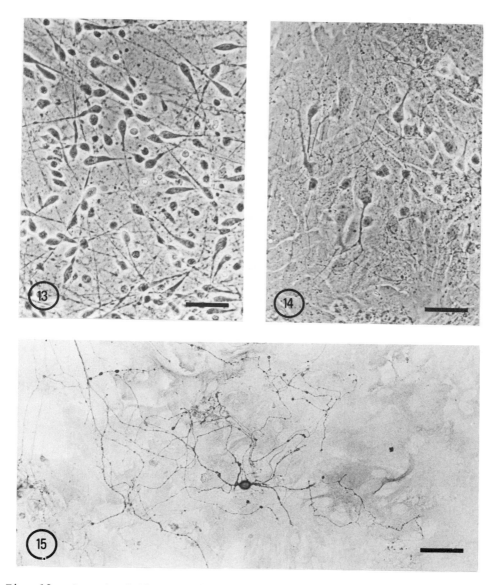

Fig. 13. Aspect of the "cortical print" from new-born cortex after one hour *in vitro*. Phase contrast microscopy. CRc have their characteristic shape. Scale bar: 50μm.

Fig. 14. Explant five days *in vitro* (5 DIV) Phase contrast microscopy. A glial carpet has developed under the neurons. Scale bar: 50μm.

Fig. 15. Explant 15 DIV. Immunostaining with antiGABA antibody diluted 1/6000. Some gabaergic neurons have developed an extensive plexus of varicose axons. Scale bar: 50μm.

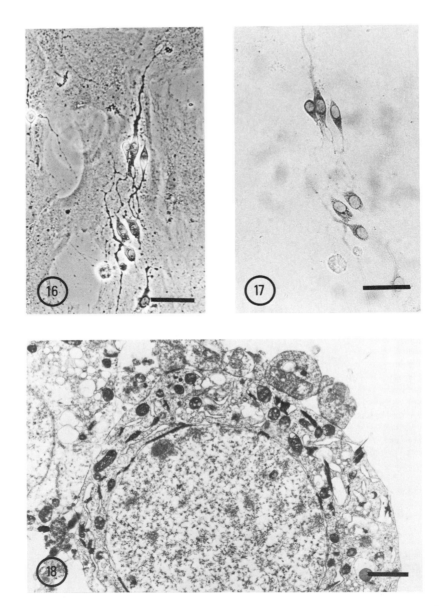

Fig. 16. Explant 40 DIV. Phase contrast microscopy. The neurons of this group have maintained their characteristic monodendritic shape. Scale bar: 50μm.

Fig. 17. Same explant as fig. 16. Koelle reaction. The above CRc retain the acetylcholinesterase activity. Scale bar: 50μm.

Fig. 18. Explant 40 DIV. This CRc, characterized by its positive Koelle reaction is in synaptic contact with numerous afferent endings, likely originating from surrounding neurons. Scale bar: 1μm.

with important swelling of cytoplasmic organelles. Usually this phenomenon is the result of a change in cellular homeostasis with modification of the osmotic activity. In the model of developing retina, necrosis was elicited by application of glutamate; this excitotoxic amino acid was able to trigger very quickly irreversible damages resulting in an important swelling of retinal neurons (Rothman and Olney 1987). These authors emphasized that the ultimate result of excitotoxic drugs is the massive influx of calcium ions into the cell, followed by water which is the cause of the cytoplasmic swelling and leaking out of the cellular content. This phenomenon was also emphasized in experiments on cortical cells (Choi et al., 1987).

Since in our material such morphological damages were also observed, it can be hypothesized that a similar process can act on CRc. The occurrence of synaptic contacts on degenerating cells seems to strengthen this hypothesis. As reviewed by Lipton and Kater (1989), glutamate can act on developing neurons through various receptors having at first a positive action on the development and maintenance of neurons, but at later stages, when other receptors are present, glutamate may become lethal. A similar mechanism could account at first for the development of CRc and later for their death. One way of impeding such an adverse effect would be to block selectively the glutamate receptors by local application of specific antagonists such as AP5 (2 amino-5 phosphovalerate) if NMDA receptors are implicated in the phenomenon (Choi et al., 1988).

Another hypothesis which may also account for nerve cell death would be the synthesis of "killer proteins" by neurons which are deprived of trophic factors, or which are transiently deprived of oxygen supply (Goto et al., 1990, Shigeno et al., 1990). A way to prevent such a suicide process would be to inhibit protein synthesis. Anisomycin was used by Martin et al. (1988) on NGF deprived sympathetic neurons in culture; and cycloheximide by Goto et al., (1990), and Shigeno et al. (1990) on hippocampal neurons which were asphyxiated. In the same way we can speculate that CRc could be sensitive to the deprivation of trophic factors, when the marginal glia limitans is progressively set up. This barrier could separate the CRc from meningeal cells known to elaborate growth factors (Matthiessen et al., 1991).

Although CRc population is numerically very small, it may have an important role in cortical structuration. From an observation made previously with HRP (Derer and Derer 1990) and found again here with Dil, it seems likely that CRc axons make contacts with immature,developing pyramidal cell dendrites. One can speculate that the inside out gradient of cortical cell deposition is influenced by this interaction. A pyramidal cell can go up all the way along radial glia during its migration (Rakic 1972, Gadisseux et al., 1990), and then become attached to the superficial network of CRc axons (by which it is probably specifically attracted). This may explain the maintenance of the radial arrangement of the cortical plate. This interaction between a homogeneous CRc population and the cortical plate neurons might give then a uniform basal tone of stimuli to all pyramidal cells, possibly to maintain all of them alive until cortical migration is completed. In turn this might also prevent cortical parcellation to begin before all cellular elements are in place, thus maintaining the cortex in an immature state.

3) Hypothesis for CRc survival *in vitro*

In vitro the CRc survived well beyond their *in vivo* lifespan. Three lines of hypothesis can be followed to explain that difference.

a) Beside its transmitter functions, glutamate is known to have toxic actions. We can speculate that *in vitro* the specific afferents that release glutamate to the CRc do not exist anymore. In culture, however, glutamate is most likely present due to the metabolic transformation of glutamine which was added to the culture medium (Hamberger et al., 1979). Nevertheless since astrocytes developed extensively in our cultures, they might constitute a sink for the exogenous glutamate (Schousboe 1981, Barbour et al., 1988; Flott and Seifert 1991), thus taking away the CRc from potential excitotoxic action as it was observed in astrocyte rich cortical culture (Rosenberg 1991).

b) If glutamate is present anyway, the excitotoxic action of the transmitter could be prevented by GABA, since it has been reported that this molecule which is known to induce hyperpolarization of target cells (Ditcher 1980), can be protective against excitotoxic brain damage only through transneuronal mechanism (Saji and Reis 1985). Usually this requirement is not reached in dispersed cell cultures where neurons are separate from one another. However, in our explants we observed that the CRc were highly synapsed and that an extensive network of GABAergic neurons was present around CRc. So it is likely that transsynaptic effect may occur through GABAergic endings thus preventing any glutamate excitotoxic CRc death.

c) As seen above, trophic factors of meningeal origin may exert influence on developing neurons (Matthiessen et al., 1991). *In vitro,* CRc survived although meninges were removed at the time of explantation. It can be speculated that identical factors could be present in the various sera used to grow the cell cultures. Determining precisely the conditions for a prolonged survival *in vitro* (using serum free media) should allow in turn a better understanding of CRc disappearance *in vivo*.

In conclusion, the CRc population may exert influences on cortical modeling during early ontogenesis. These influences could be mediated through cellular interactions which need to be more accurately defined. Otherwise, once CRc action is accomplished, cortical maturation could begin, and at the same time, CRc population disappears by a naturally occurring neuronal death. In that process, CRc appear as a neuronal model which can be manipulated, either *in situ* due to its superficial situation, or *in vitro* since we have shown that enriched cultures of CRc can be obtained.

Acknowledgements. We are grateful to P. Gaspard for improvement of the English and to P. Cloup for her excellent technical assistance.

REFERENCES

Barbour, B., Brew, H., and Attnell, D. (1988) Electrogenic glutamate uptake in glial cells is activated by intracellular potassium. Nature 335:433-335.
Baron, M., and Gallego, A. (1971) Cajal cells of the rabbit cerebral cortex. Experientia 27:430-432.
Bradford, R., Parnavelas, J.G., and Lieberman, A.R. (1977) Neurons in layer I of the developing occipital cortex of the rat. J. Comp. Neurol. 176:121-132.
Cajal Ramon y S. (1891) Sur la structure de l'écorce cérébrale de quelques mammifères. La Cellule 7:125-176.
Caviness, V,S, Jr. (1982) Neocortical histogenesis in normal and reeler mice: a developmental study based upon ^{3}H thymidine autoradiography. Dev. Brain Res. 4:293-302.

Choi, D.W., Koh, J.Y., and Peters, S. (1988) Pharmacology of glutamate neurotoxicity in cortical cell culture: attenuation by NMDA antagonists. J. Neurosci. 8:185-196.

Choi, D.W., Maulucci-Gedde, M., and Kriegstein, A.R. (1987) Glutamate neurotoxicity in cortical cell culture. J. Neurosci. 7:357-368.

Chun, J.J.M., and Shatz, C.J. (1989) The earliest-generated neurons of the cat cerebral cortex: characterization by MAP2 and neurotransmitter immunohistochemistry during fetal life. J. Neurosci. 9:1648-1667.

Chu-Wang, I.W., and Oppenheim, R.W. (1978). Cell death of motoneurons in the chick embryo spinal cord. 1. A light and electron microscopic study of naturally occurring and induced cell loss during development. J. Comp. Neurol. 177:33-58.

Cunningham, T.J. (1982) Naturally occurring neuron death and its regulation by developing neural pathways. Int. Rev. Cytol. 74:163-185.

Derer, P. (1979) Evidence for the occurrence of early modifications in the "glia limitans" layer of the neocortex of the Reeler mutant mouse. Neurosci. Lett. 13:195-202.

Derer, P. (1985) Comparative localization of Cajal-Retzius cells in the neocortex of normal and reeler mutant mice fetuses. Neurosci. Lett. 54:1-6.

Derer, P., and Derer, M. (1990) Cajal-Retzius cell ontogenesis and death in the mouse brain visualized with horseradish peroxidase and electronmicroscopy. Neuroscience 36(3):839-856.

Derer, P., and Derer, M. (1991) Identification des cellules de Cajal-Retzius durant l'ontogenese du néocortex de la souris a l'aide d'une carbocyanine fluorescente. C.R. Acad. Sci. Paris 313(111):175-181.

Dichter, M.A. (1980). Physiological identification of GABA as the inhibitory transmitter for mammalian cortical neurons in cell culture. Brain Res. 190:111-121.

Duckett, S., and Pearse, A.G.E. (1968) The cells of Cajal-Retzius in the developing human brain. J. Anat. 102:183-187.

Edmunds, S.M., and Parnavelas, J.G. (1982) Retzius-Cajal cells: an ultrastructural study in the developing visual cortex of the rat. J. Neurocytol. 11:427-446.

Ferrer, I., Bernet, E., Soriano, E., Del Rio, T., and Fonseca, M. (1990) Naturally occurring cell death in the cerebral cortex of the rat and removal of dead cells by transitory phagocytes. Neuroscience 39:451-458.

Flott, B., and Seifert, W. (1991) Characterization of glutamate uptake systems in astrocyte primary cultures from rat brain. Glia 4:293-304.

Fox, M.W, and Inman, O. (1966) Persistence of Retzius-Cajal cells in the developing dog brain. Brain Res. 3:192-194.

Gadisseux, J.F., Kadhim, H.J., Van den Bosch de Aguilar, P., Caviness, V.S., and Evrard, P. (1990) Neuron migration within the radial glial fiber system of the developing murine cerebrum: an electron microscopic autoradiographic analysis. Dev. Brain Res. 52:39-56.

Giordano, D.L., Murray, M., and Cunningham, T.J. (1980) Naturally occurring neuron death in the optic layers of superior colliculus of the postnatal rat. J. Neurocytol. 9:603-614.

Godement, P., Vanselow, J., Thanos, S., and Bonhoeffer, F. (1987) A study of developing visual systems with a new method for staining neurons and their processes in fixed tissue. Development 101:697-713.

Goto, K., Ishige, A., Sekiguchi, K., Lizuka, S., Sugimoto, A., Yuzurihara, M., Aburada, M., Hosoya, E., and Kogure, K. (1990) Effects of cycloheximide on delayed neuronal death in rat hippocampus. Brain Res.534:299-302.

Hamberger, A.C., Chiang, G.H., Nylen, E.S., Scheff, S.W., and Cotman, C.W. (1979) Glutamate as a CNS transmitter. 1. Evaluation of glucose and glutamine as precursors for the synthesis of preferentially released glutamate. <u>Brain Res.</u> 168:513-530.

Honig, M.G., and Hume, R.I. (1986) Fluorescent carbocyanine dyes allow living neuronsof identified origin to be studied in long term cultures. <u>J. Cell Biol.</u> 103:171-187.

Honig, M.G., and Hume, R.I. (1989) DiI and DiO: versatile fluorescent dyes for neuronal labelling and pathway tracing. <u>Trends Neurosci.</u> 12:333-341.

Jackson, C.A., Peduzzi, J.D., and Hickey, T.L. (1989) Visual cortex development in the ferret. 1. Genesis and migration of visual cortical neurons. <u>J. Neurosci.</u> 9:1242-1253.

König, N., and Marty, R. (1981) Early neurogenesis and synaptogenesis in cerebral cortex. <u>Biblthca. anat.</u> 19:152-160.

König, N., Valat, J., Fulcrand, J., and Marty, R. (1977) The time of origin of Cajal-Retiius cells in the rat temporal cortex. An autoradiographic study. <u>Neurosci. Lett.</u>4:21-26.

Kristt, D.A. (1978) Neuronal differentiation in somatosensory cortex of the rat. 1. Relationship to synaptogenesis in the first postnatal week. <u>Brain Res.</u> 150:467-486.

Kristt, D.A. (1979) Development of neocortical circuitry: histochemical localization of acetylcholinesterase in relation to the cell layers of rat somatosensory cortex. <u>J. Comp. Neurol.</u> 186:1-16.

Larroche, J.C. (1981) The marginal layer in the neocortex of a seven week-old human embryo. <u>Anat. Embryol.</u> 162:301-312.

Lipton, S.A., and Kater, S.B. (1989) Neurotransmitter regulation of neuronal outgrowth plasticity and survival. <u>TINS</u> 12:265-270.

Luskin, M.B., and Shatz, C.J. (1985) Studies of the earliest generated cells of the cat's visual cortex: cogeneration of subplate and marginal zones. <u>J. Neurosci.</u> 5:1062-1075.

Marin-Padilla, M. (1971) Early prenatal ontogenesis of the cerebral cortex (neocortex) of the cat (Felis domestica). A Golgi study. 1. The primordial neocortical organization. <u>Z. Anat. Entwickl.-Gesch</u> 134:117-145.

Marin-Padilla, M. (1972) Prenatal ontogenic history of the principal neurons of the neocortex of the cat (Felis domestica) a Golgi study. 11. Developmental differences and their significances. <u>Z. Anat. Entwickl.-Gesch</u> 136:125-142.

Marin-Padilia, M. (1978) Dual origin of the mammalian neocortex and evolution of the cortical plate. <u>Anat. Embryol.</u> 152:109-126.

Marin-Padilla, M. (1988) Early ontogenesis of the human cerebral cortex. <u>In:</u> "Cerebral Cortex Vol 7 Development and Maturation of Cerebral Cortex: (eds Peters, A. and Jones, E.G.), pp. 1-30. Plenum Press, New York and London.

Martin, D.P., Schmidt, R.E., DiStefano, P.S., Lowry, O.H., Carter, J.G., and Johnson Jr., E.M. (1988) Inhibitors of protein synthesis and RNA synthesis prevent neuronal death caused by nerve growth factor deprivation. <u>J. Cell Biol.</u> 106:829-844.

Matthiessen, H.P., Schmalenbach, C., and Müller, H.W. (1991) Identification of meningeal cell released neurite promoting activities for embryonic hippocampal neurons. <u>J. Neurochem.</u> 56:759-768.

Meyer, G., and Ferres-Torres, R. (1984) Postnatal maturation of nonpyramidal neurons in the visual cortex of the cat. <u>J. Comp. Neurol.</u> 228:226-244.

Noback, C.R., and Purpura, D.P. (1961) Postnatal ontogenesis of neurons in cat neocortex. <u>J. Comp. Neurol.</u> 117:291-307.

Oppenheim, R.W. (1991) Cell death during development of the nervous system. <u>Annu. Rev. Neurosci.</u> 14:453-501.

Parnavelas, J.G., and Edmunds, S.M. (1983) Further evidence that Retzius-Cajal cells transform to nonpyramidal neurons in the developing rat visual cortex. <u>J. Neurocytol.</u> 12:863-871.

Pilar, G., and Landmesser, L. (1976) Ultrastructural differences during embryonic cell death in normal and peripherally deprived cillary ganglia. J. Cell Biol. 68:339-356.

Purpura, D.P., Carmichael, M.W., and Housepian, E.M. (1960) Physiological and anatomical studies of development of superficial axodendritic synaptic pathways in neocortex. Exp. Neurol. 2:324-347.

Raedler, A., and Sievers, J. (1975) The development of the visual system of the albino rat. Adv. Anat. Embryol. Cell Biol. 50:5-88.

Raedler, A., and Sievers, J. (1976) Light and electron microscopical studies on specific cells of the marginal zone in the developing rat cerebral cortex. Anat. Embryol. 149:173-181.

Raedler, E., and Raedler, A. (1978) Autoradiographic study of early neurogenesis in rat neocortex. Anat. Embryol. 154:267-284.

Raedler, E., Raedler, A., and Feldhaus, S. (1980) Dynamical aspects of neocortical histogenesis in the rat. Anat. Embryol. 158:253-269.

Raff, M.C., Abney, E.R., Cohen, J., Lindsay, R., and Noble, M. (1983) Two types of astrocytes in cultures of developing rat white matter: differences in morphology, surface gangliosides, and growth characteristics. J. Neurosci. 3:1289-1300.

Rakic, P. (1972) Mode of cell migration to the superficial layers of fetal monkey neocortex. J. Comp. Neurol. 145:61-83.

Retzius, G. (1893) Die Cajal'schen Zellen der Grosshirnrinde bein Menschen und bei Saugetieren. Biol. Untersuch. 5:1-6.

Rickmann, M., Chronwall, B.M., and Wolff, J.R. (1977) On the development of non-pyramidal neurons and axons outside the cortical plate: the early marginal zone as a pallial anlage. Anat. Embryol. 151:285-307.

Rosenberg, P.A. (1991) Accumulation of extracellular glutamate and neuronal death in astrocyte-poor cortical cultures exposed to glutamine. Glia 4:91-100.

Rothman, S.M., and Olney, J.W. (1987) Excitotoxicity and the NMDA receptor. TINS 10:299-302.

Saji, M., and Reis, D.J. (1987) Delayed transneuronal death of substantia nigra neurons prevented by gamma-aminobutyric acid agonist. Science 235:66-69.

Sas, E., and Sanides, F. (1970) A comparative Golgi study of Cajal foetal cells. Z. mikr. anat. Forsch. 82:385-396.

Schousboe, A. (1981) Transport and metabolism of glutamate and GABA in neurons and glial cells. Int. Rev. Neurobiol. 22:1-45.

Seguela, P., Geffard, M., Buijs, R.M., and Le Moal, M. (1984) Antibodies against GABA: specificity studies and immunocytochemical results. Proc. Natl. Acad. Sci. USA 81:3888-3892.

Shigeno, T., Yamasaki, Y., Kato, G., Kusaka, K., Mima, T., Takakura, K., Graham, D.I., and Furukawa, S. (1990) Reduction of delayed neuronal death by inhibition of protein synthesis. Neurosci. Lett. 120:117-119.

Shoukimas, G.M., and Hinds, J.W. (1978) The development of the cerebral cortex in the embryonic mouse: an electron microscopic serial section analysis. J. Comp. Neurol. 179:795-830.

Valverde, F., and Facal-Valverde, M.V. (1987) Transitory population of cells in the temporal cortex of Kittens. Dev. Brain Res. 32:283-288.

Valverde, F., and Facal-Valverde, M.V. (1988) Postnatal development of interstitial (subplate) cells in the white matter of the temporal cortex of kittens: a correlated Golgi and electron microscopic study. J. Comp. Neurol. 269:168-192.

COMPARATIVE AND CELLULAR ASPECTS OF DEVELOPMENT OF CONNECTIONS IN CEREBRAL CORTEX

Giorgio M. Innocenti

Institut d'Anatomie
9 rue du Bugnon
1005 Lausanne, Switzerland

The development of cortical connections consists of both progressive and regressive events several aspects of which have been reviewed recently (Innocenti, 1986; Payne et al., 1988; Innocenti, 1991).

Developmental exuberance and selective elimination of projections may have acted as a crucially permissive mechanism in brain evolution (Katz and Lasek, 1978; Innocenti, 1990). Here we will focus on some of the basis for this hypothesis. Sufficient data have accumulated on the development of cortical connections in different species to encourage a first and provisional assessment of the stability of developmental strategies in this structure which underwent a particularly dramatic evolution. In addition, some of the cellular changes involved in the formation of cortical connections are beginning to be investigated, using callosal connections as a model.

EXUBERANT DEVELOPMENT OF CORTICAL CONNECTIONS

The notion of "developmental exuberance" was introduced in studies with retrograde transport techniques of the development of visual callosal connections in the cat to describe the existence of transient projections between brain sites destined to become completely or partially disconnected in the adult (Innocenti et al., 1977). The elimination of these projections was found to involve the selective deletion of axons, rather than neuronal death (Innocenti, 1981a).

Callosal connections were not the first example of proven or suspected transient connectivity in the developing brain. Cajal had described with clarity surpassing in some respects even the most advanced present knowledge of the phenomenon transient axons from ganglion cells in the retina (Cajal, 1929) as well as transient climbing fibers and collaterals of Purkinje cells (1911). A phase of transient multiple innervation of the motor end plate (Redfern, 1970) and of Purkinje cells in the cerebellum (Crepel et al., 1976) had been demonstrated electrophysiologically. Rakic (1976) and Hubel et al., (1977) had documented the progressive segregation of territories innervated from the two eyes in the visual cortex and in the lateral geniculate nucleus. Much of the evidence available in the mid seventies on the issue of transient connectivity was summarized by Changeux and Danchin (1976) in a

Development of the Central Nervous System in Vertebrates
Edited by S.C. Sharma and A.M. Goffinet, Plenum Press, New York, 1992

131

selectionistic hypothesis of the development of neural connections.

Transient projections are not restricted to the corpus callosum but turned out to be a general trait in cortical development (see Innocenti, 1991, for review). The cortical type of developmental exuberance had several new and interesting features. First, certain transient projections, such as those between peripheral representations of the visual field in the two hemispheres, or between auditory and visual cortex or between visual cortex and cerebellum or spinal cord, appeared to violate both functional and topographical principles of cortical organization. Second, some orderliness in the transient projections, and their large number discredited the notion that they are just developmental errors, a view which may have been introduced by Cajal (1929). In addition, the selection of connections from the juvenile stock could be modulated by several "epigenetic" factors. Therefore, the development of connections seems to be endowed with an intrinsic potential for plasticity (Innocenti, 1981b) whose specific "task" may be to remedy insufficiencies in the genetic control of brain development (for converging views on this concept see Changeux and Danchin, 1976; Innocenti, 1991).

Although the blatant topographical "inappropriateness" of certain juvenile projections allowed the discovery of developmental exuberance the concept clearly includes more subtle types of reorganization. The development of cortical connections, for example, also involves the trimming of short local collaterals (Callaway and Katz, 1990) and probably the translocation of synaptic terminals (Mates and Lund, 1983). Furthermore, in certain cases, for example in the loss of axons from the developing corpus callosum, or the pyramidal tract, it is not completely clear in which way the projections which are massively eliminated differ from those which are maintained.

Transient axonal projections were found in the development of many other brain structures (Land and Lund, 1979; Schneider et al., 1987; Bower and Payne, 1987; Mistretta et al., 1988; Jeffery, 1989; Bhide and Frost, 1991; inter alios). Therefore, some of the concepts which emerged from the study of cortical connections have broader applicability. All together, these studies prompt a revision of Sperry's hypothesis that chemical affinity between axons and their targets is a sufficient mechanism to explain the formation of connections in the central nervous system (for discussion, see Innocenti, 1988; Innocenti 1991).

The relevance of developmental exuberance is now also being explored with respect to developmental pathologies such as early brain lesions (Frost, 1986) microgyria (Innocenti and Berbel, 1991) early degenerative processes (Lyon et al., 1990) fetal alcohol syndrome (Miller, 1987), hypothyroidism (Gravel and Hawkes, 1990) epilepsy (Grigonis et al., 1991) and even schizophrenia (Feinberg, 1982), none of which can be covered within the present review.

DEVELOPMENT OF CORTICAL CONNECTIONS IN DIFFERENT SYSTEMS AND SPECIES

Efferent projections from cerebral cortex undergo exuberant development in several species some of which e.g. marsupials (Sheng et al., 1990) and lagomorphs (Chow et al., 1981) have branched from the other mammals 135-65 million year ago (Johnson, 1980), suggesting that this mode of development appeared early and was conserved in evolution (see for review Innocenti, 1991). Exuberant projections may however differ in magnitude and extent and even more interestingly in their functional role in different systems and/or species.

Regressive events may play a minor role in the development of the anterior commissure in rodents. Projections through the anterior commissure originate, in rodents, mainly from the olfactory bulbs, and nuclei, and from the entorhinal and piriform cortex. When traced with retrograde transport of DiI, the sites of origin and termination of the projections appear to undergo only minor topographical sharpening (Lent and Guimares, 1991). In addition, the number of axons in the anterior commissure, estimated by electronmicroscopic counts does not appear to decrease in development (Guadano-Ferraz et al., 1991). Before this evidence can be taken as conclusive, it is necessary to exclude the possibility that the elimination of subtly "inappropriate" projections may have failed to be identified with the retrograde tracers and may occur in synchrony with an addition of new axons to the anterior commissure. Because in rodents the anterior commissure connects territories which underwent modest evolutionary changes across the mammalian radiation, its parsimonious development would give circumstantial support to the hypothesis that developmental exuberance has been closely, possibly crucially related to cortical evolution (Innocenti, 1990). It should be added, that the anterior commissure of the rhesus monkey, which unlike that of rodents, interconnects large neocortical territories of the temporal lobes, undergoes axonal elimination in development (LaMantia and Rakic, 1984) even though this elimination, and more generally the elimination of commissural axons in the monkey (see below) has not yet found its counterpart in connectional studies. Transient projections through the anterior commissure of the ferret were also mentioned (Dehay et al., 1988b).

The considerations above stress the importance of unequivocally identifying instances, if any, in which axons grow precisely to their target, without undergoing exuberance and elimination. Unfortunately, past experience suggests that this may not be an easy task since now well documented examples of transient projections have often failed to be identified (Anker and Cragg, 1974; Lund and Mitchell, 1979; Kalil and Reh, 1981; see O'Leary and Stanfield, 1986, for discussion). More recently, the existence of transient projections spanning tangentially across area 17 has been somewhat controversial (cf. Luhmann et al., 1986 with Callaway and Katz, 1990). In more recent studies with anterogradely transported biocytin transient axons spanning the whole mediolateral extent of area 17 were identified; they could have been missed by injections of retrograde tracers restricted to the gray matter since only few of them grow into it and usually not beyond layer vi (Assal and Innocenti, 1991).

In the monkey, no conclusive evidence exists in favor or against elimination of callosal projections from area 17 (see Innocenti 1991, for discussion) and from the prefrontal cortex. In the latter, however, as in the visual cortex of the cat, transient axons, if they exist, do not appear to enter the cortical gray matter (Schwartz and Goldmann Rakic 1991). In contrast, transient projections originating in the somatosensory cortex have been unequivocally documented (Killackey and Chalupa, 1986; Chalupa and Killackey, 1989). Transient projections were demonstrated between the temporal cortex and the limbic system and may subserve important memory functions in the young (Webster et al., 1991).

Across species, several other developmental events coincide with the elimination of transient interhemispheric projections. In the cat (Fig. 1), a massive decrease in the number of callosal axons was revealed by electron microscopic investigations (Berbel and Innocenti, 1988) and is synchronous with the loss of projections revealed by retrograde transport studies; therefore the two events are probably facets of the same phenomenon. The bulk of both occurs during the fast phase of synaptogenesis in neocortex and before myelination of the corpus callosum.

These temporal relations imply that most or all the axons which are eliminated are unmyelinated and that the elimination of axons, at least in its initial phase, does not necessarily result in the elimination of synapses.

A slight decrease, or at least a pause in the growth of the sagittal section area of the corpus callosum, appears to be common to cat (Fig. 1), man (Clarke et al., 1989), monkey (see Fig. 2, based on data of LaMantia and Rakic, 1990) and rat (Berbel et al., personal communication). In all species, this growth pause is terminated by the onset of myelination, probably because the latter causes an increase in the size of individual callosal axons.

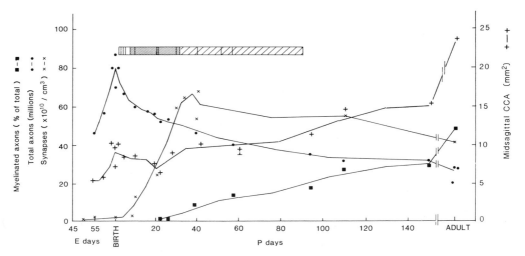

Fig 1. Time course and temporal relations of developmental events in the corpus callosum and visual cortex of the cat (from Innocenti, 1991). The horizontal bar at the top indicates the period of elimination of callosal projections originating in area 17 as shown by axon tracer experiments: each vertical line indicates the age of an animal at the time of horseradish peroxidase injection; fast and slow elimination of callosal projections are denoted by light and heavy hatching, respectively. Filled dots (each corresponding to an animal) are estimates of the total number of callosal axons and filled squares of the fraction of myelinated axons in the developing corpus callosum from Berbel and Innocenti, 1988). Crosses are measurements of the sagittal section area of the corpus callosum in the same animals. The remaining graph shows density of synapses in the visual cortex according to Cragg (1975); the peak synaptic density is reached later than indicated here i.e. at around P70, according to Winfield (1981).

In cat (Fig. 1) and monkey (Fig. 2), the growth pause corresponds to the period of elimination of transient projections revealed by retrograde transport studies. As mentioned above, in the cat, this growth pause also coincides with the massive decrease in the number of callosal axons. Because, during the same period, density of callosal axons decreases slightly and axon size increases slightly, it was argued that the loss of callosal axons actually causes the pause in the growth of the corpus callosum (Berbel and Innocenti, 1988).

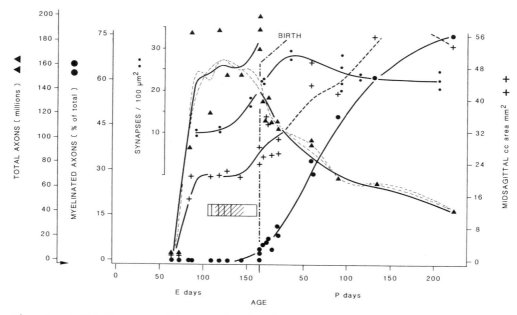

Fig. 2.   Time course and temporal relations of developmental events in the
corpus callosum and visual cortex of the rhesus monkey.   Filled triangles
are estimates of the number of callosal axons in the corpus callosum as in
Fig. 3; large filled circles show the proportion of myelinated callosal
axons; crosses are measurements of the sagittal section area of the corpus
callosum in the same animals.   The original data from LaMantia and Rakic
(1990) were fitted by splines (SAS statistics).   The interrupted line
denotes a probably unreliable (due to the lack of experimental points)
part of one of the curves.   Filled circles show density of synapses in the
somatosensory cortex according to Rakic et al., (1986).   The horizontal
bar shows with conventions similar to those in used in Fig. 1 the period
of elimination of callosal projections from areas SI and 18, as
demonstrated with retrograde transport of horseradish peroxidase by Dehay
et al., (1988) and Killackey and Chalupa (1986).

        In the monkey however, a clear decrease in the number of callosal
axon can be documented only after the end of this growth pause (Figs. 2
and 3) which, unlike in all the other species mentioned above, is a
prenatal event.   Although the waviness of data points precludes a clear
interpretation of changes in the number of callosal axons during the
prenatal period, the number of callosal axons may decrease, or possibly
remain stationary during this period (Figs. 2 and 3), while transient
callosal projections are eliminated.   The most likely possibility is that
during this pause in callosal growth new axons are added to the corpus
callosum of the monkey and the new addition balances the loss of callosal
axons.   In the rat as well, addition of new axons to the corpus callosum
may compensate the loss of transient projections (Gravel et al., 1990).   A
second possibility is that callosal axons cease to transport tracers some
time before they are eliminated.   Both are probably true.   Growth cones
are found in the corpus callosum of the monkey during the period in which
transient projections are eliminated (Fig. 3).   In the cat as well, new
axons, some of which transient, continue to be added to the corpus
callosum, while the number of callosal axons begins to decrease (Innocenti
and Assal, in preparation). On the other hand, recent studies with
anterograde transport in the cat (Innocenti and Assal, in preparation)
suggest that transient callosal axons fail to transport tracers in a

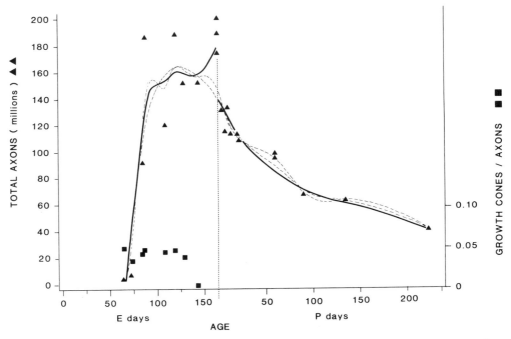

Fig. 3. Filled triangles are estimates of the number of callosal axons in
the rhesus monkey. The original data from LaMantia and Rakic, (1990) were
fitted by splines (SAS statistics) in three different ways: the
interrupted lines show the curves obtained when the spline was calculated
on the total set of data and underwent two different degrees of smoothing;
the continuous lines show the functions obtained by computing separately
pre- and postnatal data; the three animals at P0 were included in both age
groups. The filled squares show the fraction of growth cones over the
total number of axonal profiles in the corpus callosum of the same
animals. Notice that although the noisiness of the data do not allow firm
conclusions, the number of axons from around P100 onwards does not
increase proportionally to the number of growth cones. It may rather
decrease or at least remain stationary.

distal to proximal fashion and therefore may not be revealed by retrograde
transport experiments for an undetermined time before they disappear from
the corpus callosum.

     A general conclusion to be drawn from this comparative-
developmental analysis is that heterochrony (Gould, 1977; Finlay et al.,
1987) rather than changes in developmental strategies may have
characterized the evolution of neocortical development. The fact that
elimination and addition of new axons to the corpus callosum seem to
counter balance each other in monkey and rat but not in cat suggest that
the relative timing, and/or size of these morphogenetic events changed in
phylogenesis. In addition, the timing of reorganization of callosal
projections changed with respect to birth. In cat and rat, the
elimination of transient projections and the myelination of the corpus
callosum are postnatal events. In the monkey, elimination of transient
projections begins before birth and at birth callosal myelination has
already begun. In man, the pause in callosal growth that in other species
is temporally correlated with elimination of transient projections extends
over the end of gestation and the first and second month after birth.

Myelination of the corpus callosum begins during the second postnatal
month. Thus, man, as cat, is more immature at birth than the rhesus
monkey and the development of his cortical connections may be particularly
exposed to environmental influences.

CELLULAR ASPECTS OF CALLOSAL DEVELOPMENT

An array of morphological and biochemical changes coincides with the
elimination of some of the juvenile callosal projections and the
maintenance of others. These include reorganization of the dendritic
arbor of some callosal neurons, in particular the loss of apical dendrite
of neurons in the process of acquiring spiny stellate morphology (Assal et
al., 1991) as well as biochemical and morphological transformations of
cytoskeletal proteins of callosal axons (Figlewicz et al., 1988; Guadano-
Ferraz et al., 1990; Riederer et al., 1990; Berbel et al., in
preparation).

The reorganization of the dendritic and axonal arbors of callosally
projecting neurons are probably not causally related. On the contrary,
the maturation of cytoskeletal proteins may be a critical step in the
stabilization of the callosal axons. This is suggested by the nature of
the maturation, i.e. changes in proteins which cross-link neurofilaments
and microtubules such as the heavy subunit of neurofilaments (NFH) and the
microtubule associated proteins MAP5 and Tau. Furthermore, cytoskeletal
maturation follows elimination of most of the transient callosal axons and
therefore may be a distinctive trait of axons which are maintained (Fig.
4).

Till recently, one of the most serious limitations to studies of
cortical connectivity, and of callosal connectivity in particular, has
been the impossibility of visualizing individual axons of cortical origin
with anterograde tracers. The recently introduced biocytin (King et al.,
1989) has overcome many of these difficulties.

Biocytin produces localized injection sites with sharp borders,
consisting of Golgi-like stained cell bodies and their processes.
Individual axons can be followed from their site of origin to their site
of termination and be serially reconstructed using a computer system (Fig.
5). Eight kittens ranging in age between P 2.5 and P 18 where analyzed
with tracer injections restricted to the medial part of area 17.

Individual terminal or preterminal branches of callosal axons
distributed over a broad territory in the contralateral hemisphere,
including areas 17,18,19 and the lateral suprasylvian areas (LS). The
heaviest projections reached the convexity of the lateral gyrus,
corresponding approximately with the location of the border between areas
17 and 18 in the contralateral hemisphere, a site heterotopic with respect
to the injection (Fig. 5). Other axons however, reached the medial part of
area 17, as far as the suprasplenial sulcus. The overwhelming majority of
callosal axons terminated in the white matter and/or at the bottom of the
gray matter; they remained therefore associated with the subplate and/or
layer vi (Fig. 5). Only a very few axonal branches extended more
superficial in the gray matter. This topography basically confirms
previous conclusions based on anterograde transport of weat-germ
agglutinin -HRP and localized injections of retrograde tracers (Innocenti
and Clarke, 1984) and rejects different claims based on incompletely
documented evidence (Kennedy et al., 1988).

The analysis of individual axons is time consuming and therefore, at
present, based only on a limited number of axons which however share the

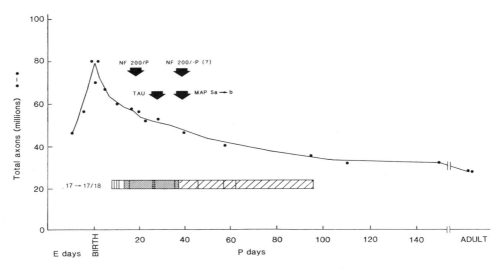

Fig. 4. Time course and temporal relations of morphological and biochemical aspects of cortical and callosal development in the cat. The curve of number of callosal axons and the bar denoting elimination of transient projections are the same as shown in Fig. 1. Arrows point to the first unequivocal appearance of four cytoskeletal proteins in callosal axons: the phosphorylated heavy subunit of neurofilaments (NF200/P), a presumably partially dephosphorylated form of the same protein (NF/200/-P (?) and the transitions of microtubule associated protein MAP5 from the a to the b isoforms and of Tau from juvenile to adult isoforms. See text for references. Modified from Innocenti (1991).

following number of features: i) At least two classes of callosal axons may exist, one projecting to areas 17, 18 and 19, and the other projecting to areas 19 and LS. Previous studies using simultaneous transport of different tracers also suggested that in the adult cat (Segraves and Innocenti, 1985) and in kittens (Innocenti and Clarke, 1983) different and distinct neuronal populations project to areas LS and to 17/18.

ii) Terminal branches of individual callosal axons (Fig. 5) do not respect functional borders between areas and can distribute to several areas. They also do not appear to aim specific retinotopic locations within one area. The territory reached by branches of one axon can span several millimeters antero-posteriorly and medio-laterally. iii) Branches of individual axons end with growth cones (Fig. 5, terminals 1,3-5,9,11) or with other endings some of which may be collapsed growth cones or axons in the process of elimination.

On the whole, these results have two possible explanations: i) callosal axons initially aim at neurons in the subplate and the formation of this connections is guided by topographical principles different from those of the adult callosal connections; ii) the growth of callosal axons, at least of the transient ones, is only poorly, if at all guided by precise target-related cues. This is not to say that precise topographic cues, possibly of a chemical nature may not guide axonal behavior in the final process of target recognition and be responsible for the elimination of some callosal axons. Both interpretations, however, support the view that the development of cortical connections cannot be understood on the basis of a single control factor. Rather, a hierarchy of crucial steps appears to be involved, each controlled by several concurring factors (Innocenti, 1988, 1990).

138

B15   P6.5 - 8.5

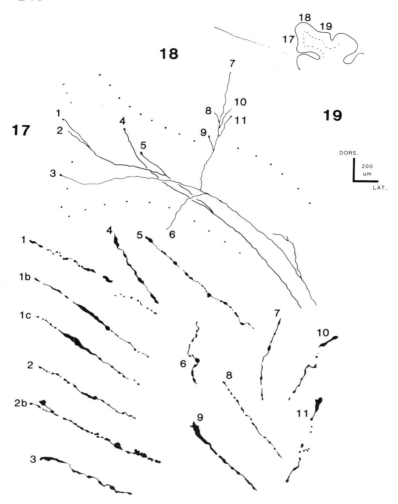

Fig. 5.   Callosal axons labeled with a biocytin injection in the medial
and transiently callosally projecting part of contralateral area 17 in a
kitten (B15) injected at P6.5, killed at P8.5.   The upper part of the
Figure shows a computer reconstruction from serial sections, corresponding
(inset) to the white/gray matter border (dotted line) of areas 17, 18 and
19, near the convexity of the lateral gyrus.   Numbers refer to camera
lucida drawings of the terminal part of an axon branch, numbers and
letters to details along the preterminal part of the same branch.   The two
axons are distinct, at least from near the callosal midline.   Notice that
the two axons ramify widely to different areas (e.g., branches 1 and 2 aim
to area 17, 4 and 5 to area 18) and/or to different retinotopic locations
within one area (e.g., branches 3 and 6, aim different visual field
locations in area 17).   The majority of the branches terminate in the
white matter or at the bottom of the gray matter with growth cones (e.g.,
1, 3, 4, 5) or with endings of more difficult identification (e.g., 2 and
6) and without further collateralizations. One of the branches forms a
terminal arbor in the deep part of the cortex between areas 18 and 19,
although it also extends a collateral (7) towards layer iii.   This complex
branching of an axon originating in medial area 17 is unique in the
material so far analyzed.

CONCLUSIONS

Callosal connections in visual area 17 and 18 of the cat appear to provide a useful model for understanding the development of patterns of cortical connections. At the level of axonal projections, but also at the level of dendritic development this system of connections adopted a strategy involving structural exuberance and regression.

This strategy was maintained across systems and species, and appears to have implications for general theories of development of connections as well as for the understanding of brain pathology and possibly evolution.

The results of cellular and biochemical approaches foreshadow a better understanding of this aspect of neuronal development.

ACKNOWLEDGMENTS

Supported by Swiss National Science Foundation Grant n. 3129948.90.

The author is grateful to the Department of Histology and the Institute for Neuroscience of the University of Alicante in Spain for the hospitality during the preparation of this paper.

REFERENCES

Anker, R.L., and Cragg, B.G. (1974) Development of the extrinsic connections of the visual cortex in the cat. J. Comp. Neurol. 154:29-42.

Assal, F., and Innocenti, G.M. (1991) Development of intraareal connections in the primary visual cortex of the cat. Europ. J. Neurosci. Suppl. 4:172.

Assal, F., Vercelli, A., and Innocenti, G.M. (1991) The morphology of immature callosal neurons in areas 17 and 18 of the cat. Europ. J. Neurosci. Suppl. 4:283.

Berbel, P., and Innocenti, G.M. (1988) The development of the corpus callosum in cats: A light- and electronmicroscopic study. J. Comp. Neurol. 276:132-156.

Bhide, P.G., and Frost, D.O. (1991) Stages of growth of hamster retinofugal axons: Implications for developing axonal pathways with multiple targets. J. Neurosci. 11:485-504.

Bower, A.J., and Payne, J.N. (1987) An ipsilateral olivocerebellar pathway in the normal neonatal rat demonstrated by the retrograde transport of True blue. Neurosci. Lett. 78:138-144.

Cajal, S.R. y (1911) Histologie du Systéme Nerveux de l'Homme et des Vertébrés, Maloine, Paris.

Cajal, S.R. y (1929) Etudes sur la Neurogenèse de quelques Vertébrés, Tipografia Artistica, Madrid.

Callaway, E.M., and Katz, L.C. (1990) Emergence and refinement of clustered horizontal connections in cat striate cortex. J. Neurosci. 10:1134-1153.

Chalupa, L.M., and Killackey, H.P. (1989) Process elimination underlies ontogenetic change in the distribution of callosal projection neurons in the postcentral gyrus of the fetal rhesus monkey. Proc. Natl. Acad. Sci. USA 86:1076-1079.

Changeux, J.P., and Danchin, A. (1976) Selective stabilisation of developing synapses as a mechanism for the specification of neuronal networks. Nature 264:705-712.

Chow, K.L., Baumbach, H.D., and Lawson, R. (1981) Callosal projections of the striate cortex in the neonatal rabbit, Exp. Brain Res. 42:122-126.

Clarke, S., Kraftsik, R., Van der Loos, H., and Innocenti, G.M. (1989) Forms and measures of adult and developing human corpus callosum: Is there sexual dimorphism? J. Comp. Neurol. 280:213-230.

Cragg, B.G. (1975) The development of synapses in the visual system of the cat. J. Comp. Neurol. 160:147-166.

Crepel, F., Mariani, J., and Delhaye-Bouchaud, N. (1976) Evidence for a multiple innervation of Purkinje cells by climbing fibres in the immature rat cerebellum, J. Neurobiol. 7:567-578.

Dehay, C., Kennedy, H., Bullier, J., and Berland, M. (1988a) Absence of interhemispheric connections of area 17 during development in the monkey. Nature 331:348-350.

Dehay, C., Kennedy, H., and Messirel, C. (1988b) A transient pathway interconnecting the cerebral hemispheres via the anterior commissure in the neonatal ferret. J. Physiol. (London) 400:45P.

Feinberg, I. (1982/83) Schizophrenia: Caused by a fault in programmed synaptic elimination during adolescence? J. Psychist. Res. 17:319-334.

Figlewicz, D.A., Gremo, F., and Innocenti, G.M. (1988) Differential expression of neurofilament subunits in the developing corpus callosum. Brain Res. 42:181-189.

Finlay, B.L., Wikler, K.C., and Sengelaub, D.R. (1987) Regressive events in brain development and scenarios for vertebrate brain evolution. Brain Behav. Evol. 30:102-117.

Frost, D.O. (1986) Development of anomalous retinal projections to nonvisual thalamic nuclei in Syrian hamsters: A quantitative study. J. Comp. Neurol. 252:95-105.

Gould, S.J. (1977) "Ontogeny and Phylogeny", Harvard University Press, Cambridge, MA.

Gravel, C., and Hawkes, R. (1990) Maturation of the corpus callosum of the rat: I. Influence of thyroid hormones on the topography of callosal projections. J. Comp. Neurol. 291:128-146.

Gravel, C., Sasseville, R., and Hawkes, R. (1990) Maturation of the corpus callosum of the rat: II. Influence of thyroid hormones on the number and maturation of axons. J. Comp. Neurol. 291:147-161.

Grigonis, A.M., Ju, B., and Murphy, E.H. (1991) Exuberant callosal cell distribution in the striate cortex of the rabbit following cortical epileptic activity during development. Soc. Neurosci. Abstr. 17:768.

Guadano-Ferraz, A., Berbel, P., Balboa, R., and Innocenti, G.M. (1991) The development of the anterior commissure in normal and hypothyroid rats. Europ. J. Neurosci. Suppl. 4:225.

Guadano-Ferraz, A., Riederer, B.M., and Innocenti, G.M. (1990) Developmental changes in the heavy subunit of neurofilaments in the corpus callosum of the cat. Dev. Brain Res. 56:244-256.

Hubel, D.H., Wiesel, T.N., and LeVay, S. (1977) Plasticity of ocular dominance columns in monkey striate cortex. Phil. Trans. R. Soc. Lond. (Biol.) 78:377-409.

Innocenti, G.M. (1981a) Growth and reshaping of axons in the establishment of visual callosal connections. Science 212:824-827.

Innocenti, G.M. (1981b) Transitory structures as substrate for developmental plasticity of the brain, in: "Developments in Neuroscience", Vol. 13, M.W. Van Hof and G. Mohn, eds., Elsevier, Amsterdam, pp. 305-333.

Innocenti, G.M. (1986) General organization of callosal connections in the cerebral cortex, in: "Cerebral Cortex", Vol. 5, E.G. Jones, and A. Peters, eds., Plenum, New York, pp. 291-353.

Innocenti, G.M. (1988) Loss of axonal projections in the development of the mammalian brain, in: "The Making of the Nervous System", J.G. Parnavelas et al., eds., Oxford University Press, Oxford, pp. 319-339.

Innocenti, G.M. (1990) Pathways between development and evolution, in: "The Neocortex", B.L. Finlay et al., eds., Plenum Press, New York, pp 43-52.

Innocenti, G.M. (1991) The development of projections from cerebral cortex. Prog. Sens. Physiol. 12:65-114.

Innocenti, G.M., and Berbel, P. (1991) Analysis of an experimental cortical network: ii) Connections of visual areas 17 and 18 after neonatal injections of ibotenic acid. J. Neural Transplant. 2:29-54.

Innocenti, G.M., and Clarke, S. (1983) Multiple sets of visual cortical neurons projecting transitorily through the corpus callosum. Neurosci. Lett. 41:27-32.

Innocenti, G.M., and Clarke, S. (1984) The organization of immature callosal connections. J. Comp. Neurol. 230:387-390.

Innocenti, G.M., Fiore, L., and Caminiti, R. (1977) Exuberant projection into the courpus callosum from the visual cortex of newborn cats. Neurosci. Lett. 4:237-242.

Jeffery, G. (1989) Shifting retinal maps in the development of the lateral geniculate nucleus. Dev. Brain Res. 46:187-196.

Johnson, J.I. (1980) Morphological correlates of specialized elaborations in somatic sensory cerebral neocortex, in: "Comparative Neurology of the Telencephalon, Ebbesson (ed.), Plenum Press, New York.

Kalil, K., and Reh, T. (1981) Establishment of cortical topography in hamster pyramidal tract neurons during development. Soc. Neurosci. Abst. 7:177.

Katz, M. J., and Lasek, R.J. (1978) Evolution of the nervous system: Role of ontogenetic mechanisms in the evolution of matching populations. Proc. Natl. Acad. Sci. USA 75:1349-1352.

Kennedy, H., Dehay, C., and Bourdet, C. (1988) Inter- and intrahemispheric transient pathways in the cat, in: "Seeing Contour and Colour", J.J. Kulikowski, C.M. Dickinson and I.J. Murray, eds, Pergamon Press, Oxford, pp. 142-145.

Killackey, H.P., and Chalupa, L.M. (1986) Ontogenetic change in the distribution of callosal projection neurons in the postcentral gyrus of the fetal rhesus monkey. J. Comp. Neurol. 244:331-348.

King, M.A., Louis, P.M., Hunter, B.E., and Walker, D.W. (1989) Biocytin: A versatile anterograde neuroanatomical tract-tracing alternative. Brain Res. 497:361-367.

LaMantia, A.-S., and Rakic, P. (1984) The number, size, myelination, and regional variation of axons in the corpus callosum and anterior commissure of the developing rhesus monkey. Neurosci. Abstr. 10:1081.

LaMantia, A-S., and Rakic, P. (1990) Axon overproduction and elimination in the corpus callosum of the developing rhesus monkey. J. Neurosci. 10:2156-2175.

Land, P.W., and Lund, R.D. (1979) Development of the rat's uncrossed retinotectal pathway and its relation to plasticity studies. Science 205:698-700.

Lent, R., and Guimaraes, R.Z.P. (1991) Development of paleocortical projections through the anterior commissure of hamsters adopts progressive, not regressive, strategies. J. Neurobiol. 22:475-498.

Luhmann, H.J., Martínez Millan, L., and Singer, W. (1986) Development of horizontal intrinsic connections in cat striate cortex. Exp. Brain Res. 63:443-448.

Lund, R.D., and Mitchell, D.E. (1979) Plasticity of visual callosal projections, in: "Aspects of Developmental Neurobiology", J.A. Ferrendelli, ed., Society for Neuroscience, Bethesda, MD, pp. 142-152.

Lyon, G., Arita, F., Le Galloudec, E., Vallé, L., Misson, J.P., and Ferriére, G. (1990) A disorder of axonal development, necrotizing myopathy, cardiomyopathy and cataracts: A new familial disease. Ann. Neurol. 27:193-199.

Mates, S. L., and Lund, J.S. (1983) Developmental changes in the relationship between type 2 synapses and spiny neurons in the monkey visual cortex. J. Comp. Neurol. 221:98-105.

Miller, M.W. (1987) Effect of prenatal exposure to alcohol on the distribution and time of origin of corticospinal neurons in the rat. J. Comp. Neurol. 257:372-382.

Mistretta, C.M., Gurkan, S., and Bradley, R.M. (1988) Morphology of chorda tympani fiber receptive fields and proposed neural rearrangements during development. J. Neurosci. 8:73-78.

O'Leary, D.D.M., and Stanfield, B.B. (1986) A transient pyramidal tract projection from the visual cortex in the hamster and its removal by selective collateral elimination. Dev. Brain Res. 27:87-99.

Payne, B.R., Pearson, H., and Cornwell, P. (1988) Development of visual and auditory cortical connections in the cat, "Cerebral Cortex", Vol. 7., "Development and Maturation of Cerebral Cortex", A. Peters, and E. G. Jones, eds., Plenum, New York, pp. 309-389.

Rakic, P. (1976) Prenatal genesis of connections subserving ocular dominance in the rhesus monkey. Nature 261:467-471.

Rakic, P., Bourgeois, J.P., Eckenhoff, M.F., Zecevic, N., and Goldman-Rakic, P.S. (1986) Concurrent overproduction of synapses in diverse regions of the primate cerebral cortex. Science 232:232-235.

Redfern, P.A. (1970) Neuromuscular transmission in new-born rats. J. Physiol. 209:701-709.

Riederer, B. M., Guadano-Ferraz, A., and Innocenti, G.M. (1990) Difference in distribution of microtubule-associated proteins 5a and 5b during the development of cerebral cortex and corpus callosum in cats: Dependence on phosphorylation. Dev. Brain Res. 56:235-243.

Schneider, G.E., Jhaveri, S., and Davis, W.F. (1987) On the development of neuronal arbors. Pont. Acad. Sci. Scr. Varia 59:31-64.

Schwartz, M.L., and Goldman-Rakic, P.S. (1991) Prenatal specification of callosal connections in rhesus monkey. J. Comp. Neurol. 397:144-162.

Segraves, M.A., and Innocenti, G.M. (1985) Comparison of the distributions of ipsilaterally and contralaterally projecting corticocortical neurons in cat visual cortex using two fluorescent tracers. J. Neurosci. 5:2107-2118.

Sheng, X.M., Marotte, L.R., and Mark, R.F. (1990) Development of connections to and from the visual cortex in the wallaby (Macropus Eugenii). J. Comp. Neurol. 300:196-210.

Webster, M.J., Ungerleider, L.G., and Bachevalier, J. (1991) Connections of inferior temporal areas TE and TEO with medial temporal-lobe structures in infant and adult monkeys. J. Neurosci. 11:1095-1116.

Winfield, D. A. (1981) The postnatal development of synapses in the visual cortex of the cat and the effects of eyelid closure. Brain Res. 206:166-171.

THE DEVELOPING MOUSE WHISKERPAD: PATTERN FORMATION AT THE PERIPHERY OF A HIGHLY ORGANIZED SOMATOSENSORY PATHWAY

W. Ourednik*, W. Wahli**, and H. Van der Loos*
*Institut d'Anatomie
Université de Lausanne
1005 Lausanne, and
** Institut de Biologie Animale
Université de Lausanne
1015 Lausanne, Switzerland

INTRODUCTION

To a recent volume of the NATO-ASI series having as subject "The Neocortex: Ontogeny and Phylogeny", our group contributed two reports on the development and plasticity of brain maps (Van der Loos et al., 1990; Welker et al., 1990). The subject of both reports was the somatosensory whisker-to-barrel pathway of rodents. In the mouse - our experimental animal - and in a number of other rodent species, one of the major characteristics of this pathway is the pattern of vibrissal follicles - sensory organs - on the animal's muzzle. This pattern finds, at the other end of the pathway, its central counterpart in a homeomorphic arrangement of multineuronal units, "barrels", in a defined region of the primary somatosensory cortex (Fig. 1 and Woolsey and Van der Loos, 1970). Today it is still not known how the geometry of the pattern is generated at the periphery, respected throughout the pathway and what the developmental mechanisms are by which periphery and brain interact, resulting in the homeomorphic relationship alluded to. In line with our earlier argument that the periphery plays a major role in the creation of the pattern in the central nervous system (Van der Loos and Dörfl, 1978; Andrés and Van der Loos, 1983; Van der Loos and Welker, 1985; Van der Loos et al., 1986), the present paper describes ideas, born here and elsewhere, about the developmental rules that guide the formation of the vibrissal pattern. And we present a project whose purpose is to find genes and gene products that are part of the molecular regulatory network that we assume to govern the formation of this pattern.

In the mouse embryo the whiskerpad region evolves through the mergence of the lateral nasal fold with the maxillary arch. At day 11 of gestation (E11; EO being the day of conception*) five horizontal ridges appear in this region, the two upper ones as part of the lateral nasal fold, the three lower ones originating from the maxillary process (Fig. 2, left pannel). While the mesenchyme in the ridges does not seem to be morphologically different from that between them, the epidermis over the ridges is thicker than that in between (Van Exan and Hardy, 1980). About simultaneously and along the ridges begins the development of individual

---

*When referring to articles of others we have, where alternative ways of designating ages were in use, made them conform to our convention.

Development of the Central Nervous System in Vertebrates
Edited by S.C. Sharma and A.M. Goffinet, Plenum Press, New York, 1992

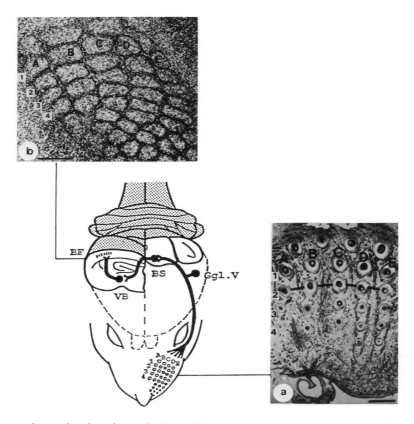

Fig. 1.   Schematic drawing of the whisker-to-barrel pathway in the mouse.
The brain is partially removed to expose the neural stations along the
pathway: the ganglion of the trigeminal (Vth cranial) nerve (Ggl.V), the
trigeminal sensory nuclei in the brainstem (BS; only one of the four
nuclei of termination is depicted), the ventrobasal nucleus of the
thalamus (VB) and the barrelfield (BF) in the primary somatosensory
cortex.   Photomicrograph **a** shows a section taken tangentially with respect
to the skin surface through a left adult whiskerpad (reduced silver stain)
indicating the five rows of follicles (A-E) and four "arcs" (1-4).   The
black line connects follicles of arc 2.   Bar: 1mm; rostral is down and
dorsal to the left.   Photomicrograph **b** shows the corresponding barrelfield
(Nissl-stain) in the right somatosensory cortex.   Letters and numbers
indicate rows and arcs of barrels corresponding to the elements shown in
a.   Bar: 250μm, rostral is down, dorsal to the right.   Both micrographs
are taken from Hoogland et al. (1987) with permission.

follicles.   The first follicular primordia to form are the caudolateral
ones, followed by the others in a developmental wave sweeping in a
rostromedial direction over the immature whiskerpad (Van der Loos et al.,
1986).   At E14 the complete pattern of the mystacial follicles on the
whiskerpad is established (Fig. 2, right pannel), consisting of five
horizontal rows of them, plus four follicles adjacent to, and straddling,
the caudal elements of each row (Woolsey and Van der Loos, 1970).

146

The whisker pattern shows some important and unique characteristics: (i) the pattern, established long before the banal fur, is hereditary, stable and obviously depending on a genetic regulation that is different from that which operates in the development of the fur pattern (even nu/nu mice carry vibrissae in the standard pattern); (ii) according to Danforth (1925), the pattern possesses *phylogenetic individuality,* i.e. its natural variation within a species amounts to less than 1%, and interspecific comparison, even between for example mouse and cat, shows a striking correspondence for vibrissal positions, something not observed with the ordinary hairs of the pelage; (iii) its early development is associated with the formation of epithelial ridges and grooves; (iv) the principal branches of the massive sensory innervation of the region conform to the vibrissal rows; (v) the pattern is an essential character of the whiskerpad, an important, cutaneous sensory organ whose receptor units, the whisker follicles, are highly organized and complex structures. The molecular and genetic basis underlying the establishment of the follicle pattern still escapes our understanding. It is not known what the positional cues are according to which a cell in the developing whiskerpad defines its spatio-temporal position and, by using this information, decides to become a cell contributing to a whisker follicle or a banal skin cell. There are at least two possible mechanisms which could generate such cues in this area: the innervation from the trigeminal ganglion and the interaction between epidermis and dermis.

The Initial Innervation of the Whiskerpad

Vibrissal follicles and sensory innervation: equivalent patterns. The whiskerpad of the mouse is the most densely innervated part of the animal's body surface and it is *a priori* well possible that the innervation arriving at the embryonic maxillary process and lateral nasal fold is involved in inducing the basic follicular pattern. Light microscopy of silver-stained sections revealed already to Tello (1923) and Cajal (1929) a concomitant appearance of follicle anlagen and arriving trigeminal nerve fibres. Basing himself on observations mainly made on E12-E13 mouse embryos, Cajal stated: " ... coinciding with the development of the [follicular] rudiment, the epithelium *en masse* strongly attracts the wandering subcutaneous bundles..." (Cajal, 1929). Indeed, similar observations recently led to the suggestion that nerve branching underneath the whiskerpad epithelium might induce follicle formation (Van Exan and Hardy, 1980). However, subsequent studies in this direction suggest this possibility to be unlikely.

Using scanning and transmission electron microscopy as well as light microscopy, Wrenn and Wessells (1984) analysed the development of the whiskerpad in mouse E10-E13 embryos for global morphogenetic changes, for the development of the innervation of the incipient whiskerpad by trigeminal axons, and for the formation of the first follicular rudiments. They draw several important conclusions: (i) during the formation of epidermal ridges on the maxillary process (at E11) there are many nerve fascicles in the underlying whiskerpad mesenchyme, whose random orientation makes an association between their course and the arrangement of the ridges very improbable; (ii) the diffuseness of the nerve fibre plexus in the E12 whiskerpad region makes it unlikely that nerve fibres are responsible for the establishment of the follicular pattern; (iii) vibrissal formation begins while the trigeminal axons are still in their maturation phase - at E11 there are less nerve endings underneath

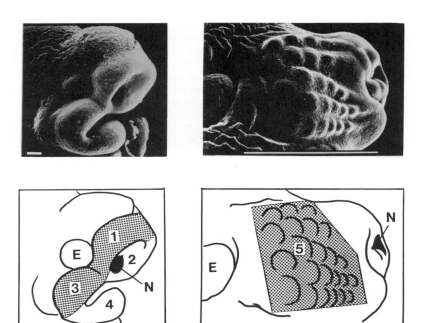

Fig. 2. Scanning electron micrographs of growing right whiskerpad regions
of E10 (to the left) and E14 (to the right) mouse embryos. Bars: O.1mm
(left) and 1mm (right), respectively; rostral is to the right, dorsal to
the top. In the two lower panels the same regions shown in the
corresponding micrographs are outlined. Stippled areas were taken for
isolation of mRNA. 1: lateral nasal fold; 2: medial nasal fold; 3:
maxillary process; 4: mandibular process; 5: whiskerpad region consisting
of five rows of follicles (the small hillocks) originating from 1 (the two
upper rows) and 3 (the three lower rows); E: eye anlage; N: nasal pit.
(Micrographs courtesy of Dr. F.L. Andrés)

the caudolateral (i.e. developmentally more advanced follicles than under
the skin of the rostromedial whiskerpad region where follicles are just
appearing; (iv) because of the continuing changes in spatial relationships
due to the extensive growth of the developing whiskerpad area it is
doubtful that a momentary correspondence between a dermal cell
condensation and the "nerve cupit (the local concentration of terminal
nerve fibres) beneath it, really reflects a direct developmental
interdependence of the two elements; (v) at E12 the growth cones are still
4-5 cell diameters away from the epithelium. Thus, Wrenn and Wessells do
not agree with the idea that the follicular arrangement on the whiskerpad
of rodents develops via a prepattern laid down by its innervation. For
them, ridges and vibrissal follicles develop independently, and even
ahead, of the nerve pattern. This independence of ridge- and follicle
formation is in line with the result of an experiment in which explants of
E9-E10 mouse whiskerpads (not yet innervated!), when cultured on
chorioallantoic membrane, were shown to develop follicle arrays akin to
those occurring in vivo (Andrés and Van der Loos, 1983). The final one-

to-one relationship between follicular rows and the mature row-nerves (nerves that contain fibres innervating the follicles of one row), together with the fact that ridges appear ahead of the fasciculation of nerve fibres in the whiskerpad, suggest that it is the ridges that govern the segregation of nerve fibres into row-nerves, and not the other way around. This speculation, discussed below in more detail, can also be found in a topographical analysis of the motor innervation of the rat whiskerpad (Klein and Rhoades, 1985): it might well be that the incoming nerve fibres would follow the epithelial ridges on their way to their targets which are the muscle slings around individual follicles, responsible for their movement. The resulting topography would later be reflected in the observed dorsoventral organization of the corresponding neurons in the lateral subnucleus of the facial motor nuclear complex.

The philosophy behind experiments investigating target-dependent behaviour of sensory nerve fibres invading the prospective whiskerpad was formulated already in 1929 in Cajal's far-sighted speculation about "trophic and orienting action" of cutaneous epithelia: "In those epithelial organs which contain specific cells that are embraced by nerve fibres, it is necessary to acknowledge two successive influences. One is global or diffuse, localized throughout the epithelium ... ; its function is to attract the general stream of embryonic nerve fibres. The other is individual, emanating from specific elements such as peripheral elements of the tactile hairs, its function is to establish an intimate symbiosis and a kind of selective attraction for strayed fibres." (Cajal, 1929).

Lumsden and Davies (1983) described a region-specific, chemotactic guidance of outgrowing sensory axons from the mouse trigeminal ganglion towards the maxillary process. In co-cultures of explants from the trigeminal ganglion together with the developing whiskerpad as proper target tissue and/or with a distal fragment of the forelimb bud of the same developmental age, the outgrowth of sensory axons was exclusively directed towards the whiskerpad when tissues were taken from E10 and E11 embryos. When tissues were taken at E12, this target preference became less pronounced and there even was sprouting towards the limb bud tissue. To test the eventual importance of nerve growth factor (NGF) in this temporary expression of target-dependence, the investigators added antiserum against isogeneric NGF to their cultures. A reduction of neurite outgrowth, more dramatic with increasing age, was observed only in tissues taken from E11 and E12 embryos. These results were in agreement with subsequent *in vivo* observations showing the NGF-production in the mouse whiskerpad to coincide with the arriving innervation and thus precede the period of neuronal death in the trigeminal ganglion (Davies and Lumsden, 1984). There should therefore exist another, as yet unidentified, agent in the maxillary process, attracting sensory fibres during the period of strong axonal outgrowth between E10 and E11, which Lumsden and Davies (1983) hypothetically called the "trigeminal neurotropic factor" (TNF). In a subsequent series of experiments, using embryonic tissue from E10 and E11 mice, Lumsden and Davies (1986) tried to localize the source of this chemotactic agent. It turned out to be the growing whiskerpad. Moreover, when epithelium and mesenchyme from the maxillary process were maintained with the trigeminal ganglion in two separate cultures, the trigeminal fibres were attracted by the epithelium and not by the mesenchyme. In the last experiments, the authors used cultures of the geniculate ganglion as controls which *in vivo,* at the age investigated, is situated close to the trigeminal ganglion and innervates the hyoid process of the second branchial arch. In these cultures,

fibres, when allowed to grow in the presence of their own and of
trigeminal target tissue, sprouted unspecifically in all directions.
Furthermore, when the geniculate ganglion was cultured in isolation,
neurite outgrowth occurred to the same extent as in the co-cultures.   Such
behaviour was not observed with the trigeminal ganglion which, when
cultured alone, never showed fibre outgrowth.

The Role of Pioneer Neurons and Merkel Cells During the Onset of
Innervation of the Whiskerpad.   Lumsden and Davies (1986) speculated that
the chemotactic attraction of trigeminal axons by TNF is necessary for
their correct target finding, because there are no motor fibres or other
pioneering elements providing guidance pathways for the sensory axons.   In
insects, the existence of early pioneer neurons in the peripheral and
central nervous system has been assumed for many years (Bate, 1976).   In
the motor system of the chick, they were proposed by Tosney and Landmesser
(1985) for spinal nerves in which motor fibres would provide a substrate
that guides the sensory ones to their destination.   Real significance in
axon guidance has been proven only recently in the sensory limb
innervation in the grasshopper embryo (Klose and Bentley, 1989) and in the
visual system of *Drosophila melanogaster* (Steller et al., 1987; Heilig et
al., 1991).   At the same time, Shatz and her group, using DiI, described
pioneer neurons in the subplate of the cerebral cortex of the cat
(McConnell et al., 1989) and identified them as cells belonging to the set
of the first postmitotic neurons in the developing cortex.   Pioneer
neurons have also been shown to be present in the central nervous system
of the E16 rat embryo (Molnar and Blakemore, 1991) and in the trigeminal
ganglion of E10 mouse embryos (Stainier and Gilbert, 1990).   In the latter
study, a novel monoclonal antibody (mAb E1.9) was used on wholemounts of
midsagittally bisected embryos for the detection of immature, primary
neurons and their outgrowing axons.   The stain revealed that already at
E9.5 nerve fibres have left the trigeminal ganglion in a dorsal direction,
forming the ophthalmic branch, while other fibres just started to leave
the ganglion in a maxillary direction.   By E10.5, mAb E1.9-positive axons
branched below the maxillary epithelium.   In all cases these fibres were
few in number and were soon followed by a second, more massive wave of
axons.   These secondary axons grew more slowly than the leading ones and
fasciculated around them.

        Referring to the observations by Stainier and Gilbert (1990) and to
the work by Lumsden and Davies (1983, 1986) we take it that the
innervation of the maxillary area occurs in two partially coincident waves
of axonal outgrowth following different modes of pathfinding: the axons
observed *in vitro* by Lumsden and Davies would be part of the second wave
and depend on chemotaxis and on contact guidance, the latter provided by
the preceding pioneer axons which were not observed by these
investigators.   To answer the question how these pioneer axons find their
target, co-culturing experiments using tissue from earlier developmental
ages (E9-E9.5) would need to be done.

        Merkel cells are specialized cells probably of epidermal origin
(Nurse and Farraway, 1988 and refs. therein) and their neuron-like
character has been demonstrated by their immunohistochemical staining for
neuron-specific enolase (Gu et al., 1981).   In the vibrissal follicle,
these cells form one of the four groups of sensory receptors described by
Andres (1966).   There are two populations of Merkel cells in the
developing whiskerpad, which, in each developing vibrissa, differentiate
at different times and at two distinct sites (Nurse and Diamond, 1984;
Nurse and Farraway, 1988):   The "collar" around the vibrissal hair shaft
begins to appear at E15 (in rat) and remains superficial, surrounding the
vibrissa in the region where it emerges from the epidermis.   The Merkel
cells here are supplied by a plexus derived from superficial skin nerves

(Dörfl, 1985; Rice et al., 1986). About two days later, when the vibrissal follicle with its hair shaft is growing and developing downwards into the mesenchyme, a second group of Merkel cells differentiates, but now forming a cylindrical "cuff" within the outer root sheath. These cells receive their innervation from the deep-lying row-nerves (Dörfl, 1985). With further development, Merkel cells are added progressively to the collars as well as to the cuffs until the end of the first postnatal week, when a collar contains about 130 Merkel cells, and a cuff 750-800 (Nurse and Farraway, 1988). Recently, Merkel cells were shown to be important producers of NGF in the whiskerpad epithelium (Vos et al., 1991). We consider this finding of particular importance in the light of Diamond's proposition from 1979 that " ... Merkel cells release a growth-promoting substance whose concentration gradient leads to directional sprouting of the nerves" and recalling the demonstration that NGF influences axonal survival and has a marked chemotropic effect on the direction of axonal growth (Letourneau, 1978; Gundersen and Barrett, 1979, 1980; Campenot, 1982a,b). Moreover, NGF production in the growing mouse whiskerpad occurs between E11 and E15 (peaking at E13), its major site of synthesis being the epidermis (Lumsden and Davies, 1986; Davies et al., 1987). These facts allow us to propose that NGF-producing Merkel cells may play a major role in axonal fasciculation by providing local trophic support whose sources, during the progressive arrangement of the developing follicles along the epithelial ridges, would gradually become concentrated in five rows. This proposal takes also into account the observation that the onset of NGF production is independent from the arrival of nerve fibres which was demonstrated in a study of isolated embryonic whiskerpads placed into culture before innervation: NGF synthesis started at a time corresponding to the developmental stage at which, *in vivo,* the first nerve fibres arrive (see Discussion in Zafra et al., 1990). Along the same line, it has been shown that intact and denervated chick limbs have the same levels of NGF (Rohrer et al., 1988). It would be interesting to see whether in the whiskerpad cultures ridge formation occurs and whether it is in the ridges that NGF production is highest.

That the arrangement of Merkel cells in the whiskerpad would serve as a template for the final nerve pattern was already suggested by Killackey (1980) and by Andrés and Van der Loos (1983). In other words, it could be the distribution of the Merkel cells that is responsible for the transfer of the follicular pattern to the brain. In this context it is necessary to point out that, although NGF synthesis by Merkel cells seems not to depend on their innervation (Zafra et al., 1990), the survival of a subset of them is. When comparing the behaviour of the two Merkel cell populations in the vibrissae of neonatal rats after transection of the infraorbital nerve - which contains the entire sensory innervation of the whiskerpad - all superficial Merkel cells degenerated, while the cells in the cuffs were unaffected (Nurse and Farraway, 1988). The authors of this study suggest that, if it could be proven that this second population of Merkel cells is nerve-independent also during development, these cells would be good candidates for early nerve targets, thus having an important organizing function for the definition of the somatotopy in the entire somatosensory pathway. In our view, this function cannot be related to the segregation of the initial nerve plexus invading the whiskerpad, as Merkel cells forming the cuffs appear, according to the same authors, only at E17. Nevertheless, the finding of these Merkel cells, whose survival is independent on innervation, still favors the notion that it is the whiskerpad integument which imposes a pattern upon its innervation and not vice versa.

After reviewing what is known about early whiskerpad innervation we consider it unlikely that it plays a role in the establishment of the follicular pattern. On the other hand we are ready to propose that the epidermal ridges, being the products of one of the earliest morphogenetic changes in the region, thus assuring the correct spatial distribution of the Merkel cell-containing vibrissal follicles, are crucial for the formation of the five row-nerves. Thus, the segregation of the initial sensory nerve plexus could occur according to the following scenario (times are based on observations in mice). At E9.5 pioneer neurons send their axons into the maxillary process reaching the whiskerpad at E10.5 (Stainier and Gilbert, 1990). At E10-E11 (probably even earlier) the whiskerpad epidermis including the ridges is producing TNF (Lumsden and Davies, 1983, 1986). Both, TNF and pioneering axons, have the same purpose to attract and guide the diffuse trigeminal nerve plexus into the incipient whiskerpad. Starting at E11, the five epidermal ridges are formed. This important morphogenetic event has two main consequences: (i) the alignment of the vibrissal follicles into five prominent rows, in turn resulting in (ii) the fasciculation of nerve fibres from the immature plexus into five row-nerves. The Merkel cells in the vibrissal follicles would thereby drive and support this "sculpting" process with their production of NGF shown to last until E15. Thus, to come back to the thoughts of Cajal, TNF and pioneer axons would stand for his first and global epithelial influence on the arriving nerve fibres, whereas the Merkel cells, concentrated along the epithelial ridges, would represent the second, precisely located source of an influence "emanating from specific elements of the tactile hairs" (Cajal, 1929).

In the aim to find the basis for the follicular pattern in the early innervation of the whiskerpad we, to the contrary, deduced from all the data presented that it are rather the epithelial ridges in this region that guide the establishment of the innervation pattern. Therefore, we now turn to another mechanism acting in this region which is likely to be responsible for the generation of the vibrissal pattern: the interaction of epidermis and dermis.

Epiderm-Derm Interactions in the Embryonic Whiskerpad

Biological considerations. The formation of integumental appendages like feathers, scales and hairs can be described using four attributes: (i) *time:* the onset of development of appendages at a defined stage; (ii) *place:* the delineation of a given region on the surface of the embryo within which appendages of a given type are to develop; (iii) *pattern:* the definition of a two-dimensional array of given geometry for individual appendages; (iv) *structure:* the development of individual appendages leading to their adult morphology.

The morphogenetic events characterizing each of these attributes need the unfolding of specific developmental programs under precise, spatio-temporal control. One possible source of such control mechanisms resides in the abundantly documented interaction of epidermis and dermis. Analyses of homo- and heterotopic epidermal-dermal tissue recombinations using intraspecies, interspecies and even interclass combinations (for reviews see Sengel, 1976; Dhouailly, 1984) helped to formulate a widely accepted model which aims at explaining how the informational exchange during this interaction leads to a proper pattern of appendage-anlagen. The model starts at a certain stage of differentiation - a stage as yet unknown - when dermal cells situated at the sites of future appendages send a signal to the overlying epidermis which responds with the formation of an epidermal "placode" (characterized by the transition from a cuboidal to a columnar epidermis) and signals back to the dermis. This second signal allows the formation of spatially restricted dermal condensations under each placode. The cells within these condensations are then the source of a third signal towards the placodal cells which now react in an appendage specific mannier which, in the case of hair formation, results in the development of dermal papillae. In the context of the present paper the first of the morphogenetic signals in this model is the most important, as it is the first and only one that provides positional information and, thus, has an instructive role in the definition of the appendage pattern. The above model, giving an attractive global picture of the morphogenetic events based on data now available, assumes that the positional information defining the pattern of appendages resides in the dermis. Sofar, however, there is no clear experimental evidence for such an assumption. Most of the studies at the origin of the model use in their recombination experiments tissues in a rather advanced developmental stage, i.e. just before or even during the appearance of the appendage anlagen (e.g. Sengel et al., 1969; Linsenmayer, 1972; Dhouailly, 1977). Therefore, as argued by Andrés and Van der Loos (1983), none of these studies rules out the possibility that the pattern is originally defined in the epidermis and subsequently transferred to the underlying mesenchyme before the recombination experiments took place.

An important contribution favoring the assumption of the model was made by Mauger (1972). Using somitic mesoderm from 2 to 2.5 day chick embryos, this author performed ortho- and heterotopic transplantation experiments in order to study the onset of regional and axial determination of the mesodermal cells. A related question was how the committed cells would influence the development of dorsal plumage which normally occurs in a medial-to-lateral sequence. Using "orthotopic" grafts, Mauger transferred somitic mesoderm, either before or after the onset of segmentation, to the contralateral side of the recipient. The original orientation of the graft in dorsoventral and in rostrocaudal sense was maintained, and, thus, the graft was inversed only with respect to its mediolateral axis. Host epiderm grew over the grafted tissue which was deprived of its own epiderm prior to grafting. When grafting was performed using as yet unsegmented mesoderm, the animals developed feathers. However, when the grafted mesoderm was already segmented, a featherless skin area extended from the medial border of the graft to the ventral side of the animal. From these results, Mauger drew three important conclusions. (i) The medial row of feather anlagen, which in normal conditions appears first in a developing dorsal pteryla (feather-forming domain), is necessary for the subsequent development of the more lateral feathers. (ii) The correct apposition of mesodermal cells and neural tube in the somitic region is crucial for the induction of the medial row of feathers; it looks as if this apposition is a prerequisite for the transfer of positional information along the medio-lateral axis within the somitic mesoderm and that this information becomes irreversibly fixed after segmentation. (iii) As the host ectoderm did not have any effect on the differentiation of the feather pattern of the dorsal pteryla, this pattern would be spatio-temporally determined by the somitic mesoderm. The work by Mauger is one of the rare studies which yield evidence supporting the idea that mesoderm is the primary source of the pattern-forming activity that defines the geometric arrangement of cutaneous appendages. Nevertheless, we cannot rule out the possible influence of the donor's ectoderm during the time it was still attached to the grafted mesoderm – a proposition which, however, would be hard to test.

During early developmental stages of vertebrates in general, global phenomena such as neural crest cell migration or determination of fate of given cell types, and morphogenetic events leading to the establishment of somitic mesoderm, pterylae, branchial arches or the nasal folds are all still in progress. To return to the mouse whiskerpad, it is unlikely that, during such early morphogenetic processes, specific genes are earmarked to govern pattern formation uniquely in this region. To the

153

contrary, one would rather evoke the implication of global phenomena such as those listed above, defining the overall head structure of which the whiskerpad is but a small part. It would, therefore, be difficult to establish, during early embryogenesis, causal relationships between the expression of single genes and defined ontogenetic events such as the formation of a follicular pattern.

Another important and often observed feature of pattern formation is its unidirectional propagation. In dorsal and femoral skin of the chick as well as in the whiskerpad of rodents, the respective patterns of feathers and of vibrissae are established progressively by morphogenetic waves proceeding in defined directions. *In vitro* experiments aimed at elucidating this phenomenon in femoral and dorsal pterylae of 4.5-7.5 day chick embryos (Linsenmayer, 1972; Novel, 1973) suggest that the onset and the direction of normal pattern formation is dependent on the intactness of the initial row of feather anlagen but, once the pattern reaches beyond that row, the latter may be removed without any effect on the propagation of the wave. The authors also demonstrated that, when dermis and epidermis of about the same age are rotated with respect to one another and recombined *in vitro,* the initial row develops always according to the orientation of the dermis, thereby defining the direction in which pattern formation advances. *Once initiated,* the progression of morphogenetic waves across tissues may be achieved by two mechanisms: through *chemical signalling* dependent on cell-cell interaction and travelling ahead of the morphogenetic wave, or through a *cell-autonomous,* temporally defined gradient of differentiation. The morphogenetic wave in dorsal pterylae was investigated in detail by Davidson (1983). In dorsal skin cultured on collagen and taken from 6 day old chick embryos, the wave was observed to cross gaps produced by the division of the pteryla into a medial and a lateral half, a fact already described for thigh skin in similar experiments by Linsenmayer (1972). Davidson, however, went beyond this and made several cuts at different distances from the midline to measure the time course describing the movement of the morphogenetic wave across the tissue gaps before reaching the lateral parts of the dorsal skin. Because this time course was the same as the one observed during differentiation of the rows of incipient feathers *in vivo,* this result destroyed the idea that a chemical, feather-inducing signal is propagated in the tissue ahead of the morphogenetic wave. Instead, it seems as if the cells building up a pteryla act in an autonomous way "knowing" the time when they have to undergo the differentiation step initiating the formation of a feather anlage. Therefore, when the spatial arrangement of these cells is changed, only the direction of movement of the morphogenetic wave may be disturbed but not the built-in time-table for differentiation of each cell.

The analyses of the formation of the feather pattern in the chick have provided useful hints for the understanding of the development of the vibrissal pattern in the mouse, as these two patterns seem to be generated according to similar rules: (i) The pattern of vibrissae is probably defined at or before E9-E10, which approximately corresponds to the age of a 3-4 day old chick embryo (Rugh, 1990). (ii) Akin to what happens during the formation of feather anlagen in pterylae, the progressive formation of follicular rows expresses itself as a morphogenetic wave moving in a defined direction across the incipient whiskerpad, starting in its caudolateral corner (Van der Loos et al., 1986). (iii) Whiskerpad explants taken at ages E9 and E10, when cultured on chorioallantoic membrane, are capable of developing an *in vivo*-like pattern of follicles (Andrés and van der Loos, 1983) which parallels the experiments performed by Linsenmayer (1972) and others in the chick. In addition, because pterylae are by far not as densely innervated as the whiskerpad, and considering what we reviewed about the pattern of follicular innervation,

we do favor the notion that epiderm-derm interaction rather than early
innervation of the whiskerpad anlage is the main mechanism responsible for
pattern formation in the whiskerpad. Tissue recombination experiments are
also supportive of our idea that the ridges are not an essential
prerequisite for the formation of the pattern. When whiskerpad mesenchyme
of E12.5 was combined with epiderm derived from the dorsum of mouse
embryos of the same age, the result was a ridge-independent induction of
whisker development in a whiskerpad-like pattern. In the intact embryo, a
similar (incidental) observation has been made in our laboratory some
years ago: follicles forming the ventralmost row of the whiskerpad are
not developing on a ridge but, close to a ridge, in a groove (see Fig.12c
in Van der Loos et al., 1986).

Models. The formation of a regular, two-dimensional pattern of skin
appendages based on epiderm-derm interactions, led not only to the tissue
recombination experiments but also to the elaboration of several
theoretical models (for a recent review on such models see Newman and
Comper, 1990). The importance of these models lies in the fact that not
only they explain how morphogenetic waves cross gaps but also they permit
to speculate about the minimal conditions necessary to achieve a regular
and stable appendage pattern and to design new concepts and strategies for
experiments.

There are two major concepts of how a biological pattern may be
generated. The "classic" concept formulated by Stern in 1968 and
concisely discussed by Tokunaga (1978) proposes the existence of a
"prepattern" characterized by Kauffman (1984) as a nonhomogeneous
distribution of a chemical substance in a developing tissue - in our case,
skin - according to which cells, responding to the concentration
differences of the chemical, may or may not start to differentiate into
integumental appendages, dependent on their responsiveness to the
prepattern. One year later, Wolpert (1969) proposed a more general and
abstract idea of pattern definition using the concept of "positional
information". Wolpert's theory has the advantage that, in contrast to
Stern's, it operates independently of any prepattern and that it may be
used to describe a large variety of patterns. According to Wolpert, every
morphogenetic area in which regularly spaced distinct units develop, may
be considered as a coordinate system or a "positional field", in which
every cell is defined by its position, i.e. has its specific "positional
value". It is only after the correct interpretation of these values by
the cells in question that a future pattern can be defined, while they -
the values - do not show a distribution that is isomorphic with that
pattern. To assign positional values to the cells, one needs to know
three parameters: (i) The boundary region(s) (having the function of an
origin in a coordinate system) serve as points of reference for positional
information, (ii) a vector providing the system with polarity, i.e.
specifying the direction of measurement and (iii) a scalar giving the
distance from the boundary region along the vector. A simple way to
obtain a positional field is therefore the establishment of a chemical
morphogenetic gradient with its source being the boundary region and
decreasing as a function of the distance from this boundary. Indeed, such
chemical gradients have been found at the level of a graded expression of
homeobox genes (Chuong et al., 1990) or in the distribution of retinoic
acid and its receptors (Eichele, 1989; Maden et al., 1989). However, as
we mentioned above, gradients need not be of chemical origin (Linsenmayer,
1972; Davidson, 1983).

Gierer and Meinhardt, (1972), applying Wolpert's definition of a
positional field together with the reaction-diffusion (RD) system of
Turing (1952), formulated a model which respects all the characteristics
of positional information and provides even the possibility that the

polarity in a positional field (the establishment of a gradient) may be achieved by self-organization. The RD-system is based on the fact that physical mechanisms like adhesion, gravity, tension, or diffusion of molecules may act as organizing principles in both non-living and living systems and may contribute to the regulation of morphogenetic events. In the model of Gierer and Meinhardt, the RD-system must meet two conditions if an ultimately stable pattern of integumental appendages is to evolve: (i) for the initiation of the pattern, a *local deviation* from a labile, near-uniform state in the positional field should have the possibility to increase, and (ii) the system must be allowed to reach a *steady state*. The simplest RD-system based on these criteria is operating by autocatalysis and lateral inhibition and is made up of two components. One of them is a local, *self-enhancing activator* and the other is a concomitantly produced *long-range inhibitor*. The identity of activator and inhibitor depends on the system. In the developing *Drosophila* eye, e.g., the product of the *scabrous* gene was recently identified as a fibrinogen-related lateral inhibitor (Baker et al., 1990). The RD-system may also be used to describe the generation of the vibrissal pattern (for an early version of such a description—advanced as a hypothesis – see Van der Loos et al., 1986). A substance of mesenchymal origin would, if present in sufficient concentration, locally induce follicular development. The inhibitor, produced together with the activator but diffusing away rapidly, would prevent follicle induction within a certain range around the activated region. Further away, where the concentration of the inhibitor would fall below a threshold value, follicular induction would reappear. Our project, i.e. the identification of developmentally regulated genes in the developing whiskerpad, has one major concrete goal: to detect molecular markers, indicating the positions at which later the follicle anlagen emerge. Were indeed the RD-system found to be at the basis of the formation of the whisker pattern, we may never find such markers. We expect that, at best, they would be present only for a brief time within the morphogenetic wave, i.e. there where self-organization of the pattern would occur. One weak point of the RD-system is that it fails to specify the character of the necessary, primary local disturbance that initiates the pattern within the positional field. The understanding of this initiation is of crucial importance and the mechanism leading to it may well depend on the embryonic structures surrounding the boundary region of the positional field in question. In the case of the whiskerpad, a candidate structure is the trigeminal ganglion, which, at that stage, is juxtaposed to the whiskerpads boundary region.

The vibrissal pattern with its remarkable constancy and regularity reminds one of patterns formed by sensory structures like ommatidia or bristles in insects. The advantage of such a periodic pattern is that even a small perturbation of its geometry is immediately detectable, which helps to identify animals with disturbed genetic control mechanisms that govern the formation of the patterns in question (Van der Loos and Dörfl, 1978). In that sense, the embryonic mouse whiskerpad might represent a unique opportunity for neurobiologists to study the molecular and genetic basis of pattern formation during the establishment of an important somatosensory pathway in higher vertebrates.

AN APPROACH TO STUDY MOLECULAR ASPECTS OF VIBRISSAL PATTERN FORMATION

In the three preceding sections we have adduced arguments for the notions that the follicular pattern is probably established prior to, and independent of, innervation, and that epiderm-derm interactions may be the main source of positional information in this area. In the hope of contributing to an explanation of the formation of the unique pattern of vibrissal follicles, we decided to generate subtractive, whiskerpadspecific hybridization probes and to use these for the identificaton of genetic control mechanisms implied specifically in the formation of the pattern.

Welker et al. (1985) demonstrated the follicle pattern to be a polygenic phenotype, a fact that,considering the structural complexity of the whiskerpad, was to be expected. Thus, one may assume that during the establishment of positional information in this area (probably around E9-E10) specific genes involved in this process are activated and/or silenced. Therefore, some of these genes may still have their peak of expression at E10 which makes them detectable in a comparative study using whiskerpad tissues of different developmental stages and tissues of different origin. These considerations guided us in the planning of experiments aiming at the characterization of E10-specific whiskerpad transcripts involved in the genetic regulation of the follicular pattern.

The Isolation of Developmentally Regulated cDNA Clones with a Subtractive Probe

One way how to detect genes which are expressed differentially during the development of a particular tissue is to compare the gene expression patterns in this tissue at two different developmental stages and to identify those genes that are expressed during one stage but not during the other. At present, a method of choice for such investigations is subtractive hybridization of nucleic acids. Two pools of nucleic acids, usually mRNA or cDNA, are hybridized and all the resulting, double-stranded hybrid molecules, which are common to both pools, are discarded. The remaining single-stranded sequences which represent differentially expressed genes are then either used to construct a subtractive cDNA library from which the clones may then be isolated and analysed or as subtractive probes for a differential screen of the two complete cDNA libraries prepared from the two pools of mRNA investigated. In neurobiology, many variations of this approach have been used with the purpose to isolate for example developmentally regulated, brain-specific genes (Rhyner et al., 1986; Miller et al., 1987; Travis and Sutcliffe, 1988; Lebeau et al., 1991 and Porteus et al., 1992).

For the subtractive and differential screens of our cDNA libraries we chose the method outlined in Fig. 3. Poly (A)$^{+}$ RNA was isolated from whiskerpad tissue of E10 and E14 embryos and from intact E14 embryo heads (Fig. 2). E10 was chosen because it is the earliest developmental stage in which the whiskerpad region can be isolated and dissected free from the rest of the embryo so that enough material can be collected in a reasonable time. As it is virtually impossible to dissect an E10 whiskerpad without bits of surrounding head tissue remaining attached to it we decided to use a combination of E14 whiskerpad and head tissue as subtractor material. Thus, sequences involved in head development outside the whiskerpad and present in both ages would be eliminated as well. The isolated RNAs were the basis for the preparation of two unidirectional cDNA libraries (an E10- and an E14-library), both in the phage $V\lambda$-derived vector Uni-ZAP XR. To obtain the subtractive probe, first strand cDNA was synthesized with the poly (A)$^{+}$ RNA from E10-whiskerpads as template. After the subsequent, random-primed ^{32}p-labeling of this cDNA, it was mixed with a tenfold excess of DNA sequences amplified from the E14-cDNA library and biotinylated by PCR (Polymerase Chain Reaction, White et al., 1989) according to Lebeau et al. (1991) and the whole was hybridized at 65°C for 24-48 hours to reach the necessary Cot value. Following this "subtractive hybridization", radioactive cDNA sequences that remained single-stranded were separated from the biotin-coupled single- and double-stranded DNAs during a repeated incubation of the hybridization mix with streptavidin, each time followed by phenol extraction. Thus, the

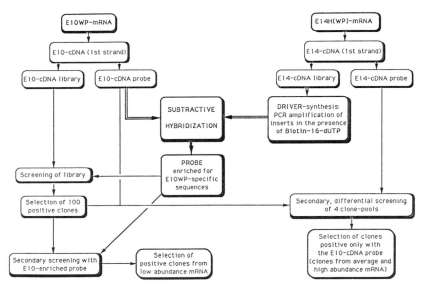

Fig. 3. Flow-diagram of the experimental strategy adopted in order to
isolate cDNA clones specific for the E10-whiskerpad. Double arrows
indicate crucial steps in the preparation of the subtractive probe. WP:
whiskerpad tissue, H(WP): tissue from total heads enriched with dissected
whiskerpads.

nonhybridized radioactive probe became concentrated in the aqueous phase
while the streptavidin/biotin-complexed cDNAs, showing a protein-like
behaviour, remained in the phenolic fraction. In our hands, about 30% of
the initial radioactivity was recovered that could be used as probe.

     After a high-density screen of our E10-library with the subtracted
probe, the approximately 100 resulting clones were analysed in two
different ways. Either they were submitted to a second round of low-
density screening with the subtracted probe, or they were taken into
several rounds of differential low-density screens, using as probes
radioactive single-stranded cDNAs synthesized on the same mRNAs that
served for the preparation of the original E10- and E14-libraries. In
these steps we eliminated false "E10-specific" clones from the first
screen by keeping only those detected with the E10- but not with the E14-
probe. Clones that resulted from this procedure, worthy candidates for
transcripts specific for the whiskerpad region of E10 embryos, are now
being characterized and submitted to a series of tests for their
developmental expression pattern in different tissues. These tests
include repeated Northern blot analyses of RNAS from tissues varying in
age and origin, which would indicate the tissue specificity, the temporal
expression pattern and transcript size of the genes represented by these
clones. A partial sequencing of the most promising clones is done as
well. The definitive proof that we have a molecular marker for the
determination of the initial follicle pattern will need histological
studies at the cellular level using *in situ* hybridization.

     The first results of this project are promising. From an initial
screen of about 250'000 clones, 100 were isolated and from these, 24
clones, varying in size from 0.3 to 2.3 kilobases, were kept as possible
representatives of stage-specific sequences (Fig. 4). In a number of
cases, Northern blot analysis with whiskerpad RNAs of E10, E12 and E14
embryos showed transcripts with a more or less pronounced expression

158

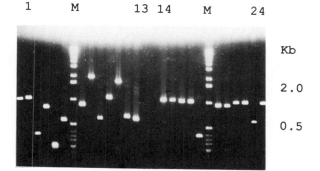

Fig. 4. The 24 final clones from subtractive and differential screening
of the E10- and E14-cDNA libraries (for details see text). Individual
phage-inserts were amplified using PCR and separated according to size on
a 1% agarose gel containing the fluorescent dye ethidiumbromide. M:
molecular size marker (BRL, 1Kb-DNA ladder).

pattern peaking at embryonic day E10. There, where the hybridization
signals were below the level of detection, the clones are to be analyzed
in more sensitive tests, like quantitative PCR or the RNAse protection
assay (Melton et al., 1984), as they probably represent mRNAs of low
abundance. In a first sequencing analysis we obtained, among several
unknown motives, the partial sequence of a protein identified as the α-
component of the mouse elongation factor EF-1. This factor is involved in
the elongation of amino acid chains during the translation of mRNAs into
proteins and consists itself of three proteins: EF-1α, β and γ (Kaziro,
1978). EF-1α is the component responsible for the GTP-dependent binding
of aminoacyl-tRNAs to the ribosomal acceptor site, and the sequence of EF-
1α was found to be highly conserved among various species (Hovemann et
al., 1988). As far as its expression in the developing whiskerpad is
concerned, our experiments are underway. As it is known that in mouse
liver and in Drosophila, there exist transcripts of this protein,regulated
with respect to age (Webster, 1985; Shepherd et al., 1989), we may find a
similar behaviour of the transcript in our region of interest as well.

It is obvious that by choosing the method of subtractive
hybridization one must be aware of its limits. There is the possibility
of losing important genes because their expression reaches its maximum
before day E10 or because their maxima persist until E14 or even further.
Also, as the dissected tissues from which the RNAs are isolated, comprise
more than just whiskerpad, we might miss genes showing developmental
regulation in sets of cells related to the whiskerpad, as the same genes
may have a high level of expression in other sets of cells, throughout the
period in question. On the other hand, this method allows one to enrich a
probe for transcripts of low abundance. This became apparent in those
Northern blots where, even with purified mRNA, no hybridization signal
could be detected. Results such as this are in agreement with our aim to
find regulative factors acting at the level of gene transcription or
intercellular signalling.

While most molecular and genetic studies of pattern formation in
vertebrates are concerned with the early segmentation of the mouse embryo
along the anteroposterior axis (Kessel and Gruss, 1990) there are now
experimental data accumulating in line with our special interest and from
which we adduce two examples. The first describes the pattern of
expression of a novel homeotic gene, Hox 7 (Benôit et al., 1989; Hill et

al., 1989). The transcript of this gene, that is homologous to the *msh* gene of *Drosophila* (Hill et al., 1989; Monaghan et al., 1991), is accumulating in rostral neural crest and is expressed in more advanced stages in various tissues among which one finds also the most rostral parts of the head and the snout of the mouse, including maxilla and mandibula. In the visceral arches its distribution seems homogeneous, without any sign of a pattern. A second example involves the expression of homeobox genes during the development of feather buds in the chick (Chuong et al., 1990). In this study, probes are used from the genes X1Hbox 1 (Xenopus laevis Homeobox 1; see Carrasco et al., 1984) and from Hox 5.2 (mouse Homeobox 5.2; see Dollé et al., 1989). To our knowledge this later study is the first to show that homeotic genes play a role in positional information concerning cutaneous appendages in vertebrates. X1Hbox 1 and Hox 5.2 form two expression gradients in opposite directions before there is any sign of feather anlagen in the field. Although in the mouse several sites of expression for both genes have been described (Oliver et al., 1988; Dollé et al., 1989) their expression pattern has not yet been investigated in the whiskerpad.

With respect to our own project, the results described in the preceding paragraph should be interpreted with caution. The observation described by Paul Hunt during this meeting that most of the transcripts of Hox genes, although expressed in migrating cranial neural crest cells, are generally not found beyond the second branchial arch during embryogenesis of the vertebrate head (Hunt et al., 1991) should remind us that the structures of the vertebrate head anterior to the tip of the notochord are considered to be profound and substantially new modifications of the head of protochordates (Gans and Northcutt, 1983; Gans, 1987; Thomson, 1987). This morphogenetic change is made possible through the parallel evolution of two tissues: the neural crest and the epidermal placodes. The evolution of the new head does not seem to involve preexisting elements. It consists rather of an addition of new tissue to the rostralmost notochordal tip and its flanking epimeres (Gans and Northcutt, 1983) and includes head structures like forebrain, cranial nerves with their sensory ganglia, nose, eyes and ears as well as the formation of a large part of the skull and other mesodermal structures due to a massive invasion of the new area by migrating neural crest cells. If this evolutionary scenario of the vertebrate head is true, we may expect that segmentation genes such as the Hox genes are not necessarily involved in it. Rather, there could be a chance for the identification of new gene families (like the POU-genes, for a review see Rosenfeld, 1991), the regulative network of which would have evolved together with the new vertebrate head. Therefore, the preparation of whiskerpadspecific, subtractive cDNA as hybridization probe to isolate cDNA clones involved in pattern formation seemed to be a reasonable experimental approach in the context of our project, so as to optimize the chances to detect new genes.

CONCLUDING REMARKS

Our project aims at answering the question: "Does the whiskerpad tell itself how to construct a follicle pattern?" This question assumes meaning in a neurobiologic context when one realizes that the developing whisker-to-barrel pathway offers, in a unique way, the possibility to address two important topics in developmental neurobiology: pattern formation at the peripheral end of a somatosensory pathway, and the translation of this pattern "inward", so that, centrally, brain maps may be established. With the identification of developmentally regulated, whiskerpad-specific genes we hope to contribute to this field, still full of enigmas.

ACKNOWLEDGMENTS

     We thank Drs. M.-C. Lebeau and S. Catsicas for helpful discussions
and advice throughout the experimental phase of this work. Support:
Swiss National Science Foundation Grant 3100.009468.

REFERENCES

Andrés, F.L. and Van der Loos, H. (1983) Cultured embryonic non-
     innervated mouse muzzle is capable of generating a whisker pattern.
     Int. J. Dev, Neurosci. 1:319-338.
Andres, K.H. (1966) Ueber die Feinstruktur der Rezeptoren an Sinushaaren.
     Z. Zellforsch. 75:339-365.
Baker, N.E., Mlodzik, M. and Rubin, G.M. (1990) Spacing differentiation
     in the developing Drosophila eye: A fibrinogen-related lateral
     inhibitor encoded by scabrous. Science 250:1370-1377.
Bate, C.M. (1976) Pioneer neurons in an insect embryo. Nature 260:54-56.
Benoît, R., Sassoon, D., Jacq, B., Gehring, W. and Buckingham, M. (1989)
     Hox-7, a mouse homeobox gene with a novel pattern of expression during
     embryogenesis. EMBO J. 8:91-100.
Cajal, S.R. (1929) "Etudes sur la neurogenèse de quelques vertébrés",
     Tipografia Artistica, Madrid. We used the version "Studies on
     vertebrate neurogenesis" translated by L. Guth (1960), Charles C.
     Thomas: Springfield, IL, USA, chapter 4:149-200.
Campenot, R.B. (1982a) Development of sympathetic neurons in
     compartmentalized cultures. I. Local control of neurite growth by
     nerve growth factor. Dev. Biol. 93:1-12.
Campenot, R.B. (1982b) Development of sympathetic neurons in
     compartmentalized cultures. II. Local control of neurite survival by
     nerve growth factor. Dev. Biol. 93:13-21.
Carrasco, A.E., McGinnis, W., Gehring, W. and De Robertis, E.M. (1984)
     Cloning of an X. laevis gene expressed during early embryogenesis
     coding for a peptide region homologous to Drosophila homeotic genes.
     Cell 37:409-414.
Chuong, C.-M., Oliver, G., Ting, S.A., Jegalian, B., Chen, H.M. and De
     Robertis, E.M. (1990) Gradients of homeoproteins in developing
     feather buds. Development 110:1021-1030.
Danforth, C.H. (1925) Hair in its relation to questions of homology and
     phylogeny. Amer. J. Anat. 36:47-68.
Davidson, D.R. (1983) The mechanism of feather pattern development in the
     chick. II. Control of the sequence of pattern formation. J.
     Embryol. Exp. Morph. 74:271-283.
Davies, A.M. and Lumsden, A. (1984) Relation of target encounter and
     neuronal death to nerve growth factor responsiveness in the developing
     mouse trigeminal ganglion. J. Comp. Neurol. 223:124-137.
Davies, A.M., Bandtlow, C., Heumann, R., Korsching, S., Rohrer, H. and
     Thoenen, H. (1987) Timing and site of nerve growth factor synthesis
     in developing skin in relation to innervation and expression of the
     receptor. Nature 326:353-358.
Dhouailly, D. (1977) Regional specification of cutaneous appendages in
     mammals. Wilhelm Roux Arch. Dev. Biol. 181:3-10.
Dhouailly, D. (1984) Specification of feather and scale patterns, in:
     "Pattern Formation: A primer in developmental biology", G.M.
     Malacinski and S.V. Bryant, eds., Macmillan: New York, 581-601.
Diamond, J. (1979) The regulation of nerve sprouting by extrinsic
     influences. In: "The Neurosciences, Fourth Study Section", F.O.
     Schmitt and F.G. Worden, eds., MIT Press: Cambridge, MA 937-955.
Dollé, P., Izpisua-Belmonte, J.-C., Falkenstein, H., Renucci, A. and
     Duboule, D. (1989) Coordinate expression of the murine Hox-5 complex

homoeobox-containing genes during limb pattern formation. Nature 342:767-772.

Dörfl, J. (1985) The innervation of the mystacial region of the white mouse: A topographical study. J. Anat. 142:173-184.

Eichele, G. (1989) Retinoids and vertebrate limb pattern formation. Trends Genet. 5:246-251.

Gans, C. (1987) The neural crest: A spectacular invention. In: "Developmental and evolutionary aspects of the neural crest", Wiley Series in Neurobiology, R.G. Northcutt and P.F.A. Maderson, eds., John Wiley & Sons: New York, etc., 361-379.

Gans, C. and Northcutt, R.G. (1983) Neural crest and the origin of vertebrates: A new head, 220:268-274.

Gierer, A. and Meinhardt, H. (1972) A theory of biological pattern formation. Kybernetik 12:30-39.

Gu, J., Polak, J.M., Tapia, F.J., Marangos, P.J. and Pearce, A.G.E. (1981) Neuron specific enolase in the Merkel cells of mammalian skin. Am. J. Pathol. 104:63-68.

Gundersen, R.W. and Barrett, J.N. (1979) Neuronal chemotaxis: Chick dorsal-root axons turn toward high concentrations of nerve growth factor. Science 206:1079-1080.

Gundersen, R.W. and Barrett, J.N. (1980) Characterization of the turning response of dorsal root neurites toward nerve growth factor. J. Cell. Biol. 87:546-554.

Heilig, J.S., Freeman, M., Laverty, T., Lee, K.J., Campos, A.R., Rubin, G.M. and Steller, H. (1991) Isolation and characterization of the disconnected gene of Drosophila melanogaster. EMBO J. 10:809-815.

Hill, R.E., Jones, P.F., Rees, A.R., Sime, C.M., Justice, M.J., Copeland, N.G., Jenkins, N.A., Graham, E. and Davidson, D.R. (1989) A new family of mouse homeobox containing genes: Molecular structure, chromosomal location and developmental expression of Hox 7. Genes Dev. 3:26-37.

Hoogland, P.V., Welker, E. and Van der Loos, H. (1987) Organization of the projections from barrel cortex to thalamus in mice studied with Phaseolus vulgaris-leucoagglutinin and HRP. Exp. Brain Res. 68:73-87.

Hovemann, B., Richter, S., Walldorf, U. and Cziepluch, C. (1988) Two genes encode related cytoplasmic elongation factors la (EF-la) in Drosophila melanogaster with continuous and stage specific expression. Nucleic Acids Res. 16:3175-3194.

Hunt, P., Wilkinson, D. and Krumlauf, R. (1991) Patterning the vertebrate head: Murine Hox 2 genes mark distict subpopulations of premigratory and migrating cranial neural crest. Development 112:43-50.

Kauffman, S.A. (1984) Pattern generation and regeneration. In: "Pattern Formation: A primer in developmental biology", G.M. Malacinski and S.V. Bryant, eds., Macmillan: New York, 73-102.

Kaziro, Y. (1978) The role of guanosine 5'-triphosphate in polypeptide chain elongation. Biochim. Biophys. Acta. 505:95-127.

Kessel, M. and Gruss, P. (1990) Murine developmental control genes. Science 249:374-379.

Killackey, H.P. (1980) Pattern formation in the trigeminal system of the rat. Trends Neurosci. 3:303-306.

Klein, B.G. and Rhoades, R.W. (1985) Representation of whisker follicle intrinsic musculature in the facial motor nucleus of the rat. J. Comp. Neurol. 232:55-69.

Klose, M. and Bentley, D. (1989) Transient pioneer neurons are essential for formation of an embryonic peripheral nerve. Science 245:982-984.

Lebeau, M.-C., Alvarez-Bolado, G., Wahli, W. and Catsicas, S. (1991) PCR driven DNA-DNA competitive hybridization: A new method for sensitive differential cloning. Nucleic Acids Res. 19:4778.

Letourneau, P.C. (1978) Chemotactic response of nerve fibre elongation to nerve growth factor. Dev. Biol. 66:183-196.

Linsenmayer, T.F. (1972) Control of integumentary patterns in the chick. Dev. Biol. 27:244-271.

Lumsden, A.G.S. and Davies, A.M. (1983) Earliest sensory nerve fibres are guided to peripheral targets by attractants other than nerve growth factor. Nature 306:786-788.

Lumsden, A.G.S. and Davies, A.M. (1986) Chemotropic effect of specific target epithelium in the developing mammalian nervous system. Nature 323:538-539.

Maden, M., Ong, D.E., Summerbell, D. and Chytil, F. (1989) The role of retinoid-binding proteins in the generation of pattern in the developing limb, the regenerating limb and the nervous system. Development 107 (supplement: The molecular basis of positional signalling):109-119.

Mauger, A. (1972) Rôle du mésoderme somitique dans le développement du plumage dorsal chez l'embryon de poulet. II. Régionalisation du mésoderme plumigène. J. Embryol. Exp. Morph. 28:343-366.

McConnell, S.K., Ghosh, A. and Shatz, C.J. (1989) Subplate neurons pioneer the first axon pathway from the cerebral cortex. Science 245:978-982.

Melton, D.A., Krieg, P.A., Rebagliati, M.R., Maniatis, T., Zinn, K. and Green, M.R. (1984) Efficient in vitro synthesis of biologically active RNA and RNA hybridization probes from plasmids containing a bacteriophage SP6 promoter. Nucleic Acid Res. 12:7035-7056.

Miller, F.D., Naus, C.C.G., Higgins, G.A., Bloom, F.E. and Milner, R.J. (1987) Developmentally regulated rat brain mRNAs: molecular and anatomical characterization. J. Neurosci. 7:2433-2444.

Molnar, Z. and Blakemore, C. (1991) Lack of regional specificity for connections formed between thalamus and cortex in coculture. Nature 351:475-477.

Monaghan, A.P., Davidson, D., Sime, C., Graham, E., Baldock, R., Bhattacharya, S. and Hill, R.E. (1991) The Msh-like homeobox genes define domains in the developing vertebrate eye. Development. 112:1053-1061.

Newman, S.A. and Comper, W.D. (1990) "Generic" physical mechanisms of morphogenesis and pattern formation. Development 110:1-18.

Novel, G. (1973) Feather pattern stability and reorganisation in cultured skin. J. Embryol. Exp. Morph. 30:605-633.

Nurse, C.A. and Diamond, J. (1984) A fluorescent microscopic study on the development of rat touch domes and their Merkel cells. Neurosnience 11:509-520.

Nurse, C.A. and Farraway, L. (1988) Development of Merkel cell populations with contrasting sensitivities to neonatal deafferentation in the rat whiskerpad. Somatosensory and Motor Res. 6:141-162.

Oliver, G., Wright, Ch.V.E., Hardwicke, J. and De Robertis, E.M. (1988) Differential antero-posterior expression of two proteins encoded by a homeobox gene in xenopus and mouse embryos. EMBO J. 7:3199-3209.

Porteus, M.H., Brice, A.E.J., Bulfone, A., Usdin, T.B., Ciaranello, R.D. and Rubenstein, J.L.R. (1992) Isolation and characterization of a library of cDNA clones that are preferentially expressed in the embryonic telencephalon. Mol. Brain Res. 12:7-22.

Rhyner, T.A., Biguet, N.F., Berrard, S., Borbely, A.A. and Mallet, J. (1986) An efficient approach for the selective isolation of specific transcripts from complex brain mRNA populations. J. Neurosci. Res. 16:167-181.

Rice, F.L., Mance, A. and Munger, B.L. (1986) A comparative light microscopic analysis of the sensory innervation of the mystacial pad. I. Innervation of vibrissal follicle-sinus complexes. J. Comp. Neurol. 252:154-174.

Rohrer, H., Heumann, R. and Thoenen, H. (1988) The synthesis of nerve growth factor (NGF) in developing skin is independent of innervation. Dev. Biol. 128:240-244.

Rosenfeld, M.G. (1991) POU-domain transcription factors: powerful developmental regulators. <u>Genes and Development</u> 5:897-907.

Rugh, R. (1990) "The mouse: Its reproduction and development", Oxford University Press: Oxford, UK, etc.

Sengel, P., Dhouailly, D. and Kieny, M. (1969) Aptitude des constituants cutanés de l'aptérie médio-ventrale à former des plumes. <u>Dev. Biol.</u> 19:436-446.

Sengel, P. (1976) "Morphogenesis of Skin", Cambridge University Press: Cambridge, UK etc.

Shepherd, J.C.W., Walldorf, U., Hug, P. and Gehring, W.J. (1989) Fruit flies with additional expression of the elongation factor EF-1a live longer. <u>Proc. Natl. Acad. Sci. USA</u> 86:7520-7521.

Stainier, D.Y.R. and Gilbert, W. (1990) Pioneer neurons in the mouse trigeminal sensory system. <u>Proc. Natl. Acad. Sci. USA</u> 87:923-927.

Steller, H., Fischbach, K.-F. and Rubin, G.M. (1987) *disconnected:* A locus required for neuronal pathway formation in the visual system of *Drosophila*. <u>Cell</u> 50:1139-1153.

Stern, C. (1968) Developmental genetics of pattern. <u>In:</u> "Genetic mosaics and other essays", Harvard University Press: Cambridge, MA 135-173.

Tello, J.F. (1923) Genèse des terminaisons motrices et sensitives II. Terminaisons dans les poils de la souris blanche. <u>Travaux du Laboratoire de recherches biologiques de l'Université de Madrid</u> 21:257-384.

Thomson, K.S. (1987) Speculations concerning the role of the neural crest in the morphogenesis and evolution of the vertebrate skeleton. <u>In:</u> "Developmental and evolutionary aspects of the neural crest", Wiley Series in Neurobiology, R.G. Northcutt and P.F.A. Maderson, eds., John Wiley & Sons: New York, etc., 301-338.

Tokunaga, C. (1978) Genetic mosaic studies of pattern formation in *Drosophila melanogaster*, with special reference to the prepattern hypothesis. <u>In:</u> "Genetic mosaics and cell differentiation", W.J. Gehring, ed., Springer-Verlag: Berlin, etc., 157-204.

Tosney, K.W. and Landmesser, L.T. (1985) Growth cone morphology and trajectory in the lumbosacral region of the chick embryo. <u>J. Neurosci.</u> 5:2345-2358.

Travis, G.H. and Sutcliffe, J.G. (1988) Phenol emulsion-enhanced DNA-driven subtractive cDNA cloning: isolation of low-abundance monkey cortex-specific mRNAs. <u>Proc. Nat. Acad. Sci. USA</u> 85:1696-1700.

Turing, A. (1952) The chemical basis of morphogenesis. <u>Phil. Trans. Roy. Soc. Lond.</u> B237:37-72.

Van der Loos, H. and Dörfl, J. (1978) Does the skin tell the somatosensory cortex how to construct a map of the periphery? <u>Neurosci. Lett.</u> 7:23-30.

Van der Loos, H. and Welker, E. (1985) Development and plasticity of somatosensory brain maps. <u>In:</u> "Development, organization, and processing in somatosensory pathways", M. Rowe and W.D. Willis Jr. eds., Alan R. Liss, Inc.: New York, NY, 53-67.

Van der Loos, H., Welker, E., Dörfl, J. and Rumo, G. (1986) Selective breeding for variations in patterns of mystacial vibrissae of mice; bilaterally symmetrical strains derived from ICR-stock. <u>J. Hered.</u> 77:66-82.

Van der Loos, H., Welker, E., Dörfl, J. and Hoogiand, P. (1990) Brain maps: Development, plasticity and distribution of signals beyond. <u>In:</u> "The Neocortex: ontogeny and phylogeny", B.L. Finlay, G. Innocenti and H. Scheich, eds., Plenum Press: New York, NY, 229-236.

Van Exan, R.J. and Hardy, M.H. (1980) A spatial relationship between innervation and the early differentiation of vibrissa follicles in the embryonic mouse. <u>J. Anat.</u> 131:643-656.

Vos, P., Stark, F. and Pittman, R.N. (1991) Merkel cells in vitro: Production of nerve growth factor and selective interactions with sensory neurons. Dev. Biol. 144:281-300.

Webster, G.C. (1985) "Molecular biology of aging, gene stability and gene expression", R.S. Sohal, L.S. Birnbaum and R.G. Culter, eds., Raven: New York, 263-289.

Welker, E., Gubbels, E.J. and Van der Loos, H. (1985) Mode of inheritance of supernumerary vibrissae and their sensory innervation as studied in a cross-breeding experiment, involving a normal and an "enriched" mouse strain. Neurosci. Lett. (Suppl.) 22:S344.

Welker, E., Van der Loos, H., Dörfl, J and Soriano, E. (1990) The possible role of GABA-ergic innervation in plasticity of adult cerebral cortex. In: "The Neocortex: ontogeny and phylogeny", B.L. Finlay, G. Innocenti and H. Scheich, eds., Plenum Press: New York, NY, 237-243.

White, T.J., Arnheim, N. and Erlich, H.A. (1989) The polymerase chain reaction. Trends in Genetics 5:185-189.

Wolpert, L. (1969) Positional information and the spatial pattern of cellular differentiation. J. Theor. Biol. 193:296-307.

Woolsey, T.A. and Van der Loos, H. (1970) The structural organization of layer IV in the somatosensory region (SI) of mouse cerebral cortex. Brain Res. 17:205-242.

Wrenn, J.T. and Wessells, N.K. (1984) The early development of mystacial vibrissae in the mouse. J. Embryol. Exp. Mornp. 83:137-156.

Zafra, F., Hengerer, B., Leibrock, J., Thoenen, H. and Lindholm, D. (1990) Activity dependent regulation of BDNF and NGF mRNAs in the rat hippocampus is mediated by non-NMDA glutamate receptors. EMBO J. 9:3545-3550.

TWO PHASES OF PATTERN FORMATION IN THE DEVELOPING

RODENT TRIGEMINAL SYSTEM

Sonal Jhaveri and Reha Erzurumlu

Department of Brain and Cognitive Sciences
Massachusetts Institute of Technology
Cambribge, MA 02139

The patterning of neural connections, as reflected by the ordered projections between functionally related groups of cells, is a hallmark of the vertebrate CNS. The precision and specificity of such organization is especially striking in the interconnections within sensory systems wherein topographic representations of the periphery are mapped onto multiple central cell groups. These features are epitomized in the rodent trigeminal system: the array of vibrissae and sinus hairs on the snout is replicated in the punctate arrangement of cells and axons along the entire trigeminal neuraxis (see Woolsey, 1989 for a review). The question of how such ordered patterns come about has been addressed at various levels, including the establishment of regional specificity (Schneider, 1973), the acquisition of positional identity (rev., Gaze, 1970; Jacobson, 1978; Lund 1978), the selection of postsynaptic partners (Purves and Lichtman,1985), and so on. In this chapter we review our studies on pattern formation in the trigeminal system within the context of two particular aspects of this issue: the conferring of axial orientation of the somatotopic map in the CNS and the emergence of modular patterning within this map.

ESTABLISHMENT OF THE AXIAL FRAMEWORK OF THE SOMATOTOPIC MAP

The infraorbital branch of the maxillary division of the trigeminal nerve innervates the vibrissal pad on the snout. In mice and rats, the vibrissae are organized in an array of 5 rows, A through E, and within each row the number of whisker follicles is remarkably constant (Yamakado and Yohro, 1979; Van Exan and Hardy, 1980). The distribution of vibrissae on the snout is reflected in the pattern of afferent axon distribution and in the clustering of postsynaptic neurons in the brainstem trigeminal nuclei, the ventrobasal thalamic nucleus (VB) and in the face representation region of the primary somatosensory (SI or barrelfield) cortex (Woolsey and Van der Loos, 1970; Van der Loos, 1976; Rice and Van der Loos, 1977; Belford and Killackey, 1979, 1980; Erzurumlu et al., 1980; Ivy and Killackey, 1982; Ma and Woolsey, 1984; Killackey and Belford, 1979; Bates and Killackey, 1985; Rice et al., 1985; Bernardo and Woolsey, 1987; Jensen and Killackey, 1987). However, despite the replicative nature of the periphery-related motif in these areas, the absolute orientation of each array, relative to the body axis of the animal, is different within each way-station (Figure 1). Previous studies have established that perturbations of the sensory

Development of the Central Nervous System in Vertebrates
Edited by S.C. Sharma and A.M. Goffinet, Plenum Press, New York, 1992

periphery during a perinatal sensitive period, or genetic selection for supernumerary whiskers, leads to corresponding alterations in each of the vibrissal representation areas of the CNS (Van der Loos and Woolsey, 1973; Belford and Killackey, 1980; Killackey and Shinder, 1981; Durham and Woolsey, 1984; Van der Loos and Welker, 1985; Welker and Van der Loos, 1986; Jeanmonod et al., 1981). However, despite the pattern of the whisker representation being abnormal, in no case is the absolute orientation of the face map shifted. These observations indicate that separate mechanisms are involved in determining the axial orientation of the map and for the punctate representation of the vibrissae.

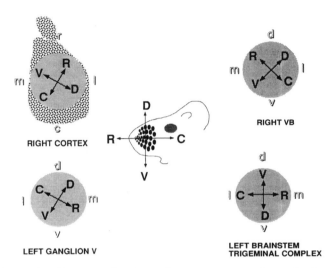

FIGURE 1. Schematic diagram showing the representation of the left whisker pad (Center) in the ipsilateral trigeminal ganglion, ipsilateral brainstem trigeminal nuclei, contralateral ventrobasal thalamic nucleus (VB) and contralateral SI cortex. The dorso-ventral (D-V) and rostrocaudal (R-C) axes of the vibrissal array in each structure are indicated in dark, capital letters. The dorsoventral (d-v), mediolateral (m-l) and rostrocaudal (r-c) body axes are indicated in open, lower case letters. The axes of the vibrissal array coincide with the body axes. Note that the axial orientation of the vibrissal array is different at each synaptic end-station.

Reviewed here are the results of two sets of experiments in which we show that distinct strategies are employed for establishing the alignment of the peripheral representation along the trigeminal pathway and for the elaboration of patterns within this representation. The former is discussed in relation to observations on the embryonic development of the trigeminal nerve and ganglion (Erzurumlu and Jhaveri, 1992a), the latter with respect to the emergence of vibrissa-related patterns in the afferents, cells and extracellular elements of the barrelfield cortex (Blue et al., 1991; Jhaveri et al., 1991; Erzurumlu and Jhaveri, 1992b).

During embryonic life, whisker rows A and B derive from the lateral nasal process, whereas rows C,D,E form on the maxillary process (Yamakado and Yohro, 1979). Using tiny implants of the lipophillic dyes DiI and DiA placed along the dorsoventral axis of the presumptive vibrissal field in aldehyde-fixed rat embryos, we were able to retrogradely label the peripheral and central extensions and the perikarya of trigeminal ganglion cells (Erzurumlu and Jhaveri, 1992a). Peripheral processes emerge from the ganglion by E11 (shortly after the first cohort of ganglion cells has become postmitotic - Forbes and Welt, 1981; Altman and Bayer, 1982; Rhoades et al., 1991) and arrive at the anlage of the snout on E12, prior to the differentiation of vibrissal follicles (English et al., 1980; Erzurumlu and Killackey, 1983). Discrete, non-overlapping applications of DiI and DiA on the upper jaw of E12 embryos result in distinct subpopulations of retrogradely labeled ganglion cells. This result is illustrated in Figure 2. Dye crystals placed (dorsally) on the nasal process label a patch of cells located dorsomedially in the ganglion whereas ventrally-placed implants (on the maxillary process) label a group of ventrolaterally located neurons. This pattern of labeling is also preserved along the cross-section of the infraorbital nerve. Furthermore, the differential labeling paradigm reveals a systematic order in the alignment of the central processes of ganglion cells: the dorsoventral axis of the face is embodied in the mediolateral distribution of the processes which course in the emerging trigeminal tract, as well as in the location of collateral arbors invading the newly-formed (Altman and Bayer, 1980 a,b,c) brainstem trigeminal nuclei. With continued development of the brain and the closing of the 4th ventricle, the hindbrain undergoes a further rotation of 90° with the result that in the mature animal, the vibrissal map within the trigeminal tract and in the hindbrain sensory nuclei is inverted 180° relative to the axis of the face. Thus, from the time trigeminal ganglion cells begin to emit processes towards their as yet undifferentiated peripheral and central targets, the topographic equivalence of their projection to the periphery, at least for the dorso-ventral axis, is delineated by the positioning of their perikarya, the trajectory of their axons and the position of their terminal arbors in central targets.

This equivalence is refined as differentiation continues. By E14, and more clearly so on E15, vibrissal rows can be distinguished on the snout. Crystals of DiI-DiA-DiI placed in vibrissal rows A, C and E respectively (caudally in rows A and E, rostrally in row C), result in 3 patches of differentially labeled axon bundles in the infraorbital nerve, of ganglion cells and of axons in the trigeminal tract. Furthermore, the delineation of the perpendicular axis can also be documented on E14: dye implants along the rostrocaudal axis of row C give rise to retrogradely filled fibers and cells segregated along the mediolateral axis of the nerve and ganglion (Erzurumlu and Jhaveri, 1992a).

Thus, our results show that the axial orientation of the peripheral map, as conveyed to trigeminal ganglion cells and to the central trigeminal tract, is hard-wired in the spatial order of ganglion cell processes. These results confirm previous reports of order within the peripheral trigeminal system (Erzurumlu and Killackey, 1983; Killackey, 1985; Rhoades et al., 1990a; Stainier and Gilbert, 1991). Furthermore, we have shown that this order is present prior to morphological differentiation of the target region. For this alignment to be transferred onto the brainstem trigeminal nuclei, the spatial arrangement of axons within the central trigeminal tract must dictate the point of entry of collateral branches, and thus the distribution of arbors, within the target zone. Our observations on the early innervation of the brainstem trigeminal nuclei show that such a plan is followed by the collaterals of primary sensory afferents as they begin to form terminal arbors in their respective projection zones in the developing hindbrain (Erzurumlu and Jhaveri, 1992b).

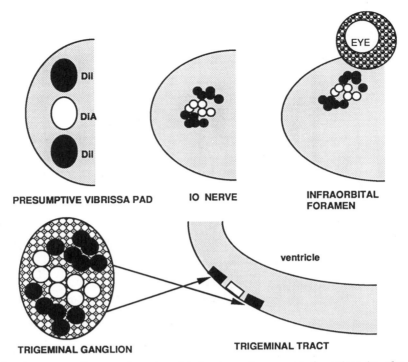

PRESUMPTIVE VIBRISSA PAD

IO NERVE

INFRAORBITAL FORAMEN

TRIGEMINAL GANGLION

TRIGEMINAL TRACT

FIGURE 2. Summary of experiments which show the spatial order in the distribution of trigeminal ganglion cells and in their central and peripheral processes. Tiny crystals of DiI (black spots) and DiA (white spots) were applied along the dorsoventral extent of the presumptive vibrissal pad. Representative cross sections through the extracranial portion of the infraorbital (IO) nerve and at the level of the infraorbital foramen show that spatial representation of the dorsoventral axis of the face is maintained in an orderly fashion by the fascicles of the nerve. Dorsally placed crystals label a patch of dorsomedially located ganglion cells which in turn project centrally, on E14, via the ventromedial part of the trigeminal tract. Dye crystals applied ventrally on the presumptive snout label vetrolaterally located ganglion cells which enter the dorsolateral part of the emerging central tract.

By extension, the axial orientation of the face map in the ventrobasal nucleus of the thalamus and in the SI cortex must also be directed by the spatial alignment of axons in the medial lemniscus and in the thalamocortical radiations, respectively. Although we do not have direct information on the presence of spatial order <u>within</u> these fiber pathways (but see Bernardo and Woolsey, 1987), there is evidence that the tangential topography of the neocortex is reflected in the ordered spatial distribution of fibers within the internal capsule (Blakemore and Molnár, 1990; Molnár and Blakemore, 1990; Erzurumlu and Jhaveri, unpublished results). Moreover, application of a tiny crystal of dye within SI cortex labels a small bundle of anterogradely and retrogradely filled fibers along the white matter and internal capsule, leading to a small patch of cells in the thalamus. This observation suggests that not only is there some order in the spatial deployment of cortical efferents, but also that for reciprocally connected regions, thalamocortical fibers follow the same trajectory as do the corticothalamic axons (see also, Molnár and Blakemore, this volume).

The resolution of the techniques we have used is limited: it is difficult to gauge the exact degree to which spatial order among axons is preserved. The possibility that strict neighbor relationships are retained at the level of single axons is unlikely: in fact, the number of axons in single fascicles varies with distance (at least over 200-300 µm) along the trigeminal nerve (Davies and Lumsden, 1986), suggesting that the relative positions of individual axons change at a local level. Nevertheless, a global order is maintained in the overall organization of the pathway. Similar observations have been made in the visual system: although individual retinofugal axons move readily from one fascicle to another within the optic nerve (Horton et al., 1979; Williams and Rakic, 1985), a coarse retinotopic order has been demonstrated along parts of the nerve and the optic tract of many species (Jhaveri, 1973; Rager, 1980; Torrealba et al. 1982; Bunt and Horder, 1983; Walsh et al., 1983; Rusoff, 1984; Walsh and Guillery, 1985; Reese and Cowey, 1990). Topographic order within fiber tracts has been reported for other systems as well (Nelson and LeVay, 1985; Ferraro and Barrera, 1936; Walker, 1937; Walker and Weaver, 1942) but it has not yet been determined whether this order is present from the outset, or occurs after "corrective" mechanisms such as cell death have been operative. Chronological gradients of neurogenesis and axon outgrowth (Horder and Martin, 1978; Rager, 1980; Walsh and Guillery, 1985; Reese and Cowey, 1990), guidance via glial channels (Silver and Sidman, 1980) and local guidance cues (Harris, 1989) are possible mechanisms implicated in the establishment of such order.

MODULAR PATTERNING OF AFFERENT AXON ARBORS IN THE BARRELFIELD CORTEX

In the rodent trigeminal system, we identify two temporally dissociable phases of map formation. In the first, described above, the general spatial configuration of axons and cells is established relative to the topography of the sensory periphery. In the second phase, vibrissa-related modules are elaborated. During the perinatal period, such modules in the SI cortex consist of thalamocortical axon arbors (Robertson, 1987; Erzurumlu and Jhaveri, 1990; Schlaggar and O'Leary, 1991) tegmentocortical serotonergic fiber ramifications (Lidov and Molliver, 1982; Rhoades et al., 1990b; Blue et al., 1991), postsynaptic cells (Rice and Van der Loos, 1977; Rice et al., 1985) and of glial cells and extracellular matrix molecules (Cooper and Steindler, 1986a,b; Steindler et al., 1989; Crossin et al., 1989; Jhaveri et al., 1991). Of these elements, the participation by serotonergic afferents, glial cells and extracellular matrix molecules appears to be transient. Our knowledge of the possible contribution of these ephemeral patterns to the construction of the barrel cortex is, at best, speculative.

In recent experiments, we have addressed the question of how this second aspect of pattern formation, the conferring of periphery-related motifs onto the undifferentiated cortical plate, comes about. We approached the issue from the point of view of the temporal progression of events occurring during development. A combination of labeling with DiI and immunostaining with antibodies directed against specific cortical elements reveals the sequence of events illustrated in Figure 3. The differentiation of the cortical plate begins on E15, prior to the arrival of brainstem afferents in the ventrolateral wall of the neocortical anlage, and proceeds along a ventrolateral to dorsomedial gradient. A day later, thalamocortical axons arrive at the intermediate zone of the cortical mantle and soon thereafter, collateral branches from these axons begin to invade the cell dense cortical plate (Erzurumlu and Jhaveri, 1990; Catalano et al., 1991; Erzurumlu and Jhaveri, 1992b). Tegmental afferents follow a different route into the telencephalon and the first tegmentocortical axons are detected

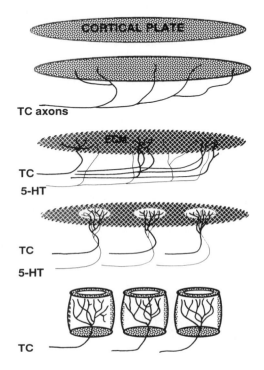

FIGURE 3. Sequence of events which results in the development of a vibrissa-related patterning of the cells and afferents of layer IV in the SI cortex. Shortly after the formation of the cortical plate, thalamocortical (TC) afferents arrive in the cortex (E16). Collaterals of the TC axons form a diffuse plexus within the cortical plate. Around the time of birth, TC axon arbors become segregated into whisker-related patches. A transiently disjunctive distribution of tegmentocortical serotonergic (5-HT) axons is observed soon after that of TC axons. This is followed by a down-regulation of extracellular matrix molecules (ECM) within the hollows of presumptive barrels. Around the same time, the clustering of layer IV granule cells into barrels becomes evident.

under the cortical plate a few days after the arrival of thalamofugal fibers (Aitken and Törk, 1988; Schlumpf et al., 1980; Wallace and Lauder, 1983; Verney et al., 1984; Erzurumlu and Jhaveri, 1992b). DiI labeling and serotonin immunoreactivity show that both corticopetal axon systems initially form a diffuse projection in the barrelfield cortex (Rhoades et al., 1990; Blue et al., 1991). By PND1, a whisker row pattern emerges and by PND2, individual whisker-related patches can be identified in each projection. Detailed examination of both afferent systems labeled simultaneously in two halves of the same brain indicates that emergence of the whisker pattern for serotonergic axons lags behind that for thalamic axons by at least half a day (Blue et al., 1991). A recent study using acetylcholinesterase histochemistry indicates that the thalamic axons are organized in whisker related patches on PND0 (Schlaggar and O'Leary, 1991), a couple of days prior to that seen by DiI labeling, underscoring the precocious nature of expression of the peripheral pattern by this system of afferents. And finally, a comparison of the distribution of the extracellular matrix molecules cytotactin and cytotactin-binding proteoglycan with the projection pattern of thalamofugal axons shows that on PND2, when thalamic axon arbors are already distributed in vibrissa-related patches, the ECM molecules are expressed uniformly across the barrelfield. It is not until PND4, when granule cells of layer IV have taken on the clustered "barrel" configuration, that the distribution of ECM molecules reflects the motif of the peripheral vibrissal array (Jhaveri et al., 1991).

The above scenario leads to specific inferences regarding the contribution of cortical elements to the manifestation of the barrel pattern:

(1) The thalamofugal afferents form the first fiber system to enter the presumptive barrelfield cortex, and are the first entities to exhibit a periphery-related pattern (Erzurumlu and Jhaveri, 1990, 1992b; Schlaggar and O'Leary, 1991). This observation fits well with previous reports that the vibrissal pattern unfolds sequentially along the trigeminal neuraxis, beginning at the periphery (Belford and Killackey, 1980), and leads to the conclusion that thalamic axons are responsible for conveying the blueprint of the peripheral pattern to the cortex. The statement is also supported by numerous earlier studies which have documented direct effects of peripheral manipulations on alterations in central patterns (Van der Loos and Woolsey, 1973; Belford and Killackey, 1980; Jeanmonod et al., 1981; Killackey and Shinder, 1981; Durham and Woolsey, 1984; Van der Loos and Welker, 1985; Welker and Van der Loos, 1986).

(2) The patterning of tegmentocortical fibers follows that of thalamocortical axons (Rhoades et al., 1990; Blue et al., 1991). The exact role of the ephemeral, patchy distribution of serotonergic afferents is not well understood. However, rats which have been administered daily doses of p-chloro-amphetamine (a potent neurotoxin selective for 5-HT containing axons) show a retardation, but not an elimination, in pattern formation by thalamic afferents (Blue et al., 1991). Thus, we hypothesize that the serotonergic axons play a trophic role, perhaps contributing to an early stabilization of the distribution of thalamic axons.

(3) A possible role for cytotactin and cytotactin binding proteoglycan, molecules which reportedly influence neurite extension (Chiquet, 1989; Wehrle & Chiquet, 1990; Lochter et al., 1991; Bartsch et al., 1992), neuronal migration (Chuong et al., 1987; Halfter et al., 1989), and glial cell distribution (Bartsch et al., 1992) has been proposed in compartmentalizing the developing cortex (Steindler et al., 1989). These compartments would set boundary conditions to subsequently direct the ingrowth and patterning of thalamic afferents and the secondary migration of nascent granule cells to form barrels (Steindler et al., 1989). Although the early schedule of pattern formation by VB axons refutes the former hypothesis, the role of the ECM molecules and the significance of their transient, patterned distribution, remains enigmatic. Several possibilities

173

can be advanced. The restricted expression of the ECM molecules along the barrel walls may serve to polarize the dendrites of granule cells inward towards the barrel centers. Alternatively, as mentioned above, the distribution of these molecules may influence the clustering of layer IV granule cells to form barrels. And finally, the possibility should be entertained that the ECM pattern, which appears to derive from a down regulation of the molecules within barrel centers, is a secondary phenomenon, resulting from the proteolytic activity (Krystosek and Seeds, 1981; Ard and Bunge, 1988; Pittman et al., 1989) of the growth cones of VB axons as they forge their way into prospective barrel centers. Ongoing experiments which involve challenging the developing barrelfield cortex with antibodies against ECM molecules (D.A. Steindler, personal communication) should further elucidate the specific contribution of these moieties in the establishment of the barrel pattern.

In conclusion, we submit that spatial ordering within fiber tracts provides a basic game plan for determining the axial framework of a topographic map. This aspect of pattern formation occurs early in development, without the directive influence of the periphery. A second stage of development involves the elaboration, positioning and differentiation of axon arbors, their target cells as well as the extracellular milieu in which they reside. It is during this second phase, while the periphery-related patterns stabilize, that their configuration is vulnerable to the influence of events occurring at the sensory periphery.

ACKNOWLEDGEMENT: This work was supported by Grant #NS27678 from the National Institutes of Health. We are grateful to Dr. G.E. Schneider for his encouragement and support during the course of these experiments.

REFERENCES

Aitken, A.R. and Törk, I., 1988, Early development of serotonin-containing neurons and pathways as seen in wholemount preparations of the fetal rat brain, J. Comp. Neurol., 274:32.
Altman, J. and Bayer, S.A., 1980a, Development of the brainstem in the rat: thymidine radiographic study of the time of origin of neurons of the lower medulla. J. Comp. Neurol., 194:1.
Altman, J. and Bayer, S.A., 1980b, Development of the brainstem in the rat: thymidine radiographic study of the time of origin of neurons of the upper medulla, excluding the vestibular and auditory nuclei. J. Comp. Neurol., 194:37.
Altman, J. and Bayer, S.A., 1980c, Development of the brainstem in the rat: thymidine radiographic study of the time of origin of neurons in the pontine region. J. Comp. Neurol., 194:905.
Altman, J. and Bayer, S.A., 1982, Development of the cranial nerve ganglia and related nuclei in the rat. Adv. Anat. Embryol. Cell Biol., 74:1.
Ard, M.D. and Bunge, R.P., 1988, Heparan sulfate proteoglycan and laminin immunoreactivity on cultured astrocytes: relationship to differentiation and neurite growth. J. Neurosci., 8:2844.
Bartsch, S., Bartsch, U., Dörries, U., Faissner, A., Weller, A., Ekblom, P. and Schachner, M., 1992, Expression of tenascin in the developing and adult cerebellar cortex. J. Neurosci., 12:736.
Bates, C.A. and Killackey, H.P., 1985, The organization of the neonatal rat's brainstem trigeminal complex and its role in the formation of central trigeminal patterns. J. Comp. Neurol., 240:265.
Belford, G.R. and Killackey, H.P., 1979, Vibrissae representation in subcortical trigeminal centers of the neonatal rat. J. Comp. Neurol., 183:305.
Belford, G.R. and Killackey, H.P., 1980, The sensitive period in the

development of the trigeminal system of the neonatal rat. J. Comp. Neurol., 193:335.

Bernardo, K.L. and Woolsey, T.A., 1987, Axonal trajectories between mouse somatosensory thalamus and cortex. J. Comp. Neurol., 258:542.

Blakemore, C. and Molnár, Z., 1990, Factors involved in the establishment of specific interconnections between thalamus and cerebral cortex. Cold Spring Harb. Symp. Quant. Biol., 55:491.

Blue, M.E., Erzurumlu, R.S. and Jhaveri, S., 1991, A comparison of pattern formation by thalamocortical and serotonergic afferents in the rat barrel field cortex. Cerebral Cortex 1:380.

Bunt, S.M. and Horder, T.J., 1983, Evidence for an orderly arrangement of optic axons within the optic nerves of the major mammalian vertebrate classes. J. Comp. Neurol., 213:94.

Catalano, S.M., Robertson, R.T. and Killackey, H.P., 1991, Early ingrowth of thalamocortical afferents to the neocortex of the prenatal rat. Proc. Natl. Acad. Sci. U.S.A., 88:2999.

Chiquet, M., 1989, Tenascin/J1/cytotactin: the potential function of hexabrachion proteins in neural development. Dev. Neurosci., 11:266.

Chuong, C.-M., Crossin, K.L. and Edelman, G.M., 1987, Sequential expression and different functions of multiple adhesion molecules during the formation of cerebellar cortical layers. J. Cell Biol., 104:331.

Cooper, N.G.F. and Steindler, D.A., 1986a, Lectins demarcate the barrel subfield in the somatosensory cortex of the early postnatal mouse. J. Comp. Neurol. 249:157.

Cooper, N.G.F. and Steindler, D.A., 1986b, Monoclonal antibody to glial fibrillary protein reveals a parcellation of individual barrels in the early postnatal mouse somatosensory cortex. Brain Res., 489:167.

Crossin, K.L., Hoffman, S., Tan, S.-S and Edelman, G.M., 1989, Cytotactin and its proteoglycan mark structural and functional boundaries in somatosensory cortex of the early postnatal mouse. Dev. Biol., 136:381.

Davies, A.M. and Lumsden, A.G.S., 1986, Fasciculation in the early mouse trigeminal nerve is not ordered in relation to the emerging pattern of whisker follicles. J. Comp. Neurol., 253:13.

Durham, D. and Woolsey, T.A., 1984, Effects of neonatal whisker lesions on mouse central trigeminal pathways. J. Comp Neurol., 223:424.

English, K.B., Burgess, P.R. and Kavka-Van Norman, D., 1980, Development of rat Merkel cells. J. Comp. Neurol., 194:475.

Erzurumlu, R.S. and Jhaveri, S., 1990, Thalamic axons confer a blueprint of the sensory periphery onto the developing rat somatosensory cortex. Dev. Brain Res., 56:229.

Erzurumlu, R.S. and Jhaveri, S., 1992a, Trigeminal ganglion cell processes are spatially ordered prior to the differentiation of the vibrissa pad. J. Neurosci., in press.

Erzurumlu, R.S. and Jhaveri, S., 1992b, Emergence of connectivity in the embryonic rat parietal cortex. Cerebral Cortex, in press.

Erzurumlu, R.S. and Killackey, H.P., 1983, Development of order in the rat trigeminal system. J. Comp. Neurol., 213:365.

Erzurumlu, R.S., Bates, C.A. and Killackey, H.P., 1980, Differential organization of thalamic projection cells in the brainstem trigeminal complex of the rat. Brain Res., 198:427.

Ferraro, A. and Barrera, S.E., 1936, Lamination of the medial lemniscus in Macaca rhesus. J. Comp. Neurol., 64:313.

Forbes, D.J. and Welt, C., 1981, Neurogenesis in the trigeminal ganglion of the albino rat: A quantitative autoradiographic study. J. Comp. Neurol., 199:133.

Gaze, R.M., 1970, "The Formation of Nerve Connections", Academic Press, NY.

Harris, W.A., 1989, Local positional cues in the neuroepithelium guide retinal axons in embryonic Xenopus brains. Nature, 339:218.

Halfter, W., Chiquet-Ehrismann, R. and Tucker, R.P., 1989, The effect of tenascin and embryonic basal lamina on the behavior and morphology of neural crest cells in vitro. Dev. Biol., 132:14.

Horder, T.J. and Martin, K.A.C., 1978, Morphogenetics as an alternative to chemospecificity in the formation of nerve connections. in, "Cell-cell recognition", v.32, Society for Exp. Biol. Symp., A.S.G. Curtis, ed., Cambridge Univ. Press, Cambridge. pp. 275.

Horton, J.C., Greenwood, M.M. and Hubel, D.H., 1979, Non-retinotopic arrangement of fibers in the cat optic nerve. Nature, 282:720.

Ivy, G.O. and Killackey, H.P, 1982, Ephemeral cellular segmentation in the thalamus of the neonatal rat. Dev. Brain Res., 2:1.

Jacobson, M., 1978, "Developmental Neurobiology", Second Edition, Plenum Press, NY.

Jeanmonod, D., Rice, F.L and Van der Loos, H., 1981, Mouse somatosensory cortex: alterations in the barrel field following receptor injury at different postnatal ages. Neuroscience, 6:1503.

Jensen, K.F. and Killackey, H.P, 1987, Terminal arbors of axons projecting to the somatosensory cortex of the adult rat. I. The normal morphology of specific thalamocortical afferents. J. Neurosci., 7:3529.

Jhaveri, S., 1973, "Altered retinal connections following partial tectal lesions in neonate hamsters." M.S. Thesis, M.I.T., Cambridge, MA.

Jhaveri, S., Erzurumlu, R.S. and Crossin, K., 1991, Barrel construction in rodent neocortex: Role of thalamic afferents versus extracellular matrix molecules. Proc. Natl. Acad. Sci. U.S.A, 88:4489.

Killackey, H.P., 1985, Intrinsic order in the developing rat trigeminal system, in: "Development, Organization, and Processing in Somatosensory Pathways," M. Rowe and W.D. Willis, eds., Liss, New York. pp. 43.

Killackey, H.P. and Belford, G.R., 1979, The formation of afferent patterns in the somatosensory cortex of the neonatal rat. J. Comp. Neurol., 183:285.

Killackey, H.P. and Shinder, A., 1981, Central correlates of peripheral pattern alterations in the trigeminal system of the rat. II. The effect of nerve section. Dev. Brain Res., 1:121.

Kristt, D.A. and Waldman, J.B., 1982, Developmental organization of acetylcholinesterase-rich inputs to somatosensory cortex of the mouse. Anat. Embryol., 164:331.

Krystosek, A. and Seeds, N.W., 1981, Plasminogen activator release at the neuronal growth cone. Science, 213:1532.

Lidov, H.G.W. and Molliver, M.E., 1982, An immunohistochemical study of serotonin development in the rat: ascending pathways and terminal fields. Brain Res. Bull., 8:389.

Lochter, A., Vaughan, L., Kaplony, A., Prochiantz, A., Schachner, M. and Faissner, A., 1991, J1/Tenascin in substrate-bound and soluble form displays contrary effects on neurite outgrowth. J. Cell Biol., 113:1159.

Lund, R.D., 1978, "Development and Plasticity of the Brain: An Introduction", Oxford Univ. Press, NY.

Ma, P.K.M. and Woolsey, T.A., 1984, Cytoarchitectonic correlates of the vibrissae in the medullary trigeminal complex of the mouse. Brain Res., 306:374.

Molnár, Z. and Blakemore, C., 1990, Relationship of corticofugal and corticopetal projections in the prenatal establishment of projections from thalamic nuclei to specific cortical areas of the rat. Proc. Physiol. Soc. (Lond.), 104P.

Pittman, R.N., Ivins, J.K. and Buettner, H.M., 1989, Neuronal plasminogen activators: cell surface binding sites and involvement in neurite outgrowth. J.Neurosci., 9:4269.

Purves, D. and Lichtman, J.W., 1985, "Principles of Neural Development", Sinauer Assoc. Press, Sunderland, MA.

Nelson, S.B. and LeVay, S., 1985, Topographic organization of the optic radiation of the cat. J. Comp. Neurol., 240:322.

Rager, G.H., 1980, Development of the retinotectal projection in the chicken. Adv. Anat. Embryol. Cell Biol., 63:1.

Reese, B.E. and Cowey, A., 1990, Fiber organization of the monkey's optic tract: I. Segregation of functionally distinct optic axons. J.Comp. Neurol., 295:385.

Rhoades, R.W., Chiaia, N.L. and MacDonald, G.J., 1990a, Topographic organization of the peripheral projections of the trigeminal ganglion in the fetal rat. Somatosens. Mot. Res., 7:67.

Rhoades, R.W., Bennett-Clark, C.A., Chiaia, N.L., White, F.A., MacDonald, G.J., Haring, J.H. and Jacquin, M.F., 1990b, Development and lesion-induced reorganization of the cortical representation of the rat's body surface as revealed by immunocytochemistry for serotonin. J. Comp. Neurol., 293:190.

Rhoades, R.W., Enfiejian, H.L., Chiaia, N.L., MacDonald, G.J., Miller, M.W., McCann, P. and Goddard, C.M., 1991, Birthdates of trigeminal ganglion cells contributing axons to the infraorbital nerve and specific vibrissal follicles in the rat. J. Comp. Neurol., 307:163.

Rice, F.L. and Van der Loos, H., 1977, Development of the barrels and barrel field in the somatosensory cortex of the mouse. J. Comp. Neurol., 171:545.

Rice, F.L., Gomez, C., Barstow, C., Burnet, A. and Sands, P., 1985, A comparative analysis of the development of the primary somatosensory cortex: interspecies similarities during barrel and lamina development. J. Comp. Neurol., 236:477.

Robertson, R.T., 1987, A morphogenic role for transiently expressed acetylcholinesterase in developing thalamocortical systems? Neurosci. Lett., 75:259.

Rusoff, A.C., 1984, Paths of axons in the visual system of perciform fish and implications of these paths for rules governing axonal growth. J. Neurosci., 4:1414.

Schlaggar, B.L. and O'Leary, D.D.M, 1991, A periphery-related pattern is evident in rat somatosensory cortex at birth. Soc. Neurosci. Abstr., 17:1126.

Schneider, G.E., 1973, Early lesions of the superior colliculus: Factors affecting the formation of abnormal retinal projections. Brain, Behav. Evol., 8:93.

Schlumpf, M., Shoemaker, W.J. and Bloom, F.E., 1980, Innervation of embryonic rat cerebral cortex by catecholamine-containing fibers. J. Comp. Neurol., 192:361.

Silver, J. and Sidman, R.L., 1980, A mechanism for the guidance and topographic patterning of retinal ganglion cell axons. J. Comp. Neurol., 189:101.

Stainier, D.Y.R. and Gilbert, W., 1991, Pioneer neurons in the mouse trigeminal sensory system. Proc. Natl. Acad. Sci. USA 87:923.

Steindler, D.A., Cooper, N.G.F., Faissner, A. and Schachner, M., 1989, Boundaries defined by adhesion molecules during development of the cerebral cortex: the J1/tenascin glycoprotein in the mouse somatosensory barrel cortical field. Dev. Biol., 131:243.

Torrealba, F., Guillery, R.W., Eysel, U., Polley, E.H. and Mason, C.A., 1982, Studies of retinal representations within the cat's optic tract. J. Comp. Neurol., 211:377.

Van der Loos, H., 1976, Barreloids in mouse somatosensory thalamus. Neurosci. Lett., 2:1.

Van der Loos, H. and Welker, E., 1985, Development and plasticity of somatosensory brain maps, in: "Development, Organization and Processing in Somatosensory Pathways," M. Rowe and W.D. Willis, eds., Liss, New York.

Van der Loos, H. and Woolsey, T.A., 1973, Somatosensory cortex: structural alterations following early injury to sense organs. Science, 179:395.

Van Exan, R.J. and Hardy, M.H., 1980, A spatial relationship between innervation and the early differentiation of vibrissa follicles in the embryonic mouse. J. Anat., 131:643.

Verney, C., Berger, B., Baulac, M., Helle, K.B. and Alvarez, C., 1984, Dopamine-β-Hydroxylase-like immunoreactivity in the fetal cerebral cortex of the rat: Noradrenergic ascending pathways and terminal fields. Int. J. Dev. Neurosci., 2:491.

Walker, A.E., 1937, Experimental anatomical studies of the topical localization within the thalamus of the chimpanzee. Proc. Kon. Ned. Akad. Wet., 40:198.

Walker, A.E. and Weaver, T.A., 1942, The topical organization and termination of the fibers of the posterior columns in Macaca mulatta. J. Comp. Neurol., 76:145.

Wallace, J.A. and Lauder, J.M., 1983, Development of the serotonergic system in the rat embryo: an immunocytochemical study. Brain Res. Bull., 10:459.

Walsh, C. and Guillery, R.W., 1985, Age-related fiber order in the optic tract of the ferret. J. Neurosci., 5:3061.

Walsh, C., Polley, E.H., Hickey, T.L. and Guillery, R.W., 1983, Generation of cat retinal ganglion cells in relation to central pathways. Nature, 302:611.

Wehrle, B. and Chiquet, M., 1990, Tenascin is accumulated along developing peripheral nerves and allows neurite outgrowth in vitro. Development, 110:401.

Welker, E. and Van der Loos, H., 1986, Quantitative correlation between barrelfield size and the sensory innervation of the whiskerpad: a comparative study in six strains of mice bred for different patterns of mystacial vibrissae. J. Neurosci., 6:3355.

Williams R.W. and Rakic, P., 1985, Dispersion of growing axons within the optic nerve of the embryonic monkey. Proc. Natl. Acad. Sci. USA., 82:3906.

Woolsey, T.A., 1989, Peripheral alterations and somatosensory development, in "Development of Sensory Systems in Mammals", J.R. Coleman, ed., John Wiley, NY. pp 462.

Woolsey, T.A. and Van der Loos, H., 1970, The structural organization of layer IV in the somatosensory region (SI) of mouse cerebral cortex. Brain Res., 17:205.

Yamakado, M and Yohro, T., 1979, Subdivision of mouse vibrissae on an embryological basis, with descriptions of variations in the number and arrangement of sinus hairs and cortical barrels in BALB/c (nu/+; nude, nu/nu) and hairless (hr/hr) strains. Am. J. Anat., 155:153.

MECHANISMS TO ESTABLISH SPECIFIC THALAMOCORTICAL CONNECTIONS IN THE DEVELOPING BRAIN

Jürgen Bolz and Magdalena Götz

Friedrich-Miescher-Labor der Max-Planck-Gesellschaft
Spemannstr. 37-39, 7400 Tübingen, Germany

The connections between the thalamus and the cerebral cortex are organized with great precision. Each sensory nucleus of the thalamus projects to a specific region of the cortex, and, in turn, receives input from the area of cortex to which it projects. Within each cortical area thalamic relay neurons contact primarily neurons located in layer 4. Over and above that, thalamic afferents form topographic connections with their cortical target cells and thereby create cortical maps, central representations of sensory sheets.

The establishment of such a precise wiring between thalamus and cortex poses several problems that must be solved during development. Growing thalamic axons have to find the correct pathway in order to reach the cortex, and they have then to select their appropriate cortical region. Once thalamic afferents arrive in their proper area, they must establish synaptic connections with their target cells in layer 4 in such a way that neighbor relationships are preserved. The development of thalamocortical connections is further complicated by the fact that thalamic axons reach the cortex before their target cells have been generated in the ventricular zone and migrated towards their final destination in the cortical plate. Thalamic fibers, however, do not invade the cortex but first grow into the subplate zone, a region situated below the cortical plate which contains the earliest generated neurons. Thalamic afferents "wait" in the subplate zone, they enter the deep cortical layers only after layer 4 cells have been generated and they arrive in layer 4 just when their target cells have reached their final position (Rakic, 1977, 1988; Shatz et al., 1988, 1990).

The development of the thalamocortical projection has been most thoroughly studied in the visual system, and a good deal is known about the sequence of events that lead to the adult pattern of connectivity. However, based on observations made in the intact animal, it is often difficult to get insights into the cellular strategies and molecular mechanisms that operate during development. This is why we have been studying the establishment of thalamocortical connections *in vitro*. Here, we will first describe a slice culture system that provides a useful model to address a number of questions pertaining to cortical development and plasticity. We will then review our *in vitro* approach to examine the developmental sequence of thalamic relationships. The main focus will be on the processes by which afferents connect with their target cells in

Development of the Central Nervous System in Vertebrates
Edited by S.C. Sharma and A.M. Goffinet, Plenum Press, New York, 1992

179

visual cortec. However, we will also present some preliminary experiments that examined the areal specificity of thalamocortical projections.

Organization and development of slice cultures from visual cortex

Slice cultures from the visual cortex of young rats were prepared using a roller culture technique (Gähwiler, 1981). These preparations survive for several months *in vitro*, and Nissl staining revealed that the cytoarchitecture is preserved in cultures prepared from animals at the day of birth (PO) up to postnatal day 11 (P11). There is almost always a sharp border between the grey matter and the underlying white matter zone, and the cortical layers are recognizable (Caeser et al., 1989; Annis et al., 1990; Behan et al., 1992). However, it is not always possible to identify the exact boundary of every cortical layer in Nissl stained cultures. Therefore, a different method was used to assess the layering of cortical slice cultures. Cells destined for the various cortical layers are born at about the same time during development. To keep track of the cells determined for a given layer, cells were labelled on their birthday by injecting time pregnant rats with bromodeoxyuridine (BrdU). Shortly after birth, slice cultures were prepared and the location of BrdU labelled cells after 1-3 weeks *in vitro* was compared with the distribution of labelled cells in littermates of the corresponding age (Götz and Bolz, 1990, 1992). As illustrated in Fig. 1, the laminar pattern of BrdU labelled cells in slice cultures is very much like the situation *in vivo*. This figure also demonstrates that most cells in layer 4, the target cells of thalamocortical projection neurons, are born at embryonic day 17 (E17). Neurons generated at E17 are located in a band in the middle of cortical slice cultures, at a similar position as *in vivo*.

In addition to the laminar organization, slice cultures are also composed of the characteristic cortical cell types. Both, pyramidal cells and different types of nonpyramidal cells with the typical morphological and neurochemical features of their *in vivo* counterparts have been identified in these preparations (Caeser et al., 1989, Götz and Bolz, 1989). At the ultrastructural level, the pattern of symmetric and asymmetric synaptic connections in slice cultures is similar to that observed in normal cortex (Wolburg and Bolz, 1991). Figure 2 illustrates some aspects of the organotypical organization of cortical slice cultures prepared from postnatal animals.

Cortical neurons are immature at birth, several of their specific properties develop postnatally. For example, in the adult animal pyramidal cells with different projection targets differ in their dendritic morphology (Katz, 1987; Hübener and Bolz, 1988; Hübener et al., 1990). This relationship between neuronal phenotype and projection target is not present their counterparts *in vivo* at the corresponding age (Bolz et al., 1991a,b). In addition to the morphological maturation, there is also evidence for neurochemical differentiation in cortical slice cultures. *In vivo*, different types of nonpyramidal cells contain neuropeptides, but it is not until 4-5 days after birth that one of these peptides, vasoactive polypeptide (VIP), is first detected immunohistochemically) in rat visual cortex (McDonald et al., 1982). In slice cultures prepared before VIP is present *in vivo,* the time course of VIP expression and the morphology of VIP-immunoreactive neurons closely matches the situation *in vivo* (Götz and Bolz, 1989).

Thus, the organotypic organization of the cortex not only remains preserved in slice cultures, the results described so far also suggest that the differentiation and maturation of cortical neurons does at least to some extend continue *in vitro*. This is an important prerequisite for studying mechanisms of neuronal development in slice cultures. However,

BrdU birthdating

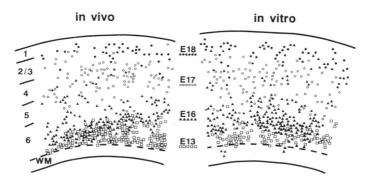

Fig. 1 Layering of cortical slice cultures determined by birthdating with BrdU. This composite drawing illustrates the distribution of BrdU immunoreactive cells *in vivo* (left) and *in vitro* (right) after BrdU injections on different embryonic days, as indicated. The dashed lines present the borders between the grey and white matter.

one has to be aware of the limitations of such preparations. In slice cultures prepared from early embryonic animals, for example, many cortical neurons do not develop their characteristic morphological features. Likewise, when slice cultures are prepared during cell migration, cells first continued to migrate, but they became arrested after about 1 week *in vitro* (Götz and Bolz, 1990, 1992). As a result, cortical layers were only formed in slice cultures from postnatal animals, whereas in embryonic slices migrating cells became scattered throughout the cortex.

Formation of thalamocortical connections in slice cultures

To examine the formation of thalamocortical connections *in vitro*, slices of visual cortex were co-cultured with slices from the lateral thalamus (Götz et al., 1990; Bolz et al., 1992). In thalamic slice cultures prepared from rats at embryonic day 16 (E16) up to postnatal day 2 (P2), as early as 2 days *in vitro* many fibers grew out of the explants. The fiber outgrowth was strongly reduced in thalamic explants taken from P3 animals, and only rarely did fibers leave explants prepared from animals after P3. The capacity of thalamic neurons in slice cultures to extend neuronal processes coincides with growth behavior of thalamic axons *in vivo*, which in rat visual cortex reach their target cells in layer 4 between P1 and P3 (Lund and Mustari, 1977).

Axons emerged from thalamic slices in all directions and grew radially away from the explants, and there was no influence of the co-cultured target tissue on the fiber outgrowth. There was neither an increased outgrowth on the side of the thalamic explant facing the cultured tissue, nor was there a directed growth of the thalamic fibers towards the cortical slice. Likewise, when thalamic explants were cultured alone, the outgrowth of thalamic fibers was about the same as in cortex-thalamus co-cultures. Thus it appears that cortical tissue *in vitro* has neither a growth-stimulating or trophic, nor an attractant or tropic effect on thalamic axons. This is different from cortical projection neurons, which are able to reorient their growing axons to innervate their co-cultured targets (Bolz et al., 1990b; Heffner et al., 1990; Novak et al., 1990; Novak and Bolz, 1992). The fact that thalamic axons are not guided by attractant cues *in vitro*, however, does not

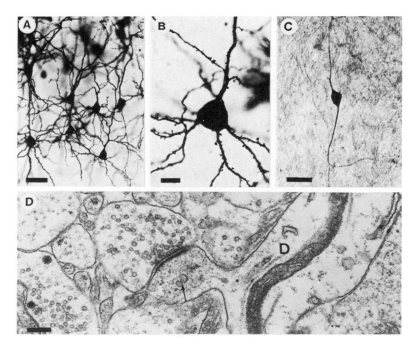

Fig. 2 Organotypic organization of cortical slice cultures. (A,B), Golgi stained pyramidal cells. (C), GABA immunoreactive non-pyramidal cell. (D), electron micrograph showing an asymmetrical synapse on a dendritic spine. The arrow points to the spine apparatus; D, dendrite. Scale bars: 200 μm in (A); 50 μm in (B), (C); 0.2 μm in (D).

exclude the possibility that such a mechanism might work *in vivo*. During development guidance factors might be released by intermediate guideposts rather than the target itself, as has been observed in the spinal cord (Tessier-Levigne et al., 1988). The internal capsule for example, the gateway between thalamus and cortex, might serve as such a guidepost for growing thalamic axons.

Thalamic axons that grew toward co-cultured cortical slices taken from postnatal animals invaded the cortical tissue, stopped in the middle of the cortical culture and often formed terminal arbors (Fig. 3A). Thalamocortical projection cells *in vitro* had the characteristic morphology of thalamic relay neurons; cells with the morphology of interneurons were present in thalamic explants, but these neurons did not project to the co-cultured cortex. When the thalamus was placed next to the pial surface of the cortical culture, thalamic fibers invaded the cortex from the pial side and again stopped in the middle of the cortical culture (Fig. 3B). In accordance with a previous study (Yamamoto et al., 1989), we found with electrophysiological techniques that thalamic axons established functional synaptic contacts in the co-cultured cortical explants (Fig. 4A). Moreover, using voltage sensitive dyes to monitor the neuronal activity over the whole cortical slice, signals with short latencies in response to stimulation in the co-cultured thalamus were recorded only in a narrow band in the middle of the cortical cultures (Fig. 4B; Götz et al., 1990; Bolz et al., 1992). These experiments

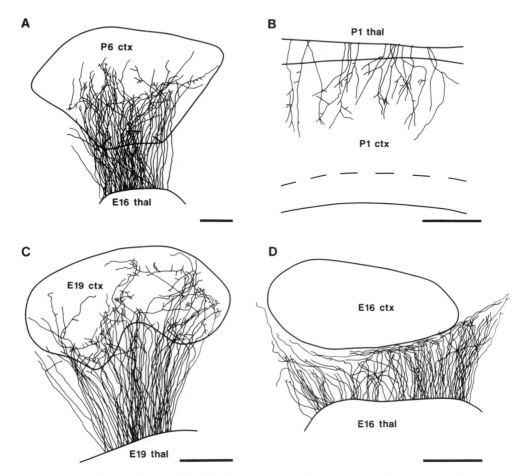

Fig. 3 Drawings of DiI labelled axons from thalamic explants (thal) co-cultured with postnatal and embryonic cortical slices (ctx). Cortical and thalamic slices were prepared at the time indicated in the figure. Scale bars: 500 μm.

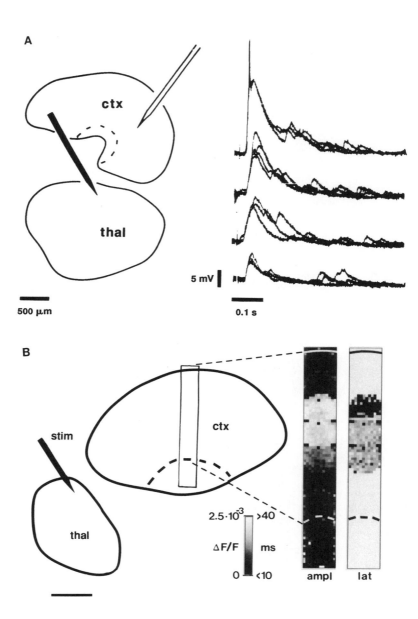

demonstrate that thalamic axons *in vitro* are able to innervate cortical slices taken from postnatal animals and to form synaptic contacts at the same laminar position, where their target cells are located. Because thalamic fibers of all ages terminated in their appropriate target layer in postnatal cortical slices, it appears that thalamic projection neurons have an intrinsic mechanisms that allows them to recognize their cortical target cells.

The pattern of thalamocortical projections *in vitro* was very different when thalamic explants were co-cultured with cortical slices prepared from animals at E19, rather than from postnatal animals (Götz et al., 1991, 1992). As mentioned in the previous section, neurons in embryonic slices that are still en route to their final position in the cortical plate stop migration after some days *in vitro*. Since cells destined for layer 4 are generated at E17, these cells have not completed their migration and became scattered throughout a cortical slice prepared at E19. In co-cultures, thalamic axons grew into E19 cortical slices, however they did not stop in the middle of such explants as in postnatal slices, but rather grew to all locations in these slices (Fig. 3C).

In view of this relationship between the position of thalamocortical afferents and their target cells in cortical slice cultures, we wished to determine where thalamic fibers would terminate if they were confronted with cortical slices where no target cells are present. For this thalamic explants were co-cultured cortical explants from E16 animals, i.e. at a time when layer 4 cells are not yet born. As illustrated in Fig. 3D, thalamic fibers did not invade an E16 cortex, regardless of whether they grew towards the ventricular of the pial surface of the cortex (Götz et al., 1991, 1992). Thus the formation of thalamocortical connections *in vitro* depends critically on the age of the cortex, but not on the age of the thalamus: thalamic fibers of all ages avoided E16 cortex, but grew into cortical explants prepared from older animals. The development of thalamocortical projections, then does not require a critical time match between axons and their target cells. Instead, the cortex seems to influence the growth of thalamic fibers irrespective of their age.

Fig. 4 Physiological recordings in cortex-thalamus co-cultures prepared from postnatal animals. (A), intracellular recordings from a cortical neuron after electrical stimulation in the thalamus with increasing stimulus intensities. At the highest stimulus intensity used a spike was elicited. In each trace 3-4 sweeps are superimposed (uppermost traces). The plot on the left shows the position of the stimulating electrode (stim) in the thalamus (thal) and the recording electrode (rec) in the co-cultured cortical slice (ctx); the dashed line marks the border between grey and white matter. (B), optical recordings from a cortical slice after electrical stimulation in the co-cultured thalamus. The recording sites were aligned in a column, running from the pial surface all the way down to the white matter of the cortical culture (open box). Optical signals were recorded with a photodiode array, the amplitudes (ampl) and latencies (lat) coated in grey levels are shown on the right. The pial surface is indicated by the continuous lines (top), the border between grey and white matter by the dashed lines (bottom). Note that optical signals were only recorded in the middle of the cortical slice cultures. Scale bar: 500 μm.

Regulation of thalamic fiber growth

The co-culture experiments demonstrated that the invasion of the cortex by thalamic axons is influenced by the age of the cortex. Which factors are responsible for these different properties of the cortex during development? Several diffusible or substrate-bound molecules have been characterized which either attract or repel growing axons (Jessel, 1988). To address the question whether substrate-bound or diffusible factors from cortical tissue affect growing thalamic fibers, cortical membranes at different stages of development were prepared and tested as substrates for fiber outgrowth (Götz et al., 1991, 1992). For this quantitative growth assay, purified cortical membranes were centrifuged onto the bottom of microwell dishes as described by Vielmetter and Stürmer (1989). When thalamic explants were placed on cortical membranes preared at P7, they were surrounded by a dense fiber network after 2-4 days *in vitro* (Fig. 5A). In contrast, thalamic explants on E16 cortical membranes showed very little, if any, fiber outgrowth (Fig. 5B). This differential effect on axonal growth was specific for thalamic fibers: cortical explants exhibited the same rate of outgrowth on embryonic and on postnatal cortical membranes (Fig. 6A). Since cortical axons are able to grow on E16 cortical membranes, embryonic cortical membranes do not prevent axonal outgrowth in general. Instead there seems to be a substrate difference between embryonic and postnatal cortical membranes which is specifically recognized by thalamic axons.

The results with this growth assay can be explained in two ways: the growth of thalamic axons may be either inhibited by molecules bound to membranes from E16 cortex, or conversely, membranes from P7 cortex may contain growth-promoting molecules for thalamic axons that are rare or absent on embryonic membranes. To address this issue, membranes prepared from E16 cortex were mixed with membranes from P7 cortex. If inhibitory molecules are associated with E16 cortical membranes, their addition should reduce the outgrowth of thalamic fibers on postnatal membranes. However, the same number of thalamic axons extended on the mixed substrate as on P7 cortical membranes alone (Fig. 6B). In other experiments, microwell dishes were coated with laminin. Thalamic fibers showed a moderate outgrowth on laminin, and the addition of E16 cortical membranes did not impair or reduce the growth of thalamic axons on laminin. However, when postnatal cortical membranes were added, the number of growing fibers exceeded the number of axons on laminin alone. These results suggest that postnatal cortical membranes possess growth-supporting molecules for thalamic axons that are not present in the early embryonic cortex. This notion was supported by additional experiments showing that trypsination had no effect on the (low) fiber outgrowth on E16 membranes, but strongly reduced the (high) rate of thalamic growth on P7 membranes, down to the level observed with embryonic membranes (Götz et al., 1991, 1992).

Developmental expression of growth-permissive molecules

The results described in the previous section indicate that the projection of thalamic axons into the cortex is guided by the differential expression of growth-supporting molecules present in cortical membrane preparations. Since almost all growth-permissive molecules known today are glycosylated, we looked at the overall glycoprotein expression during cortical development *in vivo*. To determine the distribution of glycoproteins in the cortex we used different lectins as markers (Götz et al., 1991, 1992). Figure 7 shows the pattern of peanut agglutinin (PNA) staining at different stages of development. Until E19, PNA staining was restricted to a rather narrow band in the subplate and in the intermediate zone. However, around birth the band of PNA labelling in the subplate

zone spreads into the cortical layers. Double-labelling experiments
revealed that during early development thalamic axons were precisely
restricted to those zones in the cortex where lectin-binding glycoproteins
were present, until they reach layer 4 (Fig. 7). However, once thalamic
axons arrive in their target layer, they stop and form axonal arbors,
whereas lectin staining continues to spread into the upper cortical layers
until it merges with the band labelled in the marginal zone.

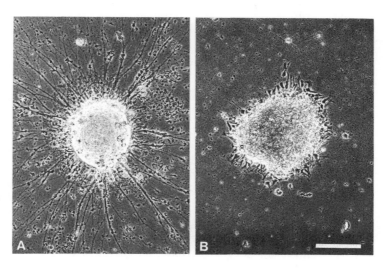

Fig. 5 Photomicrograph of thalamic explants prepared at E16 placed on
membranes prepared from (A), P7 cortex and (B), E16 cortex. Scale bar:
200 μm.

        This close relationship between the expression of lectin-labelled
glycoproteins and the growth of thalamic axons prompted us to examine the
distribution of lectin staining in cortical slice cultures. In cortical
slices prepared at B16, lectin staining was confined to two rather narrow
bands, one in the subplate zone and one in the marginal zone, at a similar
location as *in vivo*. These bands persisted throughout the whole culture
period, up to 2 weeks *in vitro*. As described above, in co-cultures almost
all thalamic axons avoided growing into E16 cortical slices, regardless of
whether thalamic fibers grew towards the white matter side or towards the
pial surface. Interestingly, however, a few thalamic fibers that
occasionally invaded the E16 cortex *in vitro* extended their axons only in
the subplate zone, the lectin-binding region. In slices from E19 cortex,
lectin staining was first restricted to the subplate deep cortical layers
and the marginal zone, but after about 1 week *in vitro* lectin labelling
was observed in all cortical layers (Götz et al., 1991, 1992). Thus
lectin-binding glycoproteins are up-regulated in E19 cortical slice
cultures, where all sources of extrinsic inputs are eliminated. As
already shown in Fig. 3C, in co-cultures, thalamic axons are able to
invade E19 cortical slices after 4-10 days *in vitro,* i.e. after lectin
binding spread in all cortical layers. Thus, as *in vivo,* the growth of
thalamic axons *in vitro* corresponds closely with the distribution of
lectin-binding molecules in slice cultures.

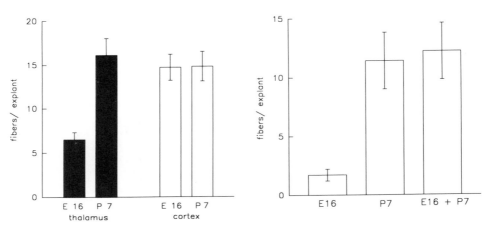

A Axonal Outgrowth on Cortical Membranes

B Thalamic Outgrowth on Cortical Membranes

Fig. 6 (A), axonal outgrowth from thalamic and cortical explants placed
on microwell dishes coated with laminin and cortical membranes prepared
from embryonic (E16) or postnatal (P7) animals. (B), outgrowth of
thalamic fibers on embryonic (E16), postnatal (P7) and mixed (E16 + P7)
cortical membranes.

Areal specificity of thalamocortical projections

The studies described so far were mainly concerned with how the
laminar specificity of the thalamocortical connections is achieved during
development, in view of the fact that there is a temporal mismatch between
the arrival of thalamic afferents near the cortex and the formation of
their cortical target layer. In most of the co-cultures prepared from
postnatal animals, thalamic slices were taken from the lateral geniculate
nucleus (LGN) while cortical slices were taken from the visual cortex.
Thus these experiments did not address the question how thalamic axons
select their appropriate cortical area. However, thalamic explants from
embryonic animals were prepared from all nuclei of the thalamus, and in
each case they established connections in layer 4 of slice cultures from
visual cortex. These findings are consistent with a study by Molnar and
Blakemore (1991), who reported that explants from LGN placed next to
explants from frontal and visual cortex innervate both cortical areas.

The areal specificity of thalamocortical projections, however, is
difficult to test in co-culture experiments. Even if explants from
different cortical areas are placed next to a given thalamic explant, an
individual thalamic axon near the inappropriate cortical region has not
much of a choice to innervate a particular cortical target, since the
appropriate cortical region might be more than 1000 growth cone diameters
away from the inappropriate cortical region. In addition, in co-cultures
it would also be difficult to see a relative preference of thalamic axons

Fig. 7 Pattern of peanut agglutinin (PNA) staining in the cortex *in vivo*
at different stages of development; (A), E17, (B), E19, (C), P7. (D),
double-staining of DiI labelled thalamic axons and PNA lectin at B19. MZ,
marginal zone; CP, cortical plate; SP, subplate; WM, white matter. Scale
bars: 100 μm.

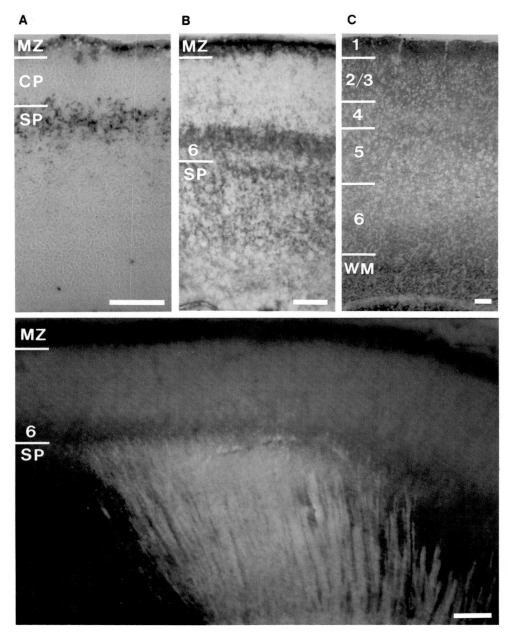

A

MZ

CP

SP

B

MZ

6
SP

C

1

2/3

4

5

6

WM

MZ

6
SP

D

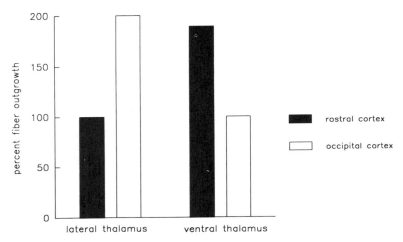

Fig. 8 Axonal outgrowth from explants of the lateral and ventral thalamus on membranes prepared from rostral and occipital cortex.

thalamic axons is an intrinsic property of the cortex. However, this by no means implies that the layer 4 neurons are themselves responsible for the developmental expression of these molecules. Since the lesion of subplate cells during early development *in vivo* also prevented thalamic fibers from innervating the cortical layers (Ghosh et al., 1990), interactions between several cortical cell types might be required for the regulation of growth-supporting moleculesb in the cortex.

It has been speculated previously that thalamic axons could fasciculate with corticothalamic axons and track along this pathway towards their appropriate cortical area (Molnar and Blakemore, 1991). In thalamus-cortex co-cultures, axons of cortical neurons often grew into thalamic explants, however thalamic fibers were never observed to fasciculate or to grow along these corticothalamic axons (Bolz et al., 1990b; Novak and Bolz, 1992). Moreover, in co-cultures with early embryonic cortical slices, thalamic fibers did not innervate the cortex even though many cells in the subplate zone of embryonic explants did project to the thalamic explants (Götz et al., 1992). Thus, the presence of a corticothalamic projection is neither necessary nor sufficient for the establishment of thalamocortical projections in vitro. This makes it unlikely that corticofugal fibers guide thalamic axons towards their appropriate target. Instead, our demonstration of a differential growth of thalamic fibers on membranes prepared form different cortical areas suggests the existence of substrate-bound guidance cues that are recognized by thalamic growth cones. It seems worth emphasizing that the preferential extension of thalamic axons on membranes from their appropriate region does not reflect the general gradients in cortical maturation from rostrocaudal and lateromedial, because axon outgrowth from explants of the LGN was higher on membranes prepared from visual (i.e. caudal) cortex than on membranes form rostral cortex. Thus differences in substrate-bound molecules between different cortical regions might be used to designate the innervation by distinct subsets of thalamic axons and thereby specify the identity of cortical areas.

REFERENCES

Annis, C.M., Edmond, J. and Robertson, R.T. (1990) A chemically-defined
    medium for organotypic slice cultures. J. Neurosci. Methods 32:63-70.
Behan, M., Kroker, A. and Bolz, J. (1991) Cortical barrel fields in
    organotypic slice cultures from rat somatosensory cortex. Neurosci.
    Lett. 133:191-194.
Bolz, J., Novak, N. and Götz, M. (1990a) Formation of efferent
    projections in organotypic slice cultures from rat visual cortex.
    Soc. Neurosci. Abstr. 16:1-128.
Bolz, J., Novak, N., Götz, M. and Bonhoeffer, T. (1990b) Formation of
    target-specific neuronal projections in organotypic slice cultures
    from rat visual cortex. Nature 346:359-362.
Bolz, J., Hübener, M., Kehrer, I. and Novak, N. (1991a) Structural
    organization and development of identified projection neurons in
    primary visual cortex. In: P. Bagnoli and W. Hodos (eds): The
    changing visual system: Maturation and aging in the central nervous
    system. New York: Plenum Press, pp. 233-246.
Bolz, J., Kehrer, I. and Novak, N. (1991b) Development of efferent
    projections in rat visual cortex in vivo and in vitro. Soc. Neurosci.
    Abstr. 17:898.
Bolz, J., Novak, N. and Staiger, V. (1992) Formation of specific afferent
    connections in organotypic slice cultures from rat visual cortex co-
    cultured with lateral geniculate nucleus. J. Neurosci. (in press).
Caeser, M., Bonhoeffer, T. and Bolz, J. (1989) Cellular organization and
    development of slice cultures from rat visual cortex. Exp. Brain Res.
    77:234-244.
Gähwiler, B.H. (1981) Organotypic monolayer cultures of nervous tissue.
    J. Neurosci. Methods 4:329-342.
Ghosh, A., Antonini, A., McConnell, S.K. and Shatz, C.J. (1990)
    Requirement for subplate neurons in the formation of thalamocortical
    connections. Nature 347:179-181.
Götz, M. and Bolz, J. (1989) Development of vasoactive intestinal
    polypeptide (VIP)-containing neurons in organotypic slice cultures
    from rat visual cortex. Neurosci. Lett. 107:6-11.
Götz, M. and Bolz, J. (1990) Formation of cortical layers in organotypic
    slice cultures of rat visual cortex. In: N. Elsner and G. Roth
    (eds): Brain - Perception - Cognition. Proceedings of the 18th
    Göttingen Neurobiology Conference. Stuttgart and New York: Georg
    Thieme Verlag, p. 282.
Götz, M., Novak, N., Staiger, V., Bonhoeffer, T. and Bolz, J. (1990)
    Formation of afferent projections in organotypic slice cultures from
    rat visual cortex. Soc. Neurosci. Abstr. 16:1128.
Götz, M., Novak, N. and Bolz, J. (1991) Development of afferent
    projections in rat visual cortex in vivo and in vitro. Soc. Neurosci.
    Abstr. 17:898.
Götz, M. and Bolz, J. (1992) Preservation and formation of cortical
    layers in slice cultures. J. Neurobiol. (in press).
Götz, M., Novak, N., Bastmeyer, M. and Bolz, J. (1992) Membrane bound
    molecules in rat cerebral cortex regulate thalamic innervation.
    Development (in press).
Heffner, C.D., Lumsden, A.G.S. and O'Leary, D.D.M. (1990) Target control
    of collateral extension and directional axon growtho in the mammalian
    brain. Science 247:217-220.
Hübener, M. and Bolz, J. (1988) Morphology of identified projection
    neurons in layer 5 of rat visual cortex. Neurosci. Lett. 94:76-81.
Hübener, M., Schwarz, C. and Bolz, J. (1990) Morphological types of
    projection neurons in layer 5 of cat visual cortex. J. Como. Neurol.
    301:655-674.
Jessell, T.M. (1988) Adhesion molecules and the hierarchy of neural
    development. Neuron 1:1-13.

Katz, L.C. (1987) Local circuitry of identified projection neurons in cat visual cortex brain slices. J. Neurosci. 7:1223-1249.

Lund, R.D. and Mustari, M.J. (1977) Development of the geniculocortical pathway in rats. J. Comp. Neurol. 173:289-306.

McDonald, J.K., Pamavelas, J.G., Karamanlidis, A.N. and Brecha, N. (1982) The morphology and distribution of peptide-containing neurons in the adult and developing visual cortex of the rat. II. Vasoactive intestinal polypeptide. J. Neurocytol. 11:825-837.

Molnar, Z. and Blakemore, C. (1991) Lack of regional specificity for connections formed between thalamus and cortex in coculture. Nature 351:475-477.

Novak, N. and Bolz, J. (1990) Target specific projection patterns in organotypic slice cultures of rat visual cortex. In: N. Elsner and G. Roth (eds): Brain - Perception Cognition. Proceeding of the 18th Göttingen Neurobiology Conference. Stuttgart and New York: Georg Thieme Verlag, p. 281.

Novak, N. and Bolz, J. (1992) Formation of specific efferent connections in organotypic slice cultures from rat visual cortex co-cultured with lateral geniculate nucleus and superior colliculus. (submitted).

Rakic, P. (1977) Prenatal development of the visual system in rhesus monkey. Phil. Trans. R. Soc. Lond. B. 278:245-260.

Rakic, P. (1988) Specification of cerebral cortical areas. Science 241:170-176.

Shatz, C.J., Chun, J.J.M. and Luskin, M.B. (1988) The role of the subplate in the development of the mammalian telencephalon. In: A. Peters and E.G. Jones (eds): Cerebral Cortex. New York: Plenum Press, pp. 35-58.

Shatz, C.J., Ghosh, A., McConnell, S.K., Allendoerfer, K.L., Friauf, E. and Antonini, A. (1990) Pioneer neurons and target selection in cerebral cortical development. Cold Spring Harbor Symp. Quant. Biol. 55:469-480.

Tessier-Lavigne, M., Placzek, M., Lumsden, A.G.S., Dodd, J. and Jessell, T.M. (1988) Chemotropic guidance of developing axons in the mammalian central nervous system. Nature 336:775-778.

Vielmetter, J. and Stuermer, C.A.O. (1989) Goldfish retinal axons respond to position-specific properties of tectal cell membranes in vitro. Neuron 2:1331-1339.

Wolburg, H. and Bolz, J. (1991) Ultrastructural organization of slice cultures from rat visual cortex. J. Neurocytol. 20:552-563.

Yamamoto, N., Kurotani, T. and Toyama, K. (1989) Neural connections between the lateral geniculate nucleus and visual cortex in vitro. Science 245:192-194.

THE REELER GENE, FORMATION OF NERVE CELL PATTERNS, AND BRAIN EVOLUTION

André M. Goffinet

Department of Physiology
FUNDP Medical School
B-5000 Namur, Belgium

SUMMARY

Reeler mutant mice are characterized by profuse anomalies of cell positioning in the telencephalic and cerebellar cortices as well as by distinct malformations in non-cortical structures such as the inferior olive, the facial nerve nucleus and other brainstem nuclei. Studies of the embryonic development of these structures reveal that the early cell patterns formed by reeler neurons is consistently affected, so that the reeler gene plays an important role in the development of nerve cell patterns.

Comparative studies of cortical development in reptiles suggest further that the mammalian type of cortical architectonics has been acquired progressively during brain evolution, and reveal some similarities in early cortical organization between reeler and reptilian, particularly chelonian, embryos, most notably the presence of an inverted gradient of cortical histogenesis. These observations point to a possible role of the reeler gene in cortical evolution.

Although the factors responsible for the formation of neural cell patterns are largely unknown, most data point to the importance of cell-cell interactions. Cell-interaction molecules have probably been acquired during brain evolution and the reeler gene could act by perturbing, directly or indirectly, such cell interactions.

The characterization and thus the cloning of the reeler gene is important for our understanding of brain development. Recent data on the fine chromosomal mapping of the mutation prior to its positional cloning are reported.

INTRODUCTION

The study of vertebrate brain development is challenging, nonetheless due to the complexity and importance of the brain. So far most of the mechanisms which govern brain development remain mysterious. Yet, it is quite obvious that a better understanding of the basic principles involved in brain development is requisite to an effective management of medical problems such as brain malformations and mental retardation.

Development of the Central Nervous System in Vertebrates
Edited by S.C. Sharma and A.M. Goffinet, Plenum Press, New York, 1992

The purpose of this paper is to show that the reeler mutation in mice defines a key step of the genetic program of brain development and evolution, thus justifying attempts to characterize the reeler gene. It Will be divided into three parts. First the reeler mutation will be presented by focusing mostly on studies of cerebellar systems. Second, comparative embryological data on cortical development in reptiles and mice will serve to introduce the reeler gene in an evolutionary perspective. Thirdly, recent progress in mapping the reeler locus will be reported.

1.   THE REELER MOUSE: A MODEL FOR DEVELOPMENTAL STUDIES

The reeler mutation is an autosomal recessive trait, first isolated by Falconer (Falconer, 1951) and mapped to the fifth chromosome. A second allele of reeler appeared in 1969 in Orléans (Guenet, personal communication). The genetic symbols are rl and rl-Orl, for the classical and the Orléans alleles, respectively. Reeler mutants have various malformations of the central nervous system (Caviness and Rakic, 1978; Goffinet, 1984; Rakic, 1985). We carried out studies on the embryonic development of the reeler nervous system, with the hope that the pathology during embryogenesis would reflect more closely the primary effect of the mutation and that comparisons of the brain malformation at various levels may help define a "common denominator" to the pleiotropic effects of the mutation. In this text, examples from studies of cerebellar systems are selected.

1.1. Cerebellar development in reeler mutant mice

The development of normal cerebellar systems is relatively well-understood. The cerebellum is thus a privileged locus for defining a possible mechanism of action of the mutation, the more so since several studies have focused on the analysis of the adult reeler cerebellum (Mariani et al., 1977; Mariani, 1982; Mikoshiba et al., 1980; Terashima et al., 1986). The mouse cerebellar anlage appears at E12 as a thickening along the rostral lip of the fourth ventricle. Before E14, the cerebellum is poorly differentiated and appears similar in normal and reeler littermates. At early stages, E14 and E15 (figure 1), the cerebellar cortex is immature and the cerebellar primordium appears nearly similar in both genotypes. An intermediate zone of radially migrating cells is found external to the ventricular zone. The contingent of neurons destined to the future central cerebellar nuclei is found at the rostromedial level of the cerebellum (Korneliussen 1968; Altman and Bayer; 1978, Goffinet, 1983, 1984). The cerebellar cortex spreads around this central mass and is composed of four concentric zones. Externally, the layer of external granule cells extends from the rhombic lip to the rostral, well-defined border of the cortex. Beneath the external granular layer lies a cell-poor marginal zone which covers the Purkinje cell layer. Purkinje cells are characteristically arranged into a multicellular array which we have named the "Purkinje cell plate" by analogy with the telencephalic cortical plate (Goffinet, 1983). The majority of Purkinje cells are generated at E12, slightly later than nuclear neurons. The morphology of embryonic Purkinje cells in Golgi and EM preparations is typical of immature bipolar neurons with a dendritic bouquet and an immature axon. In reeler embryos, Purkinje cells are not arranged into a well-defined "Purkinje cell plate" but instead are scattered at the periphery of the cortex. Despite this defective cell pattern, the various types of neurons and glia are generated at normal stages and normally differentiated (Goffinet, 1983). At late embryonic stages, from E16-E17, the cerebellar cortex grows in the

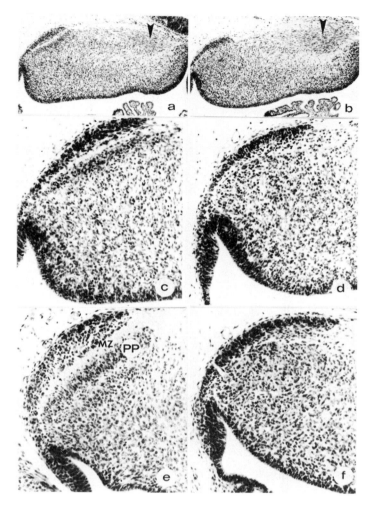

Fig. 1. Cerebellar development in normal and reeler mice. Frontal
sections in the embryonic cerebellum of normal (a,c,e) and reeler mutant
(b,d,f) mice at E14 (a-d) and E15 (e,f). In the normal embryo, the
Purkinje cell plate (PP) and incipient molecular layer (MZ) are evident at
both stage, whereas Purkinje cells fail to organize into a plate and the
MZ is poorly defined in reeler embryos. The arrowhead in a,b points to
the neurons destined to the central cerebellar nuclei.

tangential plane and begins to oberlay the mass of the central nuclei. In
parallel, the central nuclei begin to separate into their three
components. This separation proceeds normally in reeler, although the
architectonic differentiation of the dentate nucleus is not complete.
From E17, the anomaly of the reeler cerebellar cortex begins to amplify.
While the first evidence of cerebellar foliation is found in the normal
cerebellum at this stage, no such event is present in reeler. Instead,
Purkinje cells fail to become arranged into a tangential layer. Several
of them settle in ectopic positions and aggregate to form various masses.
The defect is purely one of cell patterns, and cell differentiation, by

contrast, proceeds remarkably well. The hodology of the reeler
cerebellum, particularly of olivocerebellar connections, is remarkably
preserved (Goffinet et al., 1984c; Steindler 1977; Blatt and Eisenman,
1985, 1988; Shojaeian et al., 1985). The situation is thus analogous to
that in the forebrain in that the effect of the reeler mutation can be
described as purely architectonic.

1.2. Development of the inferior olivary complex in normal and reeler mice

The embryonic development of the mouse inferior olivary complex can be
schematically divided into three stages: neuron migration, early olivary
nucleus and olivary foliation (Goffinet, 1981, 1983). Neurons destined
for the olive are generated in ventricular zones located around the fourth
ventricle, the so-called "rhombic lip". They complete their last division
at E11 and migrate tangentially along the external limiting membrane.
Some cells leave the migratory pathway to join the olivary anlage by its
lateral face; they form the deep branch of the migratory contingent.
Other cells follow the superficial pathway and enter the olive radially
from its ventral face. In the early olivary nucleus, no obvious divisions
are seen and the differentiation of olivary cells, studied by the Golgi
method and electron microscopy, proceeds similarly in normal and reeler
fetuses. However, a subtle defect in cellular arrangements is seen in
the reeler olive at E14 and E15. From E16, when neuron migration is
complete, a progressive architectonic modeling leads to the fragmentation
of the olivary mass and to the elaboration of its typical foliated shape.
This process of "olivary foliation" is markedly defective in reeler
mutants (figure 2). In the normal mouse, the olivary complex is divided
into a dorsal accessory, a principal and a medial accessory olives. Some
further divisions will not be considered here. In reeler mice, the dorsal
accessory olive is shorter and blunted. The medial accessory olive is
displaced medially and ventrally. The principal nucleus is not foliated
but appears as a "whorl" of neurons in which it is difficult to recognize
any consistent pattern. Despite the profuse architectonic anomalies, the
differentiation of individual cells, of glial cells, as well as
synaptogenesis are normal in reeler, and the topography of olivocerebellar
connections is also grossly normal in the mutant. There are, however,
subtle anomalies of olivocerebellar connectivity in reeler, such as an
abnormal persistence of multiinnervation of Purkinje cells, a feature
which is transient in normal animals but persists in the adult reeler
mouse (Mariani, 1982; Shojaeian et al., 1985; Blatt and Eisemnan, 1988).

1.3. Action of the reeler gene: role of cell-cell interactions

In addition to the well-known defect on cortical lamination and on
cerebellar systems, other targets of the reeler mutation include the
cochlear nuclei (Martin, 1981), the lateral geniculate and tectum (Derer,
Edwards, personal communications; Frost et al., 1986), the lateral
reticular nuclei, pontine nuclei, the habenula and the trigeminal complex
(Goffinet, 1984). It is thus reasonable to assume that the reeler
mutation affects the whole CNS. All the effects of the reeler gene are
consistent with the idea that the mutation acts at the end of migration,
by perturbing the early architectonic organization of postmigratory
neurons.

In other words, we are led to postulate that a specific "event"
is responsible for the early organization of nerve cell patterns in
the embryonic brain of mammals, and that this "event"

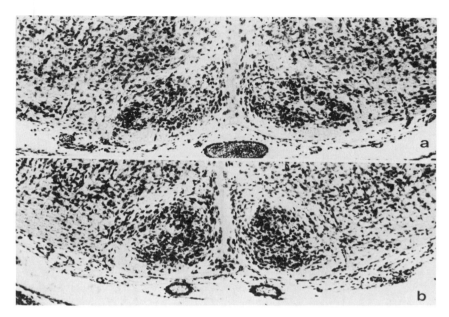

Fig. 2. Architectonics of the inferior olive in normal and reeler mice. Photomicrographs of the normal (a) and reeler (b) inferior olivary complex at a late embryonic stage (E17). Despite its abnormal foliation, the reeler olive contains a normal contingent of apparently normal cells and the relative topography of its subcomponents is preserved.

is dependent on the presence of a normal allele at the reeler locus. Several data suggest that early nerve cell patterns are not organized along morphogenetic gradients but result from an intrinsic, local property of the early neuroepithelium. Like others, we believe that the simplest hypothesis to consider is that early cell patterns result from local, intrinsic cell-cell interactions in embryonic brain tissue. The reeler gene would affect these cell-cell interactions, directly or indirectly.

There are mostly two cell types in brain tissue at an early stage, early neurons and radial neuroepithelial cells, and three types of interactions then appear particularly worth considering: neuronal-neuronal, neuronal-glial or both. Circumstantial evidence suggests that available observations are best explained by postulating homophilic interactions between immature neuronal cells at the end of migration (Goffinet, 1984b). This, however, remains to be demonstrated.

2.   COMPARATIVE EMBRYOLOGY OF THE CORTICAL PLATE

2.1. Overview of the problem

The cerebral cortex is the product of a long evolutionary process, culminating in the development of the multilaminar mammalian pallium. In all mammals studied so far, the cerebral cortex develops according to a common sequence (reviewed by Caviness and Rakic, 1978; Goffinet, 1984). As discussed above, an important event, somehow abnormal in reeler, must occur at the end of radial neuronal migration in order to "stabilize" early neural cell patterns. Although very little is known about this important morphogenetic step, the very fact that it is defective in reeler mutants suffices to show that it is submitted to a genetic control. As a corollary, the question of a possible phylogenetic control may be raised. In other terms: Is the property of radial organization in the developing cortex present in every cortex or has it been acquired during cortical evolution, independently of the appearance of the cortex itself?

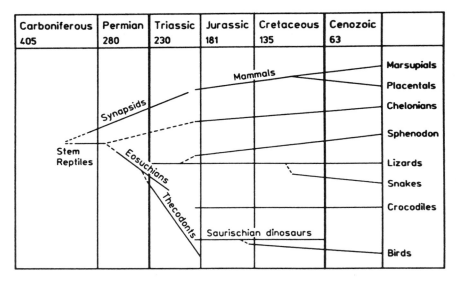

Fig. 3. Evolutionary filiations of upper vertebrates. Time in Myrs since beginning of geological period. See text for discussion.

The most elegant way to examine this question would be to compare brain development in mammals and in their reptilian ancestors. However, since mammalian ancestors are extinct, the developmental question formulated above can only be approached indirectly by comparing cortical histogenesis in the main reptilian phyla. Therefore, the results of our studies need to be understood by reference to known filiations among living reptilian groups, of which only well-established features will be considered. As a basis for discussion, we shall use the "minimal consensus" cladogram shown in figure 3. A common reptilian ancestor (probably during the Pennsylvanian) gave rise to several independent lines, four of which led to living reptiles, mammals and birds. A first branch, the synapsids, separated early and gave rise to mammals; a second branch led to chelonians, via a poorly understood lineage; a third branch led to Rhynchocephalia (of which *Sphenodon punctatus* is the only living remnant), as well as to lizards and their ophidian derivatives; the fourth branch gave rise to the crocodilians (via thecodonts) and to birds (via saurischian dinosaurs). The third and fourth branches form the diapsid lineage, the ancestors of which correspond to eosuchians. It is generally thought that chelonians (turtles) have evolved very little since the permian-triassic period and can be considered quite similar to stem reptiles, including mammalian ancestors. In order to cover the various branches of the evolutionary tree, cortical development has been examined in at least one species of turtles, squamates, crocodiles and in *Sphenodon,* and two representative species of the synapsid and squamate lineages have been analyzed in detail, using usual histological techniques, the Golgi method, electron microscopy and tritiated thymidine to determine the timing of neuronal histogenesis (Goffinet et al., 1983, 1984, 1986).

2.2. Cortical histogenesis in reptiles

It is generally admitted that the cerebral cortex (or pallium) of reptiles in composed of four divisions: the dorsomedial cortex or hippocampus, the dorsal or general cortex, the lateral or pyriform cortex, and the dorsal ventricular ridge (DVR) which will not be considered here.

For reasons mentioned above, cortical development was studied comparatively in several reptilian species belonging to the various branches of the evolutionary tree. Morphological studies at critical stages of embryonic cortical development show that important species variations are present in the degree of radial organization of the cortical plate. The architectonics of the embryonic cortex is the most primitive in turtles. In these species, the radial cytological pattern is extremely poor, either at the level of neurons or of glial cells. By contrast, all lizards have a nicely ordered cortical plate at all developmental stages. This property is best appreciated in Golgi preparations which show the radial deployment of neuronal processes as well as of radial glial fibers. The level of cortical organization in other reptilian species can be described as intermediate. For example, snakes are in this respect quite similar to lizards, whereas the crocodilian cortex is characterized by a poor architectonic pattern. In *Sphenodon,* the medial cortex is extremely well developed and organized, while the dorsal cortex is rather reminiscent of the turtle, primitive, type.

The observations demonstrate that the radial organization of the cortical plate is not a "all or nothing" property. There are various degrees of organization in the different segments of the embryonic pallium. Among living species, turtles on one hand, and lizards (and mammals) on the other hand, may be viewed as the extreme types of a spectrum of histological variations. According to the cladogram outlined above, radial cytoarchitectonics must then be regarded as a property which has been acquired gradually, independently and to variable extents after phyletic divergence. It was probably not present in the ancestral cortex of stem reptiles and has not been inherited by the different phyla from their common root. It is thus a case of homoplasy (by opposition to homology), due to evolutionary convergence. As in other cases of homoplasy, it reveals that "similar solutions to biological problems have occurred independently" (Northcutt, 1981) and presumably correspond to especially efficient solutions.

The embryological studies on the reptilian cortex have been complemented by autoradiographic analyses of neurogenesis in the cortex of a turtle (*Emys orbicularis*) and a lizard (*Lacerta trilineata*), two species selected because of their widely different types of cortical organization. The data confirm the general pattern of neurogenesis suggested by embryological studies and allow interesting comparisons between neurogenesis in mammals and reptiles, particularly regarding histogenetic gradients. In embryos injected with thymidine before the stage of neuronal generation, all cortical neurons are labeled, indicating that only precursors are present in the ventricular zones at this time. Thymidine administration later than the stages of neurogenesis results only in the labeling of glial and mesodermal cells, so that ependymal, astrocytic and satellite cells differentiate or at least continue to proliferate after the majority of the neurons are formed. In the three cortical fields (medial, dorsal and lateral cortices), neurogenesis follows a lateral to medial as well as an anterior to posterior gradients, and thus correlate with the pattern of development seen in embryological preparations of reptiles and mammals. In addition to the tangential gradients, radial histogenetic gradients are also found. In the lateral and dorsal cortices, radial histogenesis follows an outside to inside gradient. That is to say, late-generated cells settle at deeper levels in the cortex than older cells. At the level of the medial cortex, however, a difference is apparent between the primitive cortical type (turtles) and the more elaborate pattern (lizards). In turtle cortex, an outside to inside gradient is evident. By contrast, it is impossible to define any gradient in the lacertilian medial cortex.

It is worth reminding that the mammalian cortex is formed by an "inverted" histogenetic gradient (see Caviness and Rakic, 1978, for discussion). That is, younger cells traverse layers of previously established neurons to settle at progressively more superficial levels. This important property of the mammalian cortex is thus absent in reptile cortex. If the phylogenetic assumptions outlined above are acceptable, it follows that the presence of an "inverted" histogenetic gradient must be considered an acquisition, a step in the evolution of the cerebral cortex from stem reptiles to mammals (synapsid radiation). Most interestingly, in the reeler mutant mouse, histogenesis no longer follows the normal inverted gradient, but proceeds from outside to inside as it does in the primitive reptilian cortex. The data thus shows that the evolutionary acquisition of an inside to outside pattern of cortical development is contingent upon the presence of a normal gene at the reeler locus (see Goffinet, 1984 for discussion).

3.   TOWARDS THE CHARACTERIZATION OF THE REELER GENE

3.1. Introduction

       The studies summarized above point to the importance of the reeler locus during neurogenesis and brain evolution. The product of the normal allele of the *reeler* locus is unknown, so that cloning of the locus is a requisite to any understanding of the mode of action of the mutation. Although the location of *reeler* on the proximal part of chromosome 5 has been known for many years, the map of this chromosomal region remains quite imprecise. Therefore, as a first step towards establishing a genetic map of the centromeric end of chromosome 5, we assessed the localization of *reeler* relative to three markers of this region, namely the breakpoint of the translocation *T(5;12)31H*, the Pglycoprotein-1 locus (*Pgy-1*) – also called multiple drug resistance-1 (*mdr-1*) – and the engrailed-2 gene (*En-2.*). The location of *reeler* relative to nearby markers was more precisely defined by measuring recombination frequencies between *reeler*, *Pgy-1*, the sorcin locus *Sor* and *En-2*, as well as between *reeler* and *T31H* (Goffinet and Dernoncourt, 1991; Demoncourt et al., 1991).

3.2. Animal strains and crosses

       The *Orléans* allele of the *reeler* mutation is on BALB/c (C) background and noted $C-rl^{Orl}$. The original allele of *reeler* (Falconer, 1951), on C57B1/6 (B6) background, was transferred to BALB/c background by more than 10 backcrosses and the resulting congenic strain is noted C.B6-rl. The *T(5;12)31H* translocation, is a reciprocal translocation between chromosomes 5 and 12, and results into the formation of balanced carrier animals with a very long 12^5 chromosome and a very short 5^{12} chromosome. Carrier males are sterile and the translocation is maintained by mating female heterozygous carriers with normal males (Beechey et al., 1980). Carrier females also give birth to viable, sterile animals who are tertiary monosomic ($\approx 4\%$) or tertiary trisomic ($\approx 10\%$) for the small 5^{12} chromosome.

For studies of recombination between *reeler*, *Pgy-1*, *Sor* and *En-2*, backcross mice were generated as follows. Fertile homozygous rl^{Orl}/rl^{Orl} males were mated with normal C57B1/6J females, yielding F1 $rl^{Orl}/+$ offspring. 127 N2 mice were obtained by backcrossing $rl^{Orl}/+$ F1 females with homozygous rl^{Orl}/rl^{Orl} males. Recombination between reeler and the *T(5;12)31H* breakpoint was studied in another set of backcross animals obtained as follows. rl^{Orl}/rl^{Orl} males were mated with females heterozygous for the *T31H* translocation. *T31H* heterozygous F1 females, selected by karyotype analysis, were backcrossed with rl^{Orl}/rl^{Orl} males to yield N2 animals, of which 31 were available for analysis. Backcross animals were typed for the *reeler* trait by their behavior and macroscopic examination of the cerebellum. The *En-2* locus was studied with the mp2 probe (Joyner and Martin, 1987), the *Pgy-1* locus with probe pCHP-1 (Riordan et al., 1985) and the sorcin *(Sor)* locus with probe pCP7 (Van der Bliek et al., 1986).

3.3. Mapping results

The *reeler* locus is proximal to *T31H*

When crossed to mice with a normal karyotype, *T(5;12)31H/+* females produce about 4% of tertiary monosomic offspring with a chromosomal constitution of the type: $5 + 12 + 12^5$ (Beechey et al., 1980). These animals have lost the 5^{12} chromosomal segment, composed of the centromeric part of chromosome 5 and the telomeric segment of chromosome 12 distal to the breakpoint. Since the *reeler* mutation is recessive, advantage was taken from this cytogenetic peculiarity to assess whether, when mated to a *T(5;12)31H/+* female, a rl/rl male could produce or not tertiary monosomic offspring with a reeler cerebellar phenotype (rl/0 constitution). Two animals were found with the *reeler* cerebellar phenotype and were confirmed as being tertiary monosomic by karyotype of spleen cells.

Pgy-1 (Mdr-1) and *En-2* are respectively proximal and distal to the *T31H* breakpoint

In order to estimate the respective location of the *Pgy-1* and *En-2* loci relative to *T31H*, an equal amount of DNA isolated from mice who were disomic, tertiary monosomic (one dose of chromosome 5^{12}) and tertiary trisomic (three doses of 5^{12}) was dot-hybridized to the pCHP-1 and mp2 probes. A ß-actin probe was used as a control for a gene with normal dosage in all three genotypes. ß-actin and mp2 did not show any evidence of gene dosage, whereas the pCHP-1 probe for the *Pgy-1* locus clearly gave different hybridization signals with a gene-dose effect related to the diploid, tertiary haploid or tertiary triploid status of the DNA. This demonstrated that the *Pgy-1* locus is proximal, whereas the *En-2* gene is distal relative to the *T31H* translocation breakpoint.

Backcross analyses and Lenetic distances

The results of the backcross analyses are shown in tables I and II
and summarized in figure 4. Of the 127 N2 backcross mice tested, a total
of 9 recombination events were observed between reeler and *Pgy-1* and *Sor,*
while 10 recombinations occured between *reeler* and *En-2*. No recombination
between *Pgy-1* and *Sor* was observed, and the recombination between *Pgy-1*
and *Sor* on one hand, and *En-2* on the other hand were 19, the sum of
recombinants for each group separately. No double recombinant was found.
These frequencies yield distance estimates of 7.9 $\pm$ 2.4 cM between *En-2*
and *reeler,* and of 7.1 $\pm$ 2.3 cM between *Pgy-1* and *Sor,* and reeler. The
distance separating *Pgy-1* and *Sor* from *En-2* is estimated to be 15.0 $\pm$ 3.2
cM. Those recombination frequencies strongly show that *reeler* is located
in between the *Pgy-1/Sor* and the *En-2* genes, separated from these two
groups by a distance of 7 to 8 cM. Inasmuch as *reeler* and *Pgy-1* are known
to map centromeric to *En-2* (Lyon and Kirby, 1991), our results indicate
the following order: centromeric, *Pgy-1/Sor* - *reeler* - *En-2*. The strong
linkage between *Pgy-1* and *Sor* indicates that the sorcin gene lays in the
vicinity of the P-glycoprotein gene in mice as well as in hamster; this
suggests that the several genes of the hamster Multiple Drug Resistance
(*Mdr*) amplicon may be similarly linked in the mdr gene family of the mouse
(Raymond et al., 1990). The distance between reeler and *En-2* was
previously estimated indirectly to be 6 to 9 centimorgans (Hillyard et
al., 1991; Lyon and Kirby, 1991; Martin et al., 1990), in close agreement
with the present, direct estimate of ≈8 cM. On the other hand, the
present measurement of a distance of ≈7 cM between *reeler* and the *mdr*
complex suggests that the reeler locus is farther from the centromere than
the current estimate of 4 cM.

As shown in table II, no recombination was found in the 31 N2
backcross animals of the *T31H-reeler* panel. Due to difficulties in
breeding mice carrying both *reeler* and the *T(5;12)H* breakpoint, the number
of backcross animals is low. It is sufficient, however, to locate the
T31H breakpoint within 3 $\pm$ 3 cM from *reeler,* thus confirming that the *T31H*
breakpoint maps between *reeler* and *En-2* and showing that it is the closest
marker of *reeler* to date. So far as we know, however, there is no
straightforward technique to clone sequences corresponding to a
translocation breakpoint so that this marker cannot be used to approach
the *reeler* locus further.

Table I. Recombination events observed between loci in the backcross

Allelic combination	Locus				Number of Informative meioses
	Pgy-1	Sor	reeler	En-2	
Parental	C	C	rl	C	53
	B6	B6	+	B6	55
Recombinant	C	C	rl	X B6	6
	B6	B6	+	X C	4
	C	C	X +	B6	4
	B6	B6	X rl	C	5

Note: "C" and "B6" refer respectively to the *Pgy-1, Sor* and *En-2* alleles of
the BALB/c and C57BL/6 strains, respectively.

202

<u>Table II. Recombination between reeler and T31H in N2 animals</u>

brain phenotype	karyotype	
	normal	T31H/+
normal (rl/+), n=24	0	24
reeler (rl/rl), n=23	23	0

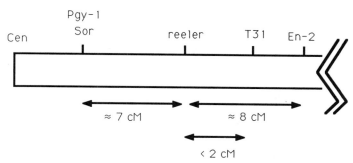

Fig. 4.   Centromeric portion of mouse chromosome 5

REFERENCES

Altman, J. and Bayer, S.A. (1978) Prenatal development of the cerebellar
    system in the rat.1. J. Comp. Neurol. 179:23-48.
Beechey, C.V., Kirk, M. and Searle, A.G. (1980) A reciprocal translocation
    induced in an oocyte and affecting fertility in male mice. Cytogenet.
    Cell Genet. 27:129-146.
Blatt, G.J. and Eisenman, L.M. (1985) A qualitative and quantitative light
    microscopic study of the inferior olivary complex of normal, reeler and
    weaver mutant mice. J. Comp. Neurol. 232:117-128.
Blatt, G.J. and Eisenman, L.M. (1988) Topographic and zonal organization of
    the olivocerebellar projection in the reeler mutant mouse. J. Comp.
    Neurol. 257:603-614.
Caviness, V.S. and Rakic, P. (1978) Mechanisms of cortical development: A
    view from mutations in mice. Ann. Rev. Neurosci. 1:297-326.
Dernoncourt, C., Ruelle, D. and Goffinet, A.M. (1991) Estimation of genetic
    distances between reeler and nearby loci on mouse chromosome 5. Genomics
    11:1167-1169.
Falconer, D.S. (1951) Two new mutants, "Trembler" and "Reeler", with
    neurological actions in the house mouse. J. Genet. 50:192-201.
Frost, D.O., Edwards, M.A., Sachs, G.M., Caviness, V.S. (1986) Retinotectal
    projection in reeler mutant mice: Relationships among axon trajectories,
    arborization patterns and cytoarchitecture. Dev. Brain Res. 28:109-120.
Goffinet, A.M. (1983) The development of the cerebellum in reeler mutant
    mice. Anat. Embryol. 168:73-86.
Goffinet, A.M. (1983) The embryonic development of the cortical plate in
    reptiles: A comparative analysis. J. Comp. Neurol. 215:437-452.
Goffinet, A.M. (1983) The embryonic development of the inferior olivary
    complex in normal and reeler mutant mice. J. Comp. Neurol. 219:10-24.
Goffinet, A.M. (1984). Abnormal development of the facial nerve nucleus in
    reeler mutant mice. J. Anat. 138:207-215.

Goffinet, A.M. (1984) Events governing the organization of postmigratory neurons. <u>Brain Res. Rev.</u> 7:261-296.

Goffinet, A.M., So, K.-F., Yamamoto, M., Edwards, M. and Caviness, V.S. (1984) Architectonic and hodological organization of the cerebellum in reeler mutant mice. <u>Brain Res.</u> 16:263-276.

Goffinet, A.M., Daumerie, Ch., Langerwerf, B., Pieau, C. (1986) H-3 thymidine autoradiographic analysis of neurogenesis in reptilian cortical structures. <u>J. Comp. Neurol.</u> 243:106-116.

Goffinet, A.M., Dernoncourt, C. (1991) Localisation of the reeler gene relative to flanking loci on mouse chromosome 5. <u>Mammalian Genome</u> 1:100-103.

Hillyard, A.L., Doolittle, D.P., Davisson, M.T. and Roderick, T.H. (1991) The locus map of the mouse. <u>Mouse Genome</u> 89:16-36.

Jenkins, N.A., Copeland, N.G., Taylor, B.A. and Lee, B.K. (1982) Organization, distribution, and stability of endogenous ecotropic reurine leukemia virus DNA sequences in chromosomes of Mus musculus. <u>J. Virol.</u> 43:26-36.

Joyner, A.L. and Martin, G.R. (1987) En-1 and En-2, two mouse genes with sequence homology to the Drosophila engrailed gene: expression during embryogenesis. <u>Genes & Dev.</u> 1:29-38.

Korneliussen, H.K. (1968) On the ontogenetic development of the cerebellum of the rat. <u>J. Hirnforsch.</u> 10:379-412.

Lyon, M.F. and Kirby, M.C. (1991) Mouse chromosome atlas. <u>Mouse Genome</u> 89:37-59.

Mariani, J. (1982) Extent of multiple innervation of Purkinje cells by climbing fibers in the olivocerebellar system of weaver, reeler and staggerer mutant mice. <u>J. Neurobiol.</u> 13:119-126.

Mariani, J., Crepel, F., Mikoshiba, K., Changeux, J.P., Sotelo, C. (1977) Anatomical, physiological and biochemical studies of the cerebellum from reeler mutant mouse. <u>Phil. Trans. Roy. Soc. (Lond.) Ser. B</u> 281:1-28.

Martin, M.R. (1981) Morphology of the cochlear nucleus of the normal and reeler mutant mouse. <u>J. Comp. Neurol.</u> 197:141-152.

Martin, G.R., Richman, M., Reinsch, S., Nadeau, J.H. and Joyner, A. (1990) Mapping of the two mouse engrailed-like genes. <u>Genomics</u> 6:302-308.

Mikoshiba, K., Nagaike, K., Koshaka, S., Takamatsu, K., Aoki, E. and Tsukada, Y. (1980) Developmental studies on the cerebellum from reeler mutant mouse in vivo and in vitro. <u>Dev. Biol.</u> 79:64-80.

Northcutt, R.G. (1981) Evolution of the telencephalon in non mammals. <u>Ann. Rev. Neurosci.</u> 4:301-350.

Rakic, P. (1971) Neuron-glia relationship during granule cell migration in developing cerebellar cortex. <u>J. Comp. Neurol.</u> 141:283-312.

Rakic, P. (1985) Contact regulation of neuronal migration. <u>In:</u> G.M. Edelman, J.P. Tiéry (Eds). The cell in contact. Wiley Intersciences, New York, pp 67-91.

Raymond, M., Rose, E., Housman, D.E. and Gros, Ph. (1990) Physical mapping, amplification, and overexpression of the mouse mdr gene family in multidrugresistant cells. <u>Mol. Cell Biol.</u> 10:1642-1651.

Riordan, J.R., Deuchars, K., Kartner, N., Alon, N., Trent, J. and Ling, V. (1985). Amplification of P-glycoprotein genes in multidrug-resistant mammalian cell lines. <u>Nature</u> 316:817-819.

Shojaeian, H., Delhaye-Bouchaud, N. and Mariani, J. (1985) Neuronal death and synapse elimination in the olivocerebellar system. <u>J. Comp. Neurol.</u> 232:309-318.

Steindler, D.A. (1977) Trigemino-cerebellar projections in normal and reeler mutant mice. <u>Neurosci. Lett.</u> 6:293-300.

Terashima, T., Inoue, K., Inoue, Y., Yokoyama, M., Mikoshiba, K. (1986) Observations on the cerebellum of normal-reeler mutant mouse chimera. <u>J. Comp. Neurol.</u> 252:264-278.

Van der Bliek, A.M., Van der Velde-Koerts, T., Ling, V. and Borst, P. (1986) Overexpression and amplification of five genes in a multidrug-resistant chinese hamster ovary cell line. <u>Mol. Cell Biol.</u> 6:1671-1678.

ANDROGEN-DEPENDENT PLASTICITY OF A NEUROMUSCULAR SYSTEM

Cecilia Cracco and Alessandro Vercelli

Department of Human Anatomy and Physiology
University of Torino, Italy

The perineal muscles and their spinal motoneurons are sexually dimorphic in adult mammals. The onset of this sexual dimorphism underlies the production of sex specific behaviors. In fact, in male rats the bulbocavernosus (BC), the ischiocavernosus (IC) and the levator ani (LA) muscles attach to the penis and participate in copulatory reflexes such as erection. In adult female rats these muscles are atrophied (Cihak et al., 1970) and made up of few muscle fibers (Tobin and Joubert, 1988). The spinal motor nuclei innervating perineal muscles in the rat are located in the lumbosacral spinal cord (Schroeder, 1980), being the homologous of Onuf's nucleus in man (Onuf, 1900). In males two distinct neuronal columns are recognizable: a dorsolateral one, generally for the IC, the external vesical sphincter and the external anal sphincter, and a dorsomedial one, for the BC and the LA muscles overall (Schroeder, 1980). In females, these motor nuclei are made up of fewer and smaller motoneurons, mostly innervating the nondimorphic anal and vesical sphincters (McKenna and Nadelhaft, 1986).

Gonadal hormones have been demonstrated to generate structural sex differences in the central nervous system, acting on neural circuits in two different modes. Early in development their "organizational" effects on differentiating pathways are permanent; later in adulthood their "activational" effects on previously organized neural circuits are transient and reversible (Gorski and Arnold, 1984). In the understanding of these processes the use of gonadal steroids as tools to perturb definite neural systems has been crucial, complemented by naturally occurring examples of "hormonal manipulation". Focusing on this sexually dimorphic neuromuscular system, for instance, the feral white-footed mouse shows androgen mediated seasonal changes both in the perineal muscle mass and morphology of their motoneurons. These changes correspond to cycles of reproductive function as a natural part of this species physiology (Forger and Breedlove, 1987).

PERINATAL DEVELOPMENT

The perineal muscles

At embryonic day 18 (E18) the blastema of the LA is similar in the two sexes (Cihak et al., 1970). Until birth perineal muscles display a

Development of the Central Nervous System in Vertebrates
Edited by S.C. Sharma and A.M. Goffinet, Plenum Press, New York, 1992

weak sexual dimorphism in terms of both number and size of muscle units (Tobin and Joubert, 1991). These data are confirmed by electrophysiological studies in newborn females still showing clear contractions in the BC on the day of birth (Rand and Breedlove, 1987). Until postnatal day 21 (P21) the LA of females shows a considerably delayed development and undergoes complete involution displaying few and thin myotubes with few myofibrils, pycnosis and regressive changes in myoblasts (Cihak et al., 1970). The result in adult females is a LA consisting of only 10% of the mean number of muscle fibers in males (Tobin and Joubert, 1988). Some authors have explained the perineal muscles atrophy in females with a perinatal increase in the total number of muscle units in males rather than with an involution of its fibers in females (Tobin and Joubert, 1991).

The neuromuscular junction

The adult pattern of single innervation contrasts with the early neonatal pattern of multiple innervation, in which muscle fibers are innervated by more than one motoneuron. During synapse elimination, multiple synaptic contacts are eliminated until the adult pattern of single innervation is established. These events, leading to the development of the adult form of neuromuscular synapses, in the androgen-sensitive LA occur later than in other muscles (P14-P28) (Jordan et al., 1988).

The spinal motor nuclei innervating the perineal muscles

Androgens are unlikely to affect the early neurogenesis of the sexually dimorphic spinal motor nucleus. In fact, bulbocavernosus motoneurons (SNB) undergo their final mitosis on E14, while testosterone production in male rats does not start until E15/E16 and does not reach different serum levels between the sexes until E18 (Breedlove et al., 1983). In fact at E18 there are no sex differences in the number of SNB motoneurons. Only later on, from the day before birth through P10, the adult sexual dimorphism in the number of SNB motoneurons is established by a differential cell death of motoneurons, normally occurring during this critical period. Females lose up 70% of their SNB motoneurons, males only about 25% (Nordeen et al., 1985). The ongoing process of perinatal sexual differentiation can also be evidentiated physiologically. Membrane current recordings from SNB motoneurons in neonatal rats showed that in females voltage-gated Ca^{++} currents are different in magnitude from males suggesting a role for high densities of sustained Ca^{++} channels in the natural cell death of these neurons (Manabe et al., 1991). After the adult range of SNB motoneurons number is reached, the maturation of their morphology is not yet complete; dendritic development requires a longer period, reaching in males exuberant length by P28 and then retracting to adult length by P49 (Goldstein et al., 1990).

EFFECTS OF EARLY HORMONAL MANIPULATION

Muscles

Following flutamide prenatal treatment and castration at birth of male rats the SNB target muscles in adulthood are absent (Breedlove and Arnold, 1983a). The androgen-insensitive rat mutant, the testicular feminized male tfm, also lack the target BC and LA (Breedlove and Arnold, 1981). Perinatal androgen treatment of female rats causes the development of a masculine number of target muscle fibers (Breedlove et al., 1982).

Neuromuscular junction

Early postnatal castration (between P7 and P20) causes a significant decrease in the level of multiply innervated muscle fibers, each of them showing a reduced number of junctional sites (Jordan et al., 1990).

Motoneurons

The spinal motoneurons innervating the perineal musculature are strongly influenced by androgen during early development. Castration of male rats at birth causes an extensive loss of the motoneurons innervating the perineal musculature and a reduced growth of the surviving ones (Breedlove and Arnold, 1981, 1983a and 1983b; Breedlove et al., 1982; Sengelaub and Arnold, 1986, 1989). Male rats prenatally treated with flutamide and castrated on the day of birth are completely sex-reversed, and display the same number and size of motoneurons as the normal females (Breedlove and Arnold, 1983a). Males castrated at P7 maintain the dendritic length typical of that day throughout their lives, instead of displaying a normal biphasic development of the dendritic arborization (Goldstein et al., 1990). All these effects are prevented by administration of exogenous testosterone. Androgen-insensitive rat mutants tfm have motoneurons feminine in both number and size (Breedlove and Arnold, 1983b). Testosterone propionate injections during the last week of gestation and from birth to P5 cause in female rats the development of masculine number and size of motoneurons (Breedlove et al., 1982; Nordeen et al., 1985).

EFFECTS OF LATE HORMONAL MANIPULATION

Muscle

Prepubertal castration causes loss of myofilaments from muscle fibers, loss of weight up to 1/3, decrease in the average diameter of the muscle fibers (Venable, 1966a and 1966b), an increase in the number of myonuclei (Galavazi and Szirmai, 1971), but no changes in the number of muscle fibers. The activities of choline acetyltrasferase (ChAT) and acetylcholinesterase (AChE) are also significantly lowered by 42% and 79% respectively (Tucek et al., 1976). The terminal AChE activity at the myotendinous junction of the IC is strong and spread, while absent in normal males (Vercelli and Cracco, 1989). Prepubertal castration also changes the pattern of adult muscle fiber types in the porcine bulbospongiosus muscle (Hughes et al., 1984). Androgen treatment of adult female rats enlarges the size of the LA without increase in the number of muscle fibers, but inducing satellite cell proliferation and increase in the number of myonuclei (Joubert and Tobin, 1989).

Neuromuscular junction

Prepubertal castration decreases the level of preterminal branching of the axons innervating the LA without affecting the level of multiple innervation (Jordan et al., 1990). Neuromuscular junctions in androgen-sensitive muscles shrink and expand as muscle fiber size is manipulated by changing testosterone levels (Vercelli and Cracco, 1989; Balice-Gordon et al., 1990).

Motoneurons

Prepubertal castration reduces the somatic and nuclear sizes of the motoneurons innervating the BC (Breedlove and Arnold, 1980) and IC muscles (Vercelli and Cracco, 1990) in the rat. Moreover some cytological

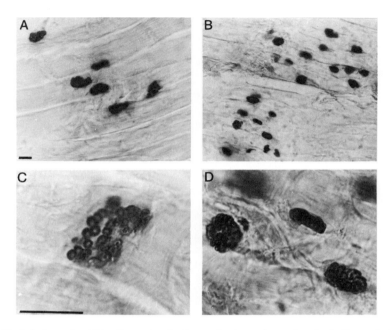

Fig. 1 – Endplates in IC of control (a and c) and castrated (b and d) rats as revealed by acetylcholinesterase reaction. Scale bars = 50 μm.

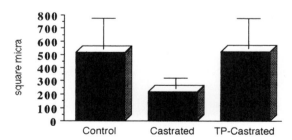

Fig.2 – Sole plate mean area in the IC of control, castrated and testosterone-treated castrated rats (bar=st.dev.).

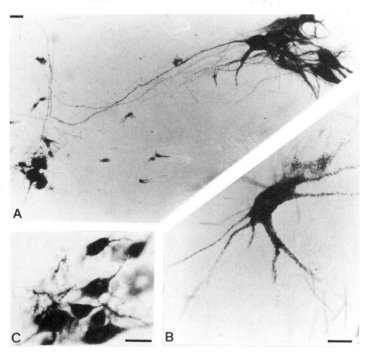

Fig. 3 – Motoneurons retrogradely labeled by HRP injection into the IC. In a, at lower magnification, motoneurons of dorsolateral (DL) and dorsomedial (DM) columns in a control rat. At higher magnification, IC motoneurons of control (b) and castrated (c) rats. Scale bars = 50 μm.

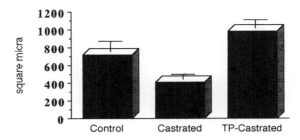

Fig. 4 – Mean somatic area of IC motoneurons in control, castrated and testosterone-treated castrated rats (bar=st.dev.).

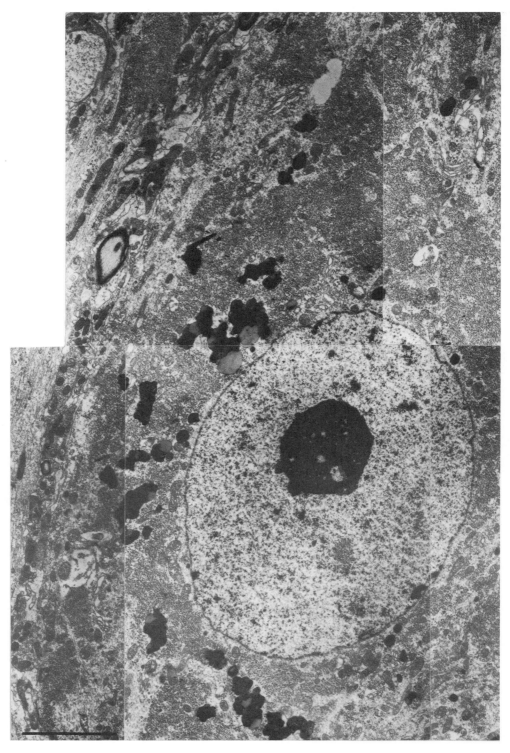

Fig. 5 - HRP labeled IC motoneuron in a control rat under electron microscopy.   Scale bar = 5 μm.

parameters vary in function of this reduction in neuronal size, and the synaptic organization as well (Cracco and Vercelli, 1991). Under electron microscopy, the reduction in neuronal size is accompanied by a uniform percent reduction of the cytoplasmic organules in the IC motoneurons of the rat (Cracco and Vercelli, 1991). Castration also induces a decrease in the percentage of somatic membrane covered by synapses both in BC (Matsumoto et al., 1988a) and IC (Cracco and Vercelli, 1991) motoneurons. This finding means that the loss of synapses is even greater than the reduction in somatic membrane area, that is the membrane available for synaptic contact. The amount of synaptic input to SNB motoneurons of prepubertally castrated rats is increased following even short-term testosterone treatment (within 48 hours), despite the lack of an increase in somatic area (Leedy et al., 1987). Androgens also regulate the expression of gap junction gene in BC motoneurons (Matsumoto et al., 1991) and therefore their number and diameter (Matsumoto et al., 1988b). It is not clear, at present, whether castration affects a particular type of connection or all of them.

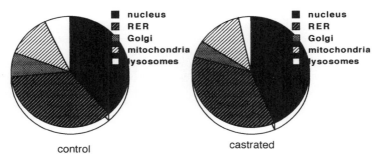

Fig. 6 - Mean percentage of somatic cross-sectional area occupied by different organules in 15 control and 15 castrated IC motoneurons.

The reduction in number and size of axosomatic synapses could be irrelevant, since it is known that 99% of synapses on a motoneuron are on its dendrites. However, it is conceivable that the same reduction occurs for axodendritic synapses and testosterone is known to affect strongly dendritic morphology. In fact, hormonal deprivation modifies the dendritic arborization of the BC motoneurons of the rat (Kurz et al., 1986). If castration is performed at P7, the dendritic arborization cess to grow, while after later castration (P28) it grows normally until P49 and shows a reduction, if compared to control animals, at P70 (Goldstein et al., 1990).

All these morphological changes have physiological consequences. Even though the passive properties of bulbospongiosus motoneurons seem to be unaffected by castration (Collins, 1991), there is evidence that androgens modulate to some extent the excitability of BC motoneurons involved in the pudendo-pudendal reflex (Tanaka and Arnold, 1991).

COMMENTS

The spinal motoneurons and their target perineal muscles are influenced both in their development and trophism in adulthood by androgens. Androgens act on fundamental ontogenetic processes, involving both progressive and regressive events. Their influence can be considered as continuous on series of discrete even though interconnected events, which may be modified by androgen manipulation at different ages.

Androgens influence prenatally the masculinization of the motoneuron number in a permanent way, without affecting their early neurogenesis, but above all regulating the entity of their naturally occurring cell death (Breedlove and Arnold, 1980). Nowadays, the strong correlation between number of neurons that survive the period of naturally occurring death and size of their target organ during development is widely accepted (Holliday and Hamburger, 1976). Developing motoneurons might compete for a target-derived trophic factor, and possibly only those obtaining sufficient amounts of the substance are able to survive (Hamburger and Levi Montalcini, 1949; Oppenheim, 1989). The same explanation might fit easily, if we accept the myogenic origin of the hormone sensitivity within this neuromuscular system. In this view, androgens could address the development of the muscle towards defined, sex-linked characteristics: subsequently, the resulting reduced size of the peripheral target in females could exacerbate neuronal death through lower levels of target-derived trophic factors (Tanaka and Landmesser, 1986).

Androgens still influence motoneuronal size and dendritic length later on, when their adult number is already established. These data confirm that the target organ continues to be important for the survival and maintenance of motoneurons, even after embryogenesis is complete (Lee Crews and Wigston, 1990), and that the size of motoneuron soma in adulthood correlates with the size of its motor unit (Henneman, 1985). Since the adult size of motor units develops during synapse elimination, it is possible that this relationship emerges exactly during that period. Once again, in fact, androgens play a role during synapse elimination and interfere in the maturation of neuromuscular endplates, by acting on the degree of multiple innervation of muscle fibers. They are also involved in the regulation of the size of the neuromuscular junctions (Vercelli and Cracco, 1989), which is known to be directly coupled to myofiber size (Balice-Gordon et al., 1990), and to the amount of neurotransmitters released at this site (Balice-Gordon and Lichtmann, 1990).

Androgens are involved in establishing the dimorphic characteristics of the target muscle, acting on myofiber number, size and histochemical pattern through different periods (Venable, 1966a and 1966b; Cihak et al., 1970; Hughes et al., 19821; Joubert and Tobin, 1989; Tobin and Joubert, 1988, 1991).

Now, the most puzzling problem does not lie in the understanding of these events, i.e. the mechanisms by which androgens effectively act on neuromuscular development and sexual differentiation, events which are essentially of the same kind as those occurring in other neural systems. We need to know which is the primary site of androgen actions, i.e. to explain the mechanisms adopted to activate the described events. The crucial role of sex hormones is indeed allowed by the interactions of androgens with their receptors. In fact, genetic XY rats affected by the androgen-receptor defect tfm have a totally feminine SNB system, despite high levels of endogenous androgens (Breedlove and Arnold, 1981).

Androgen-binding factors have been identified in the perineal muscles of neonatal male rats (by the second day of birth they display an adult array of androgen receptors), while there is no evidence that neonatal spinal motoneurons accumulate androgens (Fishman et al., 1990). Over 80% of SNB motoneurons develop the capacity to accumulate androgen

212

during the second week after birth, when also the period of synapse elimination begins (Fishman et al., 1990). In adult male rats androgen receptors have been demonstrated in both SNB motoneurons via autoradiography (Breedlove and Arnold, 1980) and in BC/LA muscles via binding assays (Krieg and Voight, 1977). About 3/4 of SNB motoneurons in adult males bind exogenous testosterone, whereas only about 1/3 do so in adult females, and very little binding occurs elsewhere in the spinal cord (Breedlove and Arnold, 1980).

The data suggest that the perineal muscles are the primary target for the androgenic masculinization of the whole neuromuscular system. Supraspinal influences in adulthood have been ruled out by transection experiments (Fishman and Breedlove, 1985). Nevertheless during development some major descending spinal tracts develop coincident with neuromuscular synapse elimination in LA, and therefore androgens might also regulate afferent inputs to SNB during that period; in any case, the importance of primary afferents in the normal development of spinal motor nuclei is also known (Okado and Oppenheim, 1984). Many results support the hypothesis of a myogenic origin of androgen action.
- When the dorsal pudendal nerve branch, innervating LA, BC and external anal sphincter, is cut and sewed on a grafted soleus muscle, castration and testosterone treatment do not affect the SNB motoneurons (Araki et al., 1991).
- Perineal muscles cross-reinnervated by a branch of sciatic nerve show atrophy after castration and hypertrophy after testosterone treatment (Hanzlikova and Gutmann, 1972).
- The wet weight of the soleus muscle reinnervated by SNB motoneurons is unaffected by castration or testosterone treatment (Hanzlikova and Gutmann, 1974).
- Androgen can spare the perineal muscles of newborn females even when the entire lumbosacral spinal cord has been removed (Fishman and Breedlove, 1988).
- Local implantation of flutamide into BC of newborn females blocks the sparing effects of androgens more effectively than the same administered systemically (Fishman and Breedlove, 1987).

The androgen action on the muscle might then be followed by a retrograde influence on motoneurons through trophic factors, as already mentioned. Although, at present, it is not known whether trophic influences from perineal muscles may also be regulated by the mechanical activity of the muscle, in addition to testosterone (Araki et al., 1991), as normally occurring in other striated muscles (Filogamo and Robecchi, 1985), or via dorsal root influences (Mills and Sengelaub, 1991).

Thus, sex hormones are a powerful tool in studying basic processes such as naturally occurring neuronal death, target dependence of motoneuron survival, and neuromuscular interrelationships.

ACKNOWLEDGEMENTS

This work was supported by Italian C.N.R. (National Research Council) and M.U.R.S.T. grants to Prof. G. Filogamo. We are grateful to Dr. P. Chandler for linguistic revision.

REFERENCES

Araki, I., Harada, Y., and Kuno, M. (1991) Target-dependent Hormonal Control of Neuron Size in the Rat Spinal Nucleus of the Bulbocavernosus. J. Neurosci. 11:3025.

Balice-Gordon, R.J., Breedlove, S.M., Bernstein, S., and Lichtman, J.W. (1990) Neuromuscular Junctions Shrink and Expand as Muscle Fiber Size is Manipulated, in vivo Observations in the Androgen-sensitive Bulbocavernosus Muscle of Mice. J. Neurosci. 10:2660.

Balice-Gordon, R.J., and Lichtman, J.W. (1990) In vivo Visualization of the Growth of Pre- and Postsynaptic Elements of Neuromuscular Junctions in the Mouse. J. Neurosci. 10:894.

Breedlove, S.M. (1985) Hormonal Control of the Anatomical Specificity of Motoneuron-to-Muscle Innervation in Rats. Science 227:1357.

Breedlove, S.M., and Arnold, A.P. (1980) Hormone Accumulation in a Sexually Dimorphic Motor Nucleus of the Rat Spinal Cord. Science 210:564.

Breedlove, S.M., and Arnold, A.P. (1981) Sexually Dimorphic Motor Nucleus in the Rat Lumbar Spinal Cord: Response to Adult Hormone Manipulation, Absence in Androgen-insensitive Rats. Brain Res. 225:297.

Breedlove, S.M., and Arnold, A.P. (1983a) Hormonal Control of a Developing Neuromuscular System: 1. Complete Demasculinization of the Male Rat Spinal Nucleus of the Bulbocavernosus Using the Anti-androgen Flutamide. J. Neurosci. 3:417.

Breedlove, S.M., and Arnold, A.P. (1983b) Hormonal Control of a Developing Neuromuscular System: 11. Sensitive Periods for the Androgen-induced Masculinization of the Rat Spinal Nucleus of the Bulbocavernosus. J. Neurosci. 3:424.

Breedlove, S.M., Jacobson, C.D., Gorski, R.A., and Arnold, A.P. (1982) Masculinization of the Female Rat Spinal Cord Following a Single Neonatal Injection of Testosterone Propionate but not Estradiol Benzoate. Brain Res. 237:173.

Breedlove, S.M., Jordan, C.L., and Arnold, A.P. (1983) Neurogenesis of Motoneurons in the Sexually Dimorphic Spinal Nucleus of the Bulbocavernosus in Rats. Devl. Brain Res. 9:39.

Cihak, R., Gutmann, E., and Hanzlikova, V. (1970) Involution and Hormone-induced Persistence of m. Sphincter (Levator) Ani in Female Rats. J. Anat. 106:93.

Collins, W.F. (1991) Passive Electrical Properties of Bulbospongiosus Motoneurons in Gonadally Intact and Castrated Adult Male Rats. Soc. Neurosci. Abstr. 16:1060.

Cracco, C., and Vercelli A. (1991) Hormone-dependent Plasticity of the Motoneurons of the Ischiocavernosus Muscle: An Ultrastructural Study. In: Plasticity and Regeneration of the Nervous System, P.S. Timiras, A. Privat, E. Giacobini, J. Lauder and A. Vernadakis, eds Plenum Press, New York.

Filogamo, G., and Robecchi, M.G. (1985) La tension mécanique régle le développement des ébouches musculaires. Bull. Ass. Anat. 69:241.

Fishman, R.B., and Breedlove, S.M. (1985) The Androgenic Induction of Spinal Sexual Dimorphism is Independent of Supraspinal Afferents. Devl. Brain Res. 23:255.

Fishman, R.B., and Breedlove, S.M. (1987) Androgen Blockade of Bulbocavernosus Muscle Inhibit Testosterone-dependent Masculinization of Spinal Motoneurons in Newborn Female Rats. Soc. Neurosci. Abstr. 13:1520.

Fishman, R.B., and Breedlove, S.M. (1988) Neonatal Androgen Maintains Sexually Dimorphic Muscles in the Absence of Innervation. Muscle and Nerve 11:553.

Fishman, R.B., Chism, L., Firestone, G.L., and Breedlove, S.M. (1990) Evidence for Androgen Receptors in Sexually Dimorphic Perineal Muscles of Neonatal Male Rats. J. Neurobiol. 21:694.

Forger, N.G., and Breedlove, S.M. (1987) Seasonal Variation in Mammalian Striated Muscle Mass and Motoneuron Morphology. J. Neurobiol. 18:155.

Galavazi, G., and Szirmai, J.A. (1971) Cytomorphometry of Skeletal

Muscle: The Influence of Age and Testosterone on the Rat m. Levator Ani. Z. Zellforsch. 121:507.

Goldstein, L.A., Kurz, E.M., and Sengelaub, D.R. (1990) Androgen Regulation of Dendritic Growth and Retraction in the Development of a Sexually Dimorphic Spinal Nucleus. J. Neurosci. 10:935.

Gorski, R. and Arnold, A.P. (1984) Gonadal Steroid Induction of Structural Sex Differences in the Central Nervous System. Ann. Rev. Neurosci. 7:413.

Hamburger, V., and Levi-Montalcini, R. (1949) Proliferation, Differentiation and Degeneration in the Spinal Ganglia of the Chick Embryo under Normal and Experimental Conditions. J. Exp. Zool. 111:457.

Hanzlikova, V., and Gutmann, E. (1972) Effect of Foreign Innervation on the Androgen-sensitive Levator Ani Muscle of the Rat, Z. Zelfforsch. 135:165.

Hanzlikova, V., and Gutmann, E. (1974) The Absence of Androgen Sensitivity in the Grafted Soleus Muscle Innervated by the Pudendal Nerve. Cell Tissue Res. 154: 121.

Henneman, E., Somjen, G., and Carpenter, D.O. (1965) Functional Significance of Cell Size in Spinal Motoneurons. J. Neurophysiol. 28:560.

Holliday, M., and Hamburger, V. (1976) Reduction of the Naturally Occurring Motor Neuron Loss by Enlargement of the Periphery. J. Comp. Neurol. 170:311.

Hughes, B.J., Bowen, J.M., Campion, D.R., and Bradley, W.E. (1982) Effect of Prepubertal Castration on Porcine Bulbospongiosus Muscle. Anat. Embryol. 168:51.

Jordan, C.L., Letinski, M.S., and Arnold, A.P. (1988) Synapse Elimination Occurs Late in the Hormone-sensitive Levator Ani Muscle of the Rat. J. Neurobiol. 19:335.

Jordan, C.L., Letinski, M.S., and Arnold, A.P. (1990) Critical Period for the Androgenic Block of Neuromuscular Synapse Elimination. J. Neurobiol. 21:760.

Joubert, Y., and Tobin C. (1989) Satellite Cell Proliferation and Increase in the Number of Myonuclei Induced by Testosterone in the Levator Ani Muscle of the Adult Female Rat. Devl. Biol. 131:550.

Krieg, M., and Voght, K.D. (1977) Biochemical Substrate of Androgenic Actions at a Cellular Level in Prostate, Bulbocavernosus and Levator Ani and in Skeletal Muscles. Acta Endocrinol. 85 (Suppl. 214):43.

Kurz, E.M., Sengelaub, D.R., and Arnold, A.P. (1986) Androgen Regulate the Dendritic Length of Mammalian Motoneurons in Adulthood. Science 232:395.

Lee Crews, L., and Wigston, D.J. (1990) The Dependence of Motoneurons on their Target Muscle during Postnatal Development of the Mouse. J. Neurosci. 10:1643.

Leedy, M.G., Beattie M.S., and Bresnahan, J.C. (1987) Testosterone-induced Plasticity of Synaptic Inputs to Adult Mammalian Motoneurons. Brain Res. 424:386.

Manabe, T., Araki, I., Takahashi, T., and Kuno, M. (1991) Membrane Currents Recorded from Sexually Dimorphic Motoneurones of the Bulbocavernosus Muscle in Neonatal Rats. J. Physiol. 440:419.

Matsumoto, A., Micevych, P.E., and Arnold, A.P. (1988a) Androgen Synaptic Input to Motoneurons of the Adult Rat Spinal Cord. J. Neurosci. 8:4158.

Matsumoto, A., Arnold, A.P., Zampighi, G.A., and Mycevych, P.E. (1988b) Androgenic Regulation of Gap Junctions Between Motoneurons in the Rat Spinal Cord. J. Neurosci. 8:4177.

Matsumoto, A., Arai, Y., Urano, A., and Hyodo, S. (1991) Androgen Regulates Gap Junction mRNA Expression in the Motoneurons of Lumbar Spinal Cords in Adult Male Rats. Soc. Neurosci. Abstr. 17:1319.

McKenna, K., and Nadelhaft, I. (1986) The Organization of Pudendal Nerve in the Male and Female Rat. J. Comp. Neurol. 248:532.

Mills, A., and Sengelaub, D.R. (1991) Development of Neuronal Number in Primary Afferents of a Sexually Dimorphic Neuromuscular System is Androgen-dependent. Soc. Neurosci. Abstr. 16:1318.

Nordeen, E.J., Nordeen, K.W., Sengelaub, D.R., and Arnold, A.P. (1985) Androgens Prevent Normally Occurring Cell Death in a Sexually Dimorphic Spinal Nucleus. Science 229:671.

Okado, N., and Oppenheim, R.W. (1984) Cell Death of Motoneurons in the Chick Embryo Spinal Cord: IX. The Loss of Motoneurons Following Removal of Afferent Inputs. J. Neurosci. 4:1639.

Onuf, B. (1900) On the Arrangement and Function of the Cell Groups in the Sacral Region of the Spinal Cord. Arch. Neurol. Psychopathol. 3:387.

Oppenheim, R.W. (1991) Cell Death during Development of the Nervous System. Annu. Rev. Neurosci. 14:453.

Rand, M.N., and Breedlove, S.M. (1987) Ontogeny of Funtional Innervation of Bulbocavernosus Muscles in Male and Female Rats. Devl. Brain Res. 33:150.

Schroeder, H.D. (1980) Organization of the Motoneurons Innervating the Pelvic Muscles of the Male Rat. J. Comp. Neurol. 192:567.

Sengelaub, D.R., and Arnold, A.P. (1986) Development and Loss of Early Projections in a Sexually Dimorphic Rat Spinal Nucleus. J. Neurosci. 6:1613.

Sengelaub, D.R., and Arnold, A.P. (1989) Hormonal Control of Neuron Number in Sexually Dimorphic Spinal Nuclei of the Rat: 1. Testosterone-regulated Death in the Dorsolateral Nucleus. J. Comp. Neurol. 280-622.

Tanaka, H., and Landmesser, L.T. (1986) Cell Death of Lumbosacral Motoneurons in Chick, Quail and Chick-Quail Chimera Embryos: A Test of the Quantitative Matching Hypothesis of Neuronal Cell Death. J. Neurosci. 6:2889.

Tanaka, J., and Arnold, A.P. (1991) Androgenic Modulation of the Excitability of Lumbar Neurons in the Rat Bulbocavernosus Reflex. Soc. Neurosci. Abstr. 17:1319.

Tobin, C., and Joubert, Y. (1988) The Levator Ani of the Female Rat: A Suitable Model for Studying the Effects of Testosterone on the Development of Mammalian Muscles. Biol. Struct. Morphog. 1:28.

Tobin, C., and Joubert, Y. (1991) Testosterone-induced Development of the Rat Levator Ani Muscle. Devl. Biol. 146:131.

Tucek, S., Kostirova, D., and Gutman, E. (1976) Testosterone-induced Changes of ChAT and ChE Activities in the Rat Levator Ani Muscle. J. Neurol. Sci. 27:353.

Venable, J.H. (1966a) Constant Cell Populations in Normal, Testosterone-deprived and Testosterone-stimulated Levator Ani Muscle. Am. J. Anat. 119:263.

Venable, J.H. (1966b) Morphology of Cells of Normal, Testosterone-deprived and Testosterone-stimulated Levator Ani Muscles. Am. J. Anat. 119:271.

Vercelli, A., and Cracco, C. (1989) Influence of Testosterone on the Development of the Ischiocavernosus Muscle of the Rat. Acta Anat. 134:177.

Vercelli, A., and Cracco, C. (1990) Effects of Prepubertal Castration on the Spinal Motor Nucleus of the Ischiocavernosus Muscle of the Rat. Cell Tissue Res. 262:551.

DEVELOPMENT OF LONGITUDINAL PATTERNS IN THE CEREBELLAR CORTEX

Jan Voogd* and Rita M. Kappel

*Department of Anatomy
Erasmus University Rotterdam and
**Dept. of Plastic Surgery
Hospital Sophia, Zwolle, The Netherlands

SUMMARY

Cerebellar Purkinje cells in the adult are arranged in longitudinal zones which differ in their connections and their biochemical properties. During early development this zonal pattern is preceded by a clustering of Purkinje cells. The topographical relationship of these clusters to the cerebellar and vestibular nuclei is similar to the cortico-nuclear relations of the adult zones. Both the adult and the embryological pattern can be considered the result of the interdigitation of two sets of Purkinje cells with different connections.

It has become increasingly clear that the Purkinje cells of the cerebellar cortex are arranged in a series of parallel longitudinal zones which differ in their efferent, corticonuclear and afferent, climbing fiber connections and in their biochemical properties. Originally this zonal pattern was recognized from the clustering of the Purkinje cell axons and the olivocerebellar climbing fiber afferents in discrete compartments of the white matter[16,17]. These compartments can be visualized with the Häggqvist myelin stain and with staining for acetylcholinesterase (AChE, Fig. 1K). The borders between the compartments contain a higher concentration of thin fibers which stain rather strongly for AChE[4,22]. There is no explanation for the preferential staining of these fibers for AChE. Cholinergic transmission is limited to certain mossy fiber systems and is not distributed in this pattern[6].

The connections of the different Purkinje cell zones are known in some detail. The diagram of Fig. 1A,C,F illustrates the principle that Purkinje cells which establish efferent connections with the rostral fastigial, the lateral vestibular, the anterior interposed (i.e. emboliform) and the rostral dentate nucleus, alternate with zones where the Purkinje cells project to the caudal fastigial and posterior interposed (globose) nuclei. These two sets of zones receive their climbing fibers from the dorsal accessory olive with the dorsal leaf of the principal olive and from the ventral leaf and the medial accessory olive respectively[19,22]. The interdigitation of two sets of Purkinje cells with different connections therefore, seems to be the most simple way to describe this pattern (Fig. 1B,D,E).

Development of the Central Nervous System in Vertebrates
Edited by S.C. Sharma and A.M. Goffinet, Plenum Press, New York, 1992

It should be appreciated that the zonal organization of the cerebellum is a highly constant one in different mammalian species. This has been well documented for the zonation of the anterior vermis. Purkinje cells with projections to the vestibular nuclei are located in two strips. One occupies the lateral part of the vermis and corresponds to the B zone projecting to Deiters' nucleus, the other is situated along the lateral border of the A-zone. The latter (A2) zone projects both to the fastigial nucleus and the medial vestibular nucleus. The B and A2 zones are separated by the wedge-shaped X zone which contains Purkinje cells projecting to the fastigial and posterior interposed nuclei[18]. The same intricate pattern is found in different mammals[21], including rodents (Fig. 1J) and primates (Fig. 1I).

The distribution of several enzymes, receptors and Purkinje cell-specific markers in the cerebellar molecular layer follows a zonal pattern. One group of these substances is present at the midline and in six or seven parasagittal strips. These substances have been mainly studied in rodents. They include the enzyme 5'-nucleotidase[14] which is present in Purkinje cell dendrites" and/or radial fibers of Bergmann glia[3]. A monoclonal antibody directed against a Purkinje cell specific protein (mabQ113 or antizebrin[2] is limited to a population of Purkinje cells, where it is expressed by the entire neuron, including dendrites and axon. The zonal pattern of zebrin-positive Purkinje cells exactly corresponds to the distribution of 5'-nucleotidase[1]. Other monoclonal antibodies, such as 192 IgG specific for the rat nerve growth factor receptor, display the same compartmentalization[15].

Fig. 1 The zonal organization of the Purkinje cells is depicted in a diagram of the flattened cerebellar cortex (A,B), with their projections to the cerebellar nuclei (C,D) and the origin of their climbing fiber afferents from the inferior olive (E,F). In (G,H) the projection method for the diagram of the inferior olive is illustrated. In A,C and F the corticonuclear and crossed olivocerebellar connections are indicated[18-23]. This pattern can be summerized the result of an interdigitation of two sets of Purkinje cell zones with different connections (B,D,E).
I,J: diagrams of the anterior lobe of monkey and rat showing the localization of Purkinje cells of the A2 and B zones retrogradely labelled from the vestibular nuclei[21].
K: compartments in the white matter of the cerebellum of a monkey stained with acetylcholinesterase. Bar represents 1 mm.
L: Purkinje cells of the A and B zones in right half of anterior vermis, retrogradely labeled with weatgerm-coupled horeseradish peroxidase (WGA-HRP) from the vestibular nuclei in the rat. Dark field. Bar represents 200 μm.
M: The WGA-HRP-labelled Purkinje cells of the A and B zones in adjacent section from Fig. 1L, alternate with immunolabelled, zebrin-positive Purkinje cells at the midline and at the site of the X zone. Zebrin-immunoreactive cells can be recognized by the staining of their dendrites. Bar represents 200 μm.
abbreviations: A-B=zones A-B; beta=group beta; DAO=dorsal accessory olive; dc=dorsal cap; dl=dorsal leaf; dmcc= dorsomedial cell column; F= fastigial nucleus; IA=anterior interposed nucleus; IP=posterior interposed nucleus; m=midline; MAO=medial accessory olive; PO=principal olive; VII-X=lobules VII-X; vl=ventral leaf, vlo=ventrolateral outgrowth.

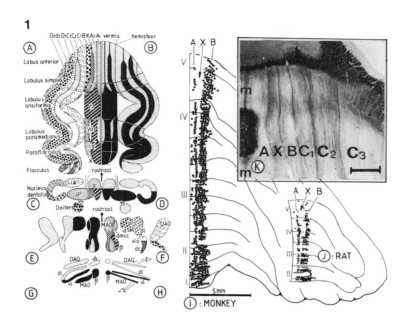

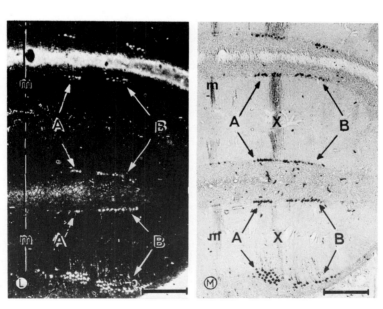

A precise correspondence has been established between the neurochemical and the projection maps in the anterior vermis[18,20]. Purkinje cells with projections to the vestibular nuclei are zebrin-negative and the intervening Purkinje cells of the X-zone, with a projection to the caudal fastigial and posterior interposed nuclei are zebrin-positive (Fig. 1L). It appears as though this observation can be generalized. The two sets of interdigitaling zones distinguished in one of the previous paragraphs and illustrated in Fig. 1B may very well correspond to the zebrin-positive and -negative zones in rodents. The zonal pattern in the corticonuclear and olivocerebellar connections is fairly constant among the mammalian species. The distribution of neurochemical markers in the cerebellum, however, is more variable. For zebrin and 5'-nucleotidase it has been established that they are expressed by most if not all Purkinje cells in carnivores and primates (Voogd, unpublished observations).

The development of this pattern occurs during an early stage, before granule cells migrate from the external- to the internal granular layer and before the transverse fissures make their appearance. After their migration from the ventricular epithelium the Purkinje cells settle in a number of discrete clusters, separated by cell-free raphes. This pattern was first recognized by Jakob[7] and well illustrated by Hochstetter.[5] More recently it was described in some detail in cetacea[9], rats[10] and primates[8]. According to Kappel[8] the final pattern arises from the interdigitation of two sets of Purkinje cell clusters, deep and superficial ones (Fig.2). The superficial clusters I, III and IV are connected, through cell strands, with the anlage of the medial cerebellar, posterior interposed and dentate nucleus respectively. They, therefore, resemble the A, C_2 and D zones of the adult anatomy. The deep clusters II and X)[*] are associated with the vestibular nuclei through the juxtarestiform body and with the anterior interposed nucleus. They resemble the adult B, C_1, and C_3 zones in this respect. Clustering of Purkinje cells in fetuses of macaque monkeys becomes visible at embryonic (E) day 48, is particularly clear between E50 and E70 and no longer can be distinguished when the Purkinje cells become arranged in a monolayer, at the time of the expansion of the cerebellar surface and the formation of fissures and the internal granular layer.

The main problem in tracing the development of the adult longitudinal zonal pattern from the Purkinje cell clusters is bridging the time-gap which separates the two formations. Moreover biochemical markers for Purkinje cell zones such as zebrinimmunoreactivity and the presence of 5'-nucleotidase are expressed late[3] during development when the Purkinje cell clusters no longer can be recognized[11,12]. Wassef and Sotelo[24] and Wassef et al., [25] found that markers which are expressed by all adult Purkinje cells such as cyclic GMP-dependent protein kinase (cGK) are only expressed by the Purkinje cells of certain clusters during early stages of development. They even suggested that cGK-expressing and cGK-non-expressing Purkinje cells would originate from different regions of the ventricular epithelium. A dual origin of Purkinje cells with different gradients of expression of cGK, which would aggregate in an interdigitating pattern of two sets of Purkinje cell clusters is in good agreement with the observations reported here. Our results, moreover, suggest a basic similarity in the cortico-nuclear relations of these Purkinje cell clusters and the adult zones.

---

[*]X was used to denote this cluster, it should not to be confused with the X zone of the anterior vermis

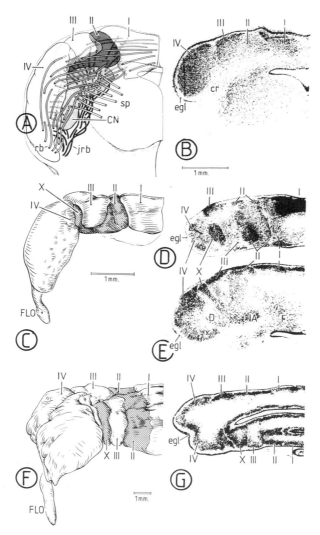

Fig. 2 A. Graphic reconstruction of the Purkinje cell clusters in an
anterior view of the cerebellum of a 54 day fetus of Macaca mulatta. The
exter granular layer (egl) is removed. The Purkinje cell clusters I-IV,
the anlage of the cerebellar nuclei (N), the superior cerebellar peduncle
(cp), the restiform body (rb) and the juxtarestiform body (jrb) are shown.
B. Transverse section through the cerebellum of the same fetus shown in
Fig. 2A. Nissl stain.
C. Graphic reconstruction of the Purkinje cell clusters in an anterior
view of the cerebellum of a 55 day fetus of Macaca mulatta.
D and E. Horizontal section through the cerebellum of the same fetus
shown in Fig. 2C. Nissl stain.
F. Graphic reconstruction of the Purkinje cell clusters in an anterior
view of the cerebellum of a 70 day fetus of Macaca mulatta.
G. Horizontal section through the cerebellum of the same fetus shown in
Fig. 2E. Nissl stain.

REFERENCES

1. Eisenman, L.M. and Hawkes, R. (1989) 5'-Nucleotidase and the mabQ113 antigen share a common distribution in the cerebellar cortex of the mouse. Neuroscience 31:231-237.

2. Hawkes, R. and Leclerc, N. (1986) Immunocytochemical demonstration of topographic ordering of Purkinje cell axon terminals in the fastigial nucleus of the rat. J. Comp. Neurol. 144:481-491.

3. Hess, D.T. and Hess, A. (1986) 5'-Nucleotidase of cerebellar molecular layer: Reduction in Purkinje cell-deficent mutant mice. Developmental Brain Res. 29:93-100.

4. Hess, D.T. and Voogd, J. (1986) Chemoarchitectonic zonation of the monkey cerebellum. Brain Res. 369:383-387.

5. Hochstetter, F. (1929) "Beiträge zur Entwicklungsgeschichte des Menschlichem Gehims. II. Die Entwicklung des Mittel- und Rautenhims". Deuticke, Vienna, Leipzig.

6. Illing, R.B. (1990) A subtype of cerebellar Golgi cells may be cholinergic. Brain Res. 522:267-274.

7. Jakob, A. (1928) Das Kleinhim, in: "Von Möllendorff's Handbuch der Mikroskopischen Anatomie des Menschen, IV/1, Nervensystem," Springer Verlag, Berlin, pp. 674-906.

8. Kappel, R.M. (1981) The development of the cerebellum in Macaca mulatta. A study of regional differences during corticogenesis. Thesis, Leiden.

9. Korneliussen, H.K. (1967) Cerebellar corticogenesis in cetacea with special reference to regional variations. J. Hirnforschung. 9:151-185.

10. Korneliussen, H.K. (1968) On the ontogenetic development of the cerebellum (nuclei, fissures and cortex) of the rat, with special reference to regional variations in corticogenesis. J. Hirnforschung. 10:379-414.

11. Leclerc, N., Gravel, C. and Hawkes, R. (1988) Development of parasagittal zonation in the rat cerebellar cortex: mabQ113 antigenic bands are created postnatally by the suppression of antigen expression in a subset of Purkinje cells. J. Comp. Neurol. 273:399-420.

12. Marani, E. (1986) Topographic histochemistry of the cerebellum. Progress Histochem. 16:1-169.

13. Marani, E. (1977) The subcellular distribution of 5'-nucleotidase activity in mouse cerebellum. Exp. Neurol. 57:1042-1048.

14. Scott, T.G. (1977) A unique pattern of localization within the cerebellum. Nature 200:793.

15. Sotelo, C. and Wassef, M. (1991) Cerebellar development: afferent organization and Purkinje cell heterogeneity. Phil. Trans. R. Soc. Lond. B. 331:307-313.

16. Voogd, J. (1964) The cerebellum of the cat. Structure and fiber connections. Van Gorcum, Assen.

17. Voogd, J. (1969) The importance of fibre connections in the comparative anatomy of the mammalian cerebellum. In: "Neurobiology of cerebellar evolution and development," Llinas R, eds. AMA/ERF, Chicago pp. 493-541.

18. Voogd, J. (1989) Parasagittal zones and compartments of the anterior vermis of the cat cerebellum. Exp. Brain Res. Series 17:3-19.

19. Voogd, J. and Bigaré, F. (1980) Topographical distribution of olivary and cortico-nuclear fibers in the cerebellum: A review. In: "The olivary nucleus. Anatomy and physiology," Courville et al., eds. Raven Press, New York, pp. 207-234.

20. Voogd, J., Eisenman, L.M. and Ruigrok, T.J.M. (1991a) Corticonuclear and -vestibular projection zones correspond to zebrin-positive and -negative in anterior vermis of rat cerebellum. Neurosci. Abstr. 17:1573.

21. Voogd, J., Epema, A.H. and Rubertone, J.A. (1991b) Cerebello-vestibular connections of the anterior vermis. A retrograde tracer study in

different mammals including primates. <u>Arch. Ital. de Biol.</u> 129:3-19.

22. Voogd, J., Gerrits, N.M. and Hess, D.T. (1987) Parasagittal zonation of the cerebellum in macaques: An analysis based on acetylcholinesterase histochemistry. <u>In:</u> "Cerebellum and Neuronal Plasticity," M. Glickstein, Chr. Yeo and J. Stein eds., Plenum Publishing Corporation, New York, NY, pp. 15-39.

23. Voogd, J., Hess, D.T. and Marani, E. (1986) The parasagittal zonation of the cerebellar cortex in cat and monkey. Topography, distribution of acetylcholinesterase and development. <u>In:</u> "New Concepts in Cerebellar Neurobiology", J.S. King and J. Courville, eds., Alan Liss, New York.

24. Wassef, M. and Sotelo, C. (1984) Asynchrony in the expression of guanosine 3:5'phosphate-dependent protein kinase by clusters of Purkinje cells during the perinatal development of rat cerebellum. <u>Neuroscience</u> 13:1217-1241.

25. Wassef, M., Zanetta, J.P., Brehier, A. and Sotelo, C. (1987) Transient biochemical compartmentation of Purkinje cells during early cerebellar development. <u>Devl. Biol.</u> 11:129-137.

NEW CONCEPTS ON THE DEVELOPMENT OF THE DENTATE GYRUS

Dieter Hartmann, Susanne Fehr* and Jobst Sievers

Anatomisches Institut, University of Kiel, Kiel, FRG
*Inst. für Klinische Neurobiologie
University of Hamburg, Hamburg, FRG

INTRODUCTION

The dentate gyrus, the medialmost extension of the mammalian
cerebral cortex, has attracted considerable interest from neurobiologists
during the past decades (see reviews by Angevine, 1975; Cowan et al.,
1980, 1981; Stanfield and Cowan, 1988). This is mostly due to the
apparent simplicity of its histological structure, with only one
prevailing cell type, and the laminated organization of its afferent and
efferent connections, which seems to make it a suitably simple model for
the analysis of cortical structure and function. Moreover, because of its
late (largely postnatal in most laboratory rodents) and protracted
development it is an easily accessible structure for various experimental
manipulations of cortical development (e.g. Altman and Bayer, 1975; Gall
and Lynch 1980; Hartmann et al., 1991).
     This review will focus on the ontogenesis of the dentate gyrus,
which in many respects differs from that of the cerebral isocortex and the
neighbouring cornu ammonis. In order to highlight these characteristics
in more detail, a short summary of some pertinent features of isocortical
development will be given first.

NEOCORTICAL ONTOGENESIS: LAMINATION AND RADIAL UNITS

Laminar Development in the Cortical Anlage

     The most characteristic feature of the developing cerebral cortex is
the early establishment of a primordial neuroepithelial lamination. The
somata of the mitotic neuroepithelial cells, which in the beginning span
the cerebral wall as a pseudostratified epithelium, become confined to the
inner surface, where they form the ventricular zone. They are separated
from the pial surface by the initially cell-sparse marginal zone. The
latter is then populated by postmitotic cells which form the preplate
('primary plexiform zone' according to Marin-Padilla 1978). Subsequently,
the anlage of the definitive laminae 11 - VI, the cortical plate, appears
within the primary plexiform zone. It consists of postmitotic neurons
that have arisen in the ventricular zone and settle within the cortical
plate along an inside-out gradient of neuro- and morphogenesis. As a
result, the preplate is split into an outer and inner (subplate) layer,
the cells of which are thought to either degenerate or to contribute to

the definitive laminae I and VIb, respectively (Marin-Padilla, 1978, 1988; Shatz et al., 1988). Concomitantly, the ventricular zone is separated from the cortical plate by the development of the intermediate zone which contains cell processes of the differentiating neurons and radial glia as well as the developing afferent and efferent axonal connections.

The Radial Unit

The early spatial segregation of cell proliferation and differentiation within distinct primordial laminae of the cerebral wall requires the regulated transport of cells from their site of origin to their laminar destination. During the early development of the cortical anlage, this transport is confined to postmitotic neurons and occurs as radial migration from the ventricular zone into the cortical plate.

A key role in the guidance of neuronal migration is attributed to the radial glial cells, a cell type transiently present during CNS development. The radial glial guidance hypothesis has been intensively proposed and substantiated by Rakic and coworkers (Rakic, 1988 a,b). According to the original concept, the radial glial cells - in contrast to the neurons - maintain both their ventricular and their pial (=basal) contacts. Their soma is situated within or adjacent to the ventricular zone, their process, the radial glial fiber, runs radially towards the pial surface, where its endfeet contribute to the glial limitans. Thus, the radial glial cells provide a point-to-point projection between the ventricular (=proliferative) zone and the pial surface, which allows the precise spatial translocation of cells deriving from the ventricular zone into the cortical plate. Tle conservation of a close topological rela-tionship within the radial developmental cell columns that consist of proliferating and migrating neuronal as well as radial glial cells, is of special importance, because these columns are thought to represent clusters of clonally related cells (Rakic 1988 a,b). For major modifications of this concept see Caviness, this volume, and Misson et al., 1988 a,b, 1991).

DEVELOPMENT OF THE DENTATE GYRUS

In the following we will review the evidence from the literature and our own work on the development of the dentate gyrus in order to show that the development of this region of the brain differs fundamentally from that of the isocortex and the hippocampus proper. Emphasis will be placed on (i) the topography of secondary proliferative matrices that give rise to the overwhelming majority of granule cells, (ii) the adaptation of the primordial radial glial scaffold of the dentate region to the development of the dentate gyrus, and (iii) the local origin and differentiation of radial glial cells that are incorporated into the granule cell layer, but are not related to the primordial radial glial scaffold of the dentate region. Additionally, we will (iv) reinterpret the morphogenetic defect of the dentate gyrus of the reeler mutant mouse in the light of the previously collected lines of evidence. These indicate, that the neuroglial interactions during dentate development are functionally different from those during neocortical ontogenesis.

The Dentate Gyrus arises from successive Germinal Matrices

The origin of the dentate anlage is the ventralmost tip of the medial hemispheral wall, immediately dorsal to the foramen of Monroe,

where the pseudostratified neuroepithelium tapers into the epithelial monolayer of the choroid plexus of the lateral ventricle. As in the rest of the
cerebral cortex, this neuroepithelium at first develops into the most primitive stage of cortical lamination, i.e. exhibiting a ventricular and a
marginal zone. With the beginning of cell emigration from the ventricular
zone, however, a unique regional development begins, which distinguishes
the dentate from the adjacent hippocampal and isocortical regions.

The first obvious difference to the 'normal' isocortical development
is the nature of the cells that leave the dentate ventricular epithelium.
The majority of these have retained their proliferative capacity, whereas
only a small minority of them are postmitotic dentate granule cells that
have been generated within the ventricular zone itself (Altman and Bayer
1975; Schlessinger et al., 1975; Bayer 1980 a,b; Altman and Bayer, 1990
a,c).

A second major difference to the neocortical anlage is the immediate
destination of these translocating cells. They do not establish a cortical
plate of differentiating neurons at the interface between marginal and
intermediate zone. By contrast, they (i) form a narrow band of radially
aligned cells across the cerebral wall dorsal to the fimbria, and (ii)
accumulate within the marginal zone immediately beneath the pial surface.
Thus, according to Altman and Bayer (1990 a,c) a 'suprafimbrial' secondary
dentate matrix, and a 'subpial' dentate migration I are established, both
of which continue cell proliferation even after the ventricular cells have
ceased to divide. Subsequently, these will generate a tertiary dentate
matrix which arises from the secondary dentate matrix, and is formed by
cells that spread within the dentate hilus and eventually reach the
innermost rows of the stratum granulosum.

According to Altman and Bayer (1990 a,c), the first dentate matrix
is the source of the earliest generated granule cells that will later
constitute the outer shell of the granular layer, while the later
migrating cells give rise in succession to the transient tertiary dentate
matrix and the enduring subgranular zone which, in turn, produce the inner
part of the granular layer. Due to the existence of the extraventricular
matrices and in contrast to the rest of the cerebral cortex that has a
rather short ontogenetic period of neurogenesis (review in Jacobson 1991),
the dentate gyrus is generated over a protracted period that continues for
a long time after the production of neurons in the hippocampus proper has
ceased (Angevine, 1965; Bayer, 1980 a,b, 1982; Bayer and Altman, 1974,
1975; Bayer et al., 1982; Schlessinger et al., 1975; Stanfield and Cowan,
1979 a,b; Cowan et al., 1980, 1981; Nowakowski and Rakic, 1981; Eckenhoff
and Rakic, 1988), and, on a small scale, even extends into rodent
adulthood (Kaplan and Hinds, 1977; Kaplan and Bell, 1983, 1984; Crespo et
al., 1986).

The concept of dentate development proposed by Altman and Bayer
(1990 a,c) thus emphasizes that successive generations of proliferative
cell pools generate different subpopulations of the cells of the dentate
gyrus. It also extends earlier concepts which attributed the prolongation
of dentate neurogenesis to the translocation of stem cells from the
ventricular zone into the dentate secondary proliterative zone (Altman and
Das, 1965, 1966; Schlessinger et al., 1975; Stanfield and Cowan, 1979 a,b;
Bayer, 1980 a,b) which appears as a small cluster of cells below the pial
surface, dorsomedially to the emerging fimbria (Cowan et al., 1980, 1981),
and which corresponds to the dentate migration I of Altman and Bayer (1990
a,c). Additionally, the formerly held concept of an exclusively radial
cell translocation from an extraventricular proliferative zone delineating
the future hilar region into the definitive granule cell layer (e.g. Cowan
et al., 1980, 1981) has been differentiated into a more precise model,

which describes the intercalation of different developmental gradients operative from successively formed proliferative cell groups (Gaarskjaer 1985, 1986; Altman and Bayer 1990 a,c).

Is the Dentate Anlage formed within a Radial Glial Scaffold ?

While isocortical development is assumed to involve the primordial radial glial scaffold as a guidance structure for the laminar deposition of neurons from the ventricular zone (Rakic, 1988 a,b), the contribution of glial cells to the development of the dentate gyrus is less clear. Several attempts to analyze the morphology and distribution of glial cells during dentate development in order to look for the applicability of the radial glial guidance hypothesis to this region of the cortex have led to conflicting results.

Thus, Woodhams et al. (1981) have identified radial glial cells in the developing hippocampal formation of the mouse from E 16 onward. In the dentate gyrus however, the authors have focussed on the description of the glial cells only after the formation of the granule cell layer. In these late ontogenetic stages they described unipolar radial glial cells – somewhat reminiscent to the cerebellar Bergmann glia – in the stratum granulosum, with basal processes traversing the packed rows of granule cells and branching within the molecular layer. The primordial radial glial scaffold of this region and its relationship to the cells of the early dentate anlage, i.e. before and during granule cell layer formation, was not described, possibly because technical limitations precluded the visualization of these cells in the early ontogenetic stages.

According to Eckenhoff and Rakic (1984) the development of the dentate gyrus in Rhesus monkeys begins with the appearance of a "dentate plate" at the interface of a dentate intermediate and marginal zone, which they take to be the regional analog of the cortical plate of the hippocampal region, a finding never observed in number of investigations of dentate development in many mammalian species including man (Humphrey 1966, 1967; Schlessinger et al., 1975; Stanfield and Cowan 1979 b; Cowan et al., 1980, 1981). This "dentate plate" is proposed to develop within the primordial radial glial scaffolding of the hippocampal anlage whose "radial fibers stretch and curve to accomodate the tectogenetic shifts as the dentate gyrus rotates and acquires its characteristic horseshoe shape". No comment was made concerning the unusual topography of cell proliferation and the superficial route of cell translocation depicted in an earlier paper by the same group (Nowakowski and Rakic 1981).

By contrast, Rickmann et al. (1987) emphasize the existence of two distinct sets of radial glial processes involved in the assembly of the rat dentate gyrus. The primordial radial glial scaffold is thought to direct the migration of the dentate stem cells in a similar fashion as described by Eckenhoff and Rakic (1984). It is supplemented with a second set of glial cells that arise from the "hilar secondary proliferative zone". These cells are assumed to intercalate with the basal portions of the primordial radial glial fibers and, thus, to amplify and extend the primordial glial template for the development of the definitive dentate gyrus. However, it remains unclear from the evidence presented, how the primary and secondary radial glial scaffolds intercalate, and how the granule cells select their migratory routes within the two different sets of radial glial processes. Moreover, both interpretations, which are largely drawn from data on postmitotic cell migration in the isocortex, do not offer an explanation for the unusual tangential trajectory of cell migration (Stanfield and Cowan 1988) and the intercalation of additional proliferative zones within the migratory pathway.

The presence of extraventricular proliferative matrices is the central feature distinguishing the development of the dentate gyrus from that of the rest of the cerebral cortex. This includes the establishment of a different type of transitory lamination and neuro-glial relationships that are only found in the dentate anlage. To analyze these unusual patterns of cortical development in more detail, we have investigated the ontogenesis of the dentate gyrus in Syrian hamsters (Mesocricetus auratus, Hausmann et al., 1987; Sievers et al., 1987, Hartmann et al., 1991; Sievers et al., 1991). This species is particularly well suited for experimental studies because of its ontogenetically early date of birth after only 16 days of gestation, and the very early expression of glial fibrillary acidic protein (GFAP) (starting on E 13) which, in comparison to other rodents, allows the unequivocal identification of glial cells during embryogenesis at significantly earlier stages.

Formation of the Secondary Dentate Matrices: Early Presence of Glial Cells

In the hamster, the first cells leaving the dentate segment of the ventricular zone are visible on E 13. In contrast to the neighbouring anlage of the CA 3 region, where a cortical plate is emerging, these cells do not form a condensed cell layer at the interface between marginal zone and intermediate zone, but populate the marginal zone. Here, the formerly radially oriented cells become aligned tangentially to the pial surface, and subsequently form the subpial dentate matrix (Fig. I A,C).

In the following days the fundamental regional differences in the histological structure of the medial cerebral wall become even more obvious. The dorsal region with the emerging cornu ammonis exhibits the typical lamination of a cortical anlage with a condensed cortical plate and a cell-sparse molecular zone. In the ventral tip the continuously growing accumulation of cells of the subpial dentate matrix collects within the marginal zone. It is in continuity with a 'stream' of radially oriented cells above the fimbria, the suprafimbrial dentate matrix, which itself lies adjacent to the ventral part of the ventricular zone (Fig. I B,D).

The subsequent growth of the subpial dentate matrix by both intrinsic proliferation, and -during early development- a continuous influx of cells from the ventricular zone and the suprafimbrial matrix fills the marginal zone, and bulges the pial surface. At the same time the ammonic cortical plate is progressively indented. In this process the region of the future stratum oriens of CA 3 and the medial surface of the area dentata are established.

The first evidence of glial cells is found on E 13, when a weakly vimentin-positive scaffold of radial glial cells appears throughout the medial and lateral hemispheral wall. Starting on E 14 this scaffold is supplemented with GFAP-positive cells in a restricted region immediately dorsal to the fimbria. Morphologically, two different types of glial cells are present. The first type corresponds to typical bipolar radial glial cells with cell bodies within or adjacent to the ventricular zone, and basal processes extending up to the pial surface. These cells form a narrow bundle immediately dorsal to the developing fimbria (Fig. I E), connecting the dentate ventricular zone with the pial surface in the region of the forming fimbriodentate sulcus (Sievers et al., 1992).

The second type of GFAP-positive cells is a short bipolar cell which is closely associated with the processes of the radial glial cells of the dentate region. These cells are visible at all horizons between the ventricular zone and the pial surface, i.e. they lie in the region of the suprafimbrial dentate matrix (Fig. 1E, 3, 4D). Like their GFAP-negative (presumably neuronal) counterparts, they also accumulate in the marginal zone within the subpial dentate matrix which extends along the pial surface up to the entrance of the hippocampal fissure (Sievers et al., (1992).

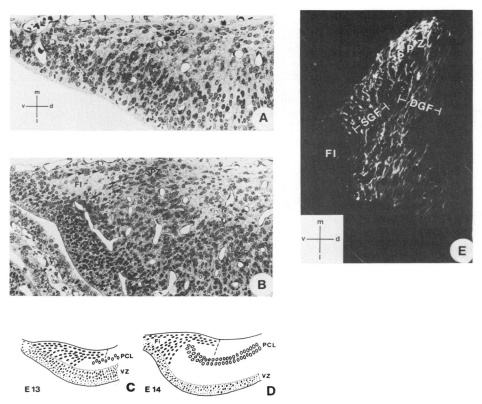

Fig. 1. Frontal sections of the dentate anlage on E 13 (A,C) and E 14
(B,D). Note the accumulation of undifferentiated cells within the
marginal zone (arrowheads) forming the subpial proliferative zone (SPZ).
The SPZ is connected to the ventricular neuroepithelium by a continuous
stream of cells dorsal (black arrows) and initially also medial
(arrowheads) to the forming fimbria (FI). (E) Visualization of glial cells
in the same region by GFAP-immunohistochemistry at a slightly later
developmental stage (E 15). The basal processes have started to diverge
into a suprafimbrial (SGF) and dorsal (DGF) glial bundle bracketing the
SPZ. The subpial proliferative zone itself is densely populated by short,
bipolar GFAP-positive cells, visible by their fluorescent rings of
cytoplasm surrounding the unstained nuclear region. PCL : Pyramidal cell
layer. Magnification in A and B x150, E x200.

230

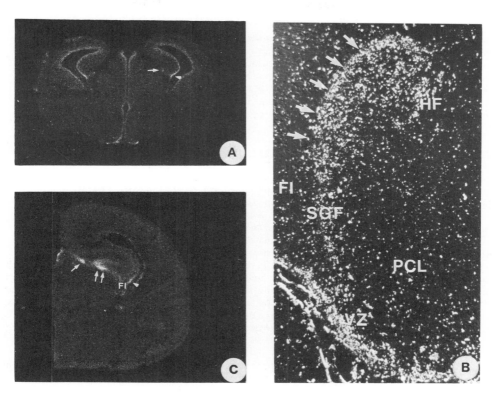

Fig. 2. Negative prints of film autoradiographs after in-situ-hybridization with a cRNA-probe against GFAP-mRNA on E 15 (A) and P 7 (C) and standard autoradiograph on P 0 (B). Initially, the mRNA signal is almost exclusively confined to the ventricular lining (A), most probably due to the presence of radial glial cell bodies. In the dentate anlage, a small cluster of mRNA-reactivity is visible at the medial hemispheral surface (arrow in (A)) in addition to an locally augmented signal in the ventricular zone (arrowhead). At birth (B), the distribution of GFAP-MRNA is coincident with the ventricular zone (VZ), the suprafimbrial glial bundle (SGF), the subpial proliferative zone (arrows) and the region of the forming suprapyramidal blade beneath the hippocampal fissure (HF), indicating the presence of actively synthesizing glial cell somata in this region in contrast to the radial glial scaffold dorsally (PCL:pyramidal cell layer), where only the ventricular zone is mRNA-positive (compare with Fig. 3 A). During later development, the peak of GFAP-mRNA-reactivity is shifted into the infrapyramidal blade (double arrow) and the entrance of the hippocampal fissure (arrow). Magnification in A and C x 8, B x 140.

These data on the early appearance of GFAP-positive astroglial cells outside of the ventricular zone correlate well with findings from in-situ-hybridization experiments using a 35S-labelled cDNA probe against GFAP-mRNA. With this method, GFAP-mRNA-positive cells are demonstrable as early as E 13. They appear within the ventricular zone of the whole circumference of the hemispheres. By contrast, the expression of the derivative protein, GFAP, is almost completely confined to the dentate anlage, and only later extends further dorsally. From E 14 onward, a thin strip of GFAP-mRNA reactivity extends radially above the fimbria between the dentate ventricular zone and the pial surface of the hemisphere. It is localized in the suprafimbrial dentate matrix. A signal of similar intensity is also seen in the subpial dentate matrix. During the subsequent days, the subpial GFAP-mRNA signal becomes more intense, exceeding that of the suprafimbrial region, thereby reflecting the progressive accumulation of glial cells in this region (Fig. 2 A-C).

Ultrastructure of the Subpial Dentate Matrix

In contrast to the rest of the immature cerebral cortex which is uninterruptedly covered with the endfeet of radial glial cells, the subpial dentate matrix features an incomplete glial limiting membrane during the whole time span of its existence, exhibiting gaps of various sizes between individual glial endfeet. Within these gaps, both undifferentiated glial and neuronal cells and/or their processes are in direct contact to the basement membrane (Sievers et al., 1992). In 3D-reconstructions both cell types exhibit the same overall morphology, with a small round to ovoid cell soma, and one or two short processes. Contact to the basement membrane is made by a cell process (either a 'leading' or 'trailing' one) or sometimes by the cell body itself (Fig. 3 A-C, A'-C'). Most of the cells are oriented parallel to the basement membrane, however, near the termination of the suprafimbrial radial glial bundle cells with 'trailing' processes that point into the direction of the ventricle are also present.

These variable morphologies and orientations of cell contacts to the basal lamina could be indicative for a surface - associated cell movement in a tangential direction. Thereby, the cell soma could move relative to its 'leading' process which thus would be transformed into a 'trailing' one, which is then replaced by a newly formed basal lamina contact ahead of the soma.

Development of the Primordial Radial Glial Scaffold in Dentate Area

The establishment of a proliferating cell population within the marginal zone and its subsequent enlargement parallel to the brain surface together with the increasing indentation of the ammonic cortical plate has a profound effect on the topography of the bipolar radial glial fibers in this region.

With the appearance and rapid growth of the subpial dentate matrix the basal portion of the primordial radial glial scaffold dorsal to the fimbria is split into (i) the suprafimbrial bundle which originates from that region of the ventricular zone that gives rise to the dentate gyrus, and (ii) the dorsal glial bundle which originates from that portion of the ventricular zone that gives rise to the ventralmost tip of future CA 3 (Fig. 4 A). The latter takes a radial course initially, but then turns dorsally and terminates in the lateral section of the hippocampal fissure, forming a mediodorsally open angle with the suprafimbrial bundle. Thus, beneath the pial surface a roughly triangular region devoid of radial glial processes is formed, corresponding to the region of the secondary proliferative zone.

232

Orientation and course of the 'dorsal' group of glial fibers correspond well to the 'supragranular' glial bundle described by Rickmann et al. (1987) in the rat (Fig. 4 A,B). In contrast to their findings, the application of various methods (see Hartmann et al., 1992; and Sievers et al., 1992, for details) clearly demonstrates that the 'ventral' (or 'fimbrial' according to Rickmann et al., 1987) radial glial cells do not run through the subpial region up to the forming granule cell layer, but terminate at the dorsomedial border of the fimbria. Within the subpial proliferative zone, GFAP reactivity is bound to numerous small cells oriented parallel to the basal lamina (Fig. 5 A-C, 4 D). Since a contact of the radial glial fiber system to the developing granule cell layer could not be demonstrated, its local radial glial scaffold has to be formed by an entirely different mechanism as compared to the isocortex (see below).

With the continuous growth of the subpial dentate matrix, and, later, the suprapyramidal blade, the dorsal glial fiber bundle is progressively displaced laterally into the cerebral wall, giving way to the growing primordial stratum granulosum (Fig. 4 A-C). With the possible exception of the ventralmost (after rotation of the tip of CA 3, the medialmost) the dorsal glial fibers do not pass through the suprapyramidal blade. Instead, their basal parts are distorted into a sigmoid course with their terminal parts running around the lateral pole of the suprapyramidal blade and then along the hippocampal fissure. Thus, it seems, as if the primordial radial glial scaffold does not take part in the organization of the dentate gyrus except delimiting the borders of the region of the cerebral wall, where it is to be established, i.e. between the fimbria and the hippocampal fissure.

However, there is some evidence that the primordial radial glial scaffold could be involved in the initiation of the suprapyramidal blade. The first columns of granule cells and their associated secondary radial glial cells appear directly adjacent to or among the basal portions of the ventralmost dorsal glial fibers which have been rotated into a position at right angle to the original ventricular-pial axis. Thus, the radial organization of the stratum granulosum seems to begin as an extension of the rotated basal part of the original radial glial scaffold. The subsequent propulsion of this radial organization seems to be the result of the addition of the constituent cells from the subpial dentate matrix to the growing end of the stratum granulosum.

Establishment of the Granule Cell Layer: Cortical Morphogenesis from Local Proliferative Matrices

The assembly of the definitive stratum granulosum is the result of at least two different developmental steps. First, the v-shaped outline of the dentate gyrus, corresponding to the outer cell layers of the adult granular layer, is formed along a transverse gradient of morphogenesis, i.e. from the lateral pole of the suprapyramidal blade to the medial crest to the lateral pole of the infrapyramidal blade, whereby the granule cells are thought to be derived from the subpial proliferative zone (Bayer, 1980 a,b; Cowan et al., 1980 1981; Altman and Bayer, 1990 a,c). This unusual pattern of morphogenesis along a transverse gradient covers a period of about 7 to 10 days in most laboratory rodents. Concomitantly, the cells of the secondary dentate matrices change their position relative to the granule cell layer and are shifted into the subgranular zone of the hilar region, and, eventually, into the innermost part of the granule cell layer itself. These intrahilar and subgranular matrices then contribute to the enlargement of the stratum granulosum by adding cells along an outside-in gradient to its hilar aspect (Gaarskjaer 1985, 1986; Altman and Bayer 1990 a,c).

233

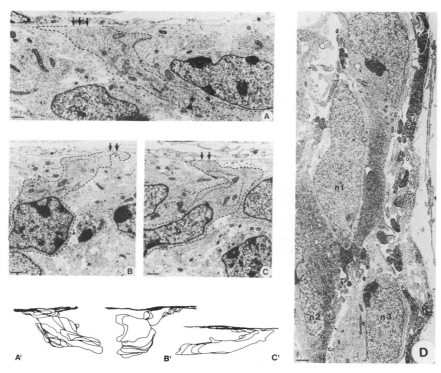

Fig. 3. Ultrastructure of the subpial proliferative zone. Figures 3 A to 3 C demonstrate direct contacts of the undifferentiated cells (the dashed lines follow the contour of the cell body) to the basal lamina (black arrows). Three-dimensional reconstructions of the same cells made from ultrathin serial sections are shown in 3 A' to 3 C'. Figure 3 D is an immunoperoxidase visualization of glial cells (nuclei n1 to n3) in the subpial proliferative zone in direct apposition to the basal lamina. In three dimensional reconstructions, these cells exhibit the same morphology as shown in 3 A' to 3 C'. Magnification in A-C x 3300, D x 3465.

Thus, unlike the horizontal waves of postmitotic neurons that migrate from the ventricular zone along the primordial radial glial scaffold to aggregate into the hippocampal pyramidal cell layer without major lateromedial temporal differences (Nowakowski and Rakic 1981; Eckenhoff and Rakic, 1984, but see also Altman and Bayer, 1990b), the aggregation of neurons and glial cells into the primordial stratum granulosum occurs along an entirely different, i.e. transverse temporospatial gradient. The sequential establishment of spatially separated pools of proliferative cells and the successive assembly of neurons and glia along a nonradial morphogenetic gradient are difficult to explain with concepts drawn from the analysis of neocortical development (Eckenhoff and Rakic, 1984; Rickmann et al., 1987), and could imply developmental mechanisms characteristic of dentate granule cells and their associated glia, that differ from those found in the rest of the cerebral cortex.

In the hamster the first columns of differentiating granule cells appear between E 15 and E 16 at the dorsolateral extreme of the subpial dentate matrix, below the anlage of the hippocampal fissure. They are always associated with short, unipolar radial glial fibers that originate

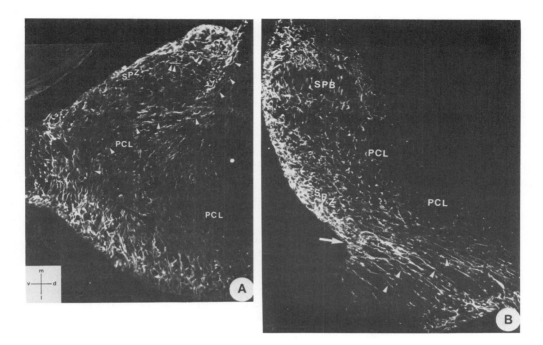

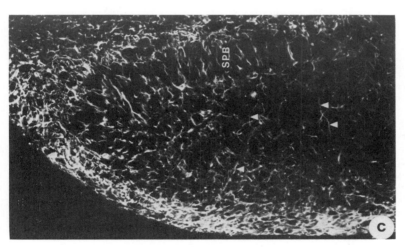

Fig. 4. Morphology and distribution of glial cells in the dentate anlage
on P 0 (A), P (B) and P 3 (C). At birth, the dorsal glial fiber bundle
has been shifted dorsally to terminate in the lateral part of the
hippocampal fissure (white arrowheads in (A)) and is separated from the
surface by the developing suprapyramidal blade (SPB). Within the
hippocampal fissure, small bipolar glial cells are aligned within these
fiber group (open arrows), that seem to have arisen from the dorsal pole
of the subpial proliferative zone. The suprafimbrial radial glial fibers
terminate in the vicinity of the fimbriodentate sulcus (white arrow in
03). Within the subpial proliferative zone (SPZ), GFAP-reactivity is bound
to numerous small cells aligned parallel to the pial surface (A–C).
Monopolar radial glial cells reappear in the forming granule cell layer
itself. Additionally, single fibers arise at right angles from the SPZ
traversing the hilar region, possibly reaching the suprapyramidal blade
(double arrowheads in (A), arrowheads in (C)). Magnification in A and B
x 150, C x 205.

from somata situated immediately beneath the granule cell layer, and that branch within the incipient molecular zone (Fig. 5 A; Sievers et al., 1992). The glial cells within the emerging stratum granulosum do not have contact to the ventricular zone, in contrast to similar cells within the cortical plate of the isocortex that appear to be unipolar forms of astrocytes transforming from radial glial cells (Schmechel and Rakic, 1979; Voigt, 1989; Misson et al., 1991) as suggested by Eckenhoff and Rakic (1984).

On the contrary, the row of these 'local' radial glial cells merges directly with the densely packed population of GFAP-positive cells in the subpial dentate matrix. Here, at the site of elongation of the primordial stratum granulosum, glial cells of a 'transitory' morphology are found, the cell bodies of which are situated at various distances from the pial surface, whereas their single cell process runs obliquely into the growing granule cell layer, sometimes crossing the prospective hilar region (Fig. 4 A,C).

When the primordial suprapyramidal blade and the dentate crest have been formed and the infrapyramidal blade begins to emerge, the involvement of the locally generated unipolar radial glial cells in the establishment of the stratum granulosum becomes even more obvious. In the suprapyramidal blade whose long axis initially runs at right angles to the pial surface, the local radial glial cells are added from the subpial dentate matrix to the columns of aggregating granule cells while both are in a position parallel to the pial surface (Fig. 4 A,B). Thus, the glial cells that are incorporated between the columns of granule cells do not have to change their orientation. In the infrapyramidal blade, however, whose long axis from the beginning runs parallel to the pial surface, the radial glial cells of the subpial dentate matrix have to erect from their initially surface-parallel position into an orientation perpendicular to the pia (Fig. 4 C), when they aggregate with the granule cells (Sievers et al., 1992).

The integration of cells from the subpial proliferative matrix into the forming stratum granulosum and the intrahilar and subgranular matrices is also reflected in the distribution of the GFAP-mRNA - signal in the dentate anlage. The peak intensity, that has earlier been shifted from the ventricular into the subpial proliferative zone, now labels the site of collateral cell addition to the growing granule cell layer. The hilar region exhibits a comparatively reduced mRNA signal, whereas the subgranular zone and the hippocampal fissure are visible as thin positive bands. The formerly intense signal dorsal to the fimbria becomes reduced by the end of the first postnatal week.

The remaining cells of the subpial and hilar dentate matrices are shifted into the developing dentate hilus, where they are situated in the subgranular region. Here they continue to proliferate and to generate additional granule cells (Bayer, 1980 a,b; Altman and Bayer, 1990 a,c). However, a significant proportion of these cells are astroglial cells of the short bipolar type. By contrast to their counterparts in the subpial dentate matrix, these cells have a different orientation, their leading processes pointing at various angles towards the hilar side of the granule cell layer. In many cases, ascending processes of these glial cells are seen to be partially inserted into the deep layer of the stratum granulosum. This observation indicates that not only granule cells are added to the preformed stratum granulosum, but that the increase in the number of neuronal cells is accompanied by a similar growth in the number of astroglial cells. These apparently also arise locally from the dentate matrices, and supplement the preexistent local radial glial scaffold of the granule cell layer (Rickmann et al., 1987; Sievers et al., 1992; Hartmann et al., 1992).

The changing topographical relationship between the dentate matrices and the granule cell layer determines the direction of growth of the stratum granulosum. While in the early stages the growth along the transverse axis is predominant, the later stages are characterized by the increase of the radial width of the granule cell layer. In contrast to the isocortex, the radial growth of the stratum granulosum follows an outside-in gradient of cytogenesis and maturation, since the newly formed cells are added to the hilar aspect of the stratum granulosum, without bypassing their predecessors along glial guides, as is the case in the cortical plate of the developing isocortex. This late addition of cells occurs at roughly the same rate in both the supra- and intrapyramidal blade (Bayer, 1980 a,b; Gaarskjaer 1985, 1986; Altman and Bayer, 1990 a,c).

Thus, it seems to be clear that the primordial radial glial scaffold of the dentate region has either no or a completely different relationship to the stratum granulosum as compared to that of the isocortical radial glia to the cortical plate. The evidence collected from the study of the hamster dentate gyrus indicates that the lamination within the area dentata is the result of a selforganizing process involving the secondary dentate matrices and their descendant neuronal and glial cells. This process involves the regulation in time and space of the aggregation of cell columns consisting at least of maturing granule cells and unipolar 'secondary' radial glial cells which possibly are supplemented with neuronal and glial stem cells from the adjacent secondary dentate matrices. The exact mechanisms controlling the assembly of the stratum granulosum which we have proposed to designate 'collateral aggregation', remain to be elucidated. However, data from our work described below provide evidence for the involvement of the meningeal fibroblasts covering the early dentate anlage in the control of secondary radial glia formation. Additionally, analysis of the effect of the reeler mutation on glial cell morphology in the dentate gyrus points towards an important role for neuron-glia interactions on radial glial cell orientation and differentiation, an effect not observed in the isocortex (review in Caviness et al., 1988).

INVOLVEMENT OF THE MENINGES IN THE DEVELOPMENT OF THE DENTATE GYRUS

We have summarized the evidence that the dentate gyrus originates almost exclusively from secondary dentate matrices established by proliferating cells that have left the ventricular zone. The most conspicuous of these, the subpial dentate matrix, contains a collection of neuronal and glial cells many of which are intercalated between the endfeet of the primordial radial glia and have contact to the basal lamina (Fig. 3). Thus, on the basis of their surface relationships, the cells of the subpial dentate matrix have some characteristics of a typical epithelium (Hausmann et al., 1987; Sievers et al., 1987, 1992), whereas the rest of the cortical anlage is characterized by an 'intraepithelial' development of neuronal cells that are isolated from the surrounding mesenchyme by glial cells. A similar situation is found in the early ontogenetic stages of the cerebellar cortex (Hausmann and Sievers 1985).

Selective Destruction of Meningeal Cells as a Tool for Investigation of Influences of Meningeal Cells on Brain Development

To clarify the question, if these morphologically demonstrable contacts of the cells within the subpial proliferative zone to the pial surface represent a functionally significant interaction with the surrounding mesenchyme, the meninges, we have recently developed a pharmacological method to selectively destroy meningeal cells by the intracranial injection of the catecholaminergic neurotoxin 6-hydroxydopamine (6-OHDA). This drug is accumulated into meningeal cells (Sievers, H. et al., 1983) by the extraneuronal uptake for catecholamines (Sievers et al., 1985) and destroys the meningeal cells within a few hours after administration (Sievers et al., 1980, 1983, 1985). Using inhibitors of the neuronal and extraneuronal uptake for catecholamines for control experiments, the selectivity of the action of 6-OHDA on meningeal cells was confirmed (Sievers et al., 1985; Pehlemann et al., 1985).

Destruction of Meningeal Cells with 6-Hydroxydopamine (6-OHDA)

Within 6 hours after birth, newborn hamsters received one injection of 25 ug free base 6-OHDA-HCl (Sigma, Munich, FRG) in 5 ul 0.9% Nacl, containing   mg/ml ascorbate, into the interhemispheric fissure, to the left of the superior sagittal sinus, just anterior to the transverse sinus. Controls received injections of the saline-ascorbate vehicle without 6-OHDA. Additionally, untreated animals were used.

In order to ascertain, that the alterations in dentate development were caused by the selective destruction of meningeal cells, we performed a pharmacological control experiment in which the extraneuronal uptake of 6-OHDA into meningeal cells was blocked with normetanephrine (NMN) (Sievers et al., 1985; Pehlemann et al., 1985). Newborn hamsters were first given a subcutaneous injection of 100 mg/kg body weight NMN (Boehringer, Ingelheim, FRG) (free base) in 25 μl ascorbate-saline, and 30 minutes later an interhemispheric injection of 25 μg 6-OHDA (free base) plus 333 ug NMN (free base) in 5 ul ascorbate-saline. In intervals of 30 min, the animals received two more interhemispheric injections of 167 ul NMN (free base) in ascorbate-saline vehicle. 24 hr and 30 days p.i. treated and control animals (which had received the same injections of NMN but without 6-OHDA) were killed, in order to evaluate the effects of the uptake inhibitor NMN on the action of 6-OHDA on meningeal cells and dentate development.

Effects of Meningeal Cell Destruction on the Development of the Dentate Anlage

The early morphological changes in the anlage of the dentate gyrus after treatment with 6-OHDA involve (i) the meningeal cells that are directly affected by the toxin, as well as their associated extracellular matrix on the surface of the dentate gyrus and the underlying diencephalon, and (ii) the cells within the subpial dentate matrix. The later developing alterations of the architecture of the dentate gyrus itself seem to be the indirect consequences of these initial effects of the treatment.

The destruction of meningeal cells covering the medial hemispheral wall and the lateral diencephalic surface is complete after 24h p.i. (Fig. 5 A,B). The alterations are similar to those seen over the cerebellar anlage after administration of 6-OHDA into the IVth ventricle as described in detail previously (Sievers et al., 1980, 1981, 1983; v. Knebel Doeberitz et al., 1986). Within 2 or 3 days the cellular debris over the medial cerebral hemisphere and the dorsolateral diencephalon are removed, leaving the basal laminae at the surfaces exposed to the subarachnoid space.

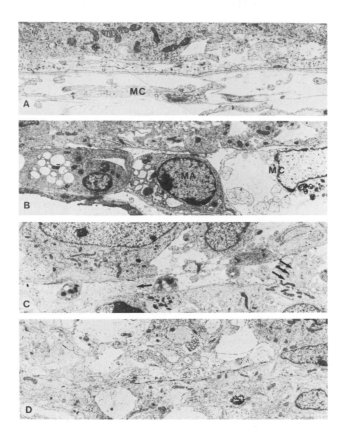

Fig. 5. Effects of administration of 6-OHDA into the subarachnoid space of
a newborn hamster. In (A) the normal structure of the pial surface is
shown, with a continuous basal lamina covered by interdigitating meningeal
cells (MC). Fig. 5 B demonstrates the acute effects of the toxin. The
continuous layer of fibroblasts has vanished, remaining meningeal cells
(MC) are degenerating and are contacted by macrophages (MA), that already
exhibit signs of phagocytosis. Concomitant with the degeneration and
removal of meningeal cells the basal lamina becomes thinned and ruptures
focally, allowing for protrusions of neuropil to extend into the subarachnoid space (arrows) in C). At later stages, a basal lamina persists or
becomes reestablished only in the vicinity of regenerating meningeal cells
(dashed line in (D)). Otherwise, a complete fusion of diencephalic and
hemispheral neuropil develops. Magnification in A x 7700, B-C x 3850.

Subsequent to the removal of the meningeal cells the dentate basement membrane becomes thinned, and the amount of collagen fibrils declines. The thinning of the basement membrane continues over the next few days and discontinuities and breaks appear. When similar ruptures also develop in the basement membrane of the diencephalon, the dentate gyrus and the diencephalon may fuse focally, obliterating the fissure that normally separates these two brain parts (Fig. 5 C,D). Regeneration of the meningeal cell layer starts at about 5 days p.i.. The fibroblasts reappear over those parts of the dentate surface that have not fused with the underlying diencephalon. Here the basement membrane regains its normal thickness and morphological appearance (Fig. 5 D; Hartmann et al., 1992).

Concomitant with the changes at the surface of the dentate gyrus described above, alterations of the development of the various components of the dentate anlage appear, which become recognizable already within 24 hr p.i. of 6-OHDA, and which are accentuated in later developmental stages. They are best seen in GFAP-preparations in which the subpial dentate matrix is readily recognizable. Here, the intensive GFAP-immunoreactivity associated with the densely aggregated cells of the subpial dentate matrix is strikingly reduced by 24 hr p.i.. Instead of the punctate accentuation of the fluoresceing reaction product characteristic for cell body staining, elongated, filiform structures are present which are reminiscent of glial processes. Thus, it seems, as if the astroglial cells that are present in great numbers in the subpial dentate matrix in control animals have either lost their GFAP-immunoreactivity, or have left their subpial position. However, there are two regions of the dentate anlage which obviously contain an increased amount of GFAP-immunoreactivity, i.e. the prospective hilus and the entrance of the hippocampal fissure, where a prominent cluster of cells collects (Hartmann et al., 1992).

In semi-thin light microscopic sections the alterations seen so strikingly in the GFAP-preparations are less obvious. Nevertheless, it is evident that the number of cells within the surface-associated subpial dentate matrix, especially its dorsalmost pole, has decreased considerably. In some regions the internal surface of the basement membrane is completely devoid of those cells, which in controls are attached to it. By contrast, the number of cells, especially darkly staining 'immature' ones, has increased in the prospective hilus, most conspicuously below the anlage of the suprapyramidal blade, and at the entrance of the hippocampal fissure. The latter cell cluster seems to merge with the tip of the growing suprapyramidal blade which subsequently is drawn out dorsomedially to the surface of the cerebral cortex.

By 3 days p.i. the subpial dentate matrix as seen by GFAP-immunohistochemistry has completely disappeared. In the subsurface region, where in controls the infrapyramidal blade has begun to develop, there are few, loosely scattered GFAP-positive cells below the glia limitans. Similar cells are present within the hilus and the emerging stratum oriens which contains cells of the suprafimbrial dentate matrix. The cell columns of the suprapyramidal blade extend up to the pial surface of the medial cerebral wall. In some cases the dentate gyrus and the diencephalon have fused in this region (Fig. 6). During the subsequent days up to P 7, the deviation from the normal developmental schedule becomes even more obvious due to the complete nondevelopment of the infrapyramidal granule cell layer. As can be demonstrated by immunohistochemical preparations, the dentate radial glial scaffold also has not formed, the subsurface region being mostly devoid of GFAP-positive cells, even exhibiting discontiniuities of several cell diameters in its glial limiting membrane, where fusion zones between diencephalon and hemisphere have developed (Fig. 6 D; see also Fig. 7 D).

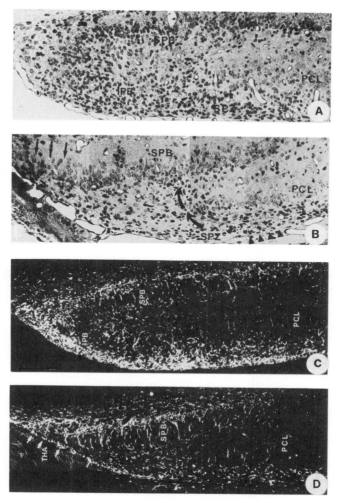

Fig. 6. Subpial proliferative zone and forming granule cell layer on P 3.
Control animals are shown in (A) and (C), whereas photomicrographs (B) and
(D) are taken from animals after meningeal cell destruction on P 0. The
treated animals exhibit a gross reduction of cell density in the subpial
proliferative zone (SPZ). Whereas the suprafimbrial cell group
(arrowheads in (B)) has an almost normal configuration, the cells seem to
turn dorsally (curved arrows) instead of moving along the defective basal
lamina. Medially, the suprapyramidal blade runs up to the hemispheral
surface (straight arrows) but does not form the normal crest covered by
the molecular zone. The anlage of the infrapyramidal blade (IPB) is
completely missing. These striking changes are even more pronounced in
immunohistochemical preparations using antibodies against GFAP (C, D).
The loss of GFAP positive cells from the SPZ is almost complete,
additionally, the glial limiting membrane exhibits large gaps (arrows in
(D)), where the hemisphere is opposed to the thalamus (THA). Monopolar
radial glial cells are only visible in the suprapyramidal blade (SPB), but
not in the region, where the crest and the medial third of the
infrapyramidal blade have developed in control animals. PCL:pyramidal
cell layer. Magnifications in A and C x 105, B and D x 94.

First traces of the infrapyramidal blade are emerging after P 7 and become more prominent about P O. Like the two different forms seen in the adult hamsters (Fig. 7, B,C), two different types of recovery take place. In the larger proportion of animals, a blunt crest and a very short fragment of a normal appearing infrapyramidal blade, attached to the medial extremity of the suprapyramidal blade, appears. In the smaller proportion of hamsters, small groups of "immature" cells and differen- tiating granule cells collect beneath restricted regions of the pial surface, while the medial extremity of the suprapyramidal blade extends far medially, up to the surface of the diencephalon. At later stages, the fragments of the infrapyramidal blade generated earlier have increased in size and begun to differentiate into the laminar structure typical of the adult dentate gyrus. In contrast to control animals, the 'undifferentiated' cells in the hilar matrix and the subgranular zone are still very conspicuous, and some cells can still be seen in the position of the former suprafimbrial matrix, below the pial surface of the stratum oriens of CA3. Within the hilus long thin glial fibers are present that extend radially into the stratum granulosum.

The emergence of fragments of the infrapyramidal blade is in either case correlated with the repopulation of the respective regions of the dentate pial surface with meningeal cells. By contrast, in those regions in which the infrapyramidal blade does not develop, the pial surface is not repopulated with meningeal cells, but, instead, the glia limitans superficialis is incomplete, and the dentate gyrus has fused with the underlying diencephalon (Fig. 7 A-D).

It is important to emphasize that those parts of the primordial radial glial scaffold - both the suprafimbrial and the dorsal glial fiber bundles - that can be demonstrated with GFAP-immunohistochemistry in our material, seem to be unaffected by the destruction of meningeal cells at any time after the treatment.

THE REELER DEFECT OF THE DENTATE GYRUS

The reeler defect of mouse brain development, originally described by Falconer (1951), exerts its influence during cortical plate formation. Whereas the kinetics of cell proliferation and initial migration are normal (Caviness 1973; Stanfield and Cowan 1979 b), the postmitotic neurons in the neocortex seem to be unable to leave their radial glial guide to become integrated into the forming laminae (Pinto-Lord et al., 1982; Goffinet 1984). Consequently, the preplate cells are pushed outward instead of being split into two sublaminae, whereas the immigrating cells destined for the cortical plate pile up along their glial fibers along an ill-defined outside-in gradient. The morphology of the glial fibers themselves exhibits only minor defects, i.e. a reduction in the number of pial endfeet formed by an individual fiber and the absence of defasciculation of fibers from the originally formed bundles, that is normally associated with neuronal migration. Establishment and overall orientation of the glial scaffold is not altered (review in Caviness et al., 1988).

In the dentate gyrus, by contrast, an entirely different pathomorphology evolves. The establishment of the extraventricular proliferative matrices as well as the subpial cell translocation seem to be undisturbed (Stanfield and Cowan 1979 a,b). The deviation from the normal developmental schedule becomes visible during the integration of granule cells into the stratum granulosum. Instead of forming the typical

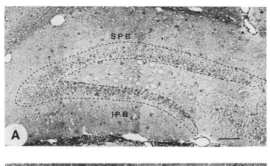

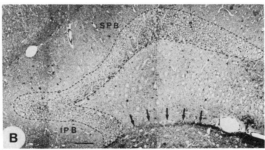

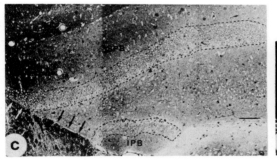

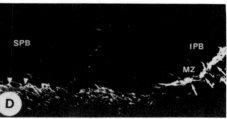

Fig. 7. Hamster dentate gyri at P 30, control animal shown in (A), two
examples of animals with meningeal cell destruction on P 0 in (B) and (C).
A belated formation of an rudimentary infrapyramidal blade (IPB) is
dependent on the repopulation of the hemispheral surface with meningeal
cells. Where fusion zones have developed between hemisphere and
diencephalon (arrows in (B) and (C)) a granule cell layer remains
definitively absent. The same is true for the formation of its medial tip
('crest'), which is then replaced by a direct contact of the
suprapyramidal granule cell layer (SPB) to the fusion zone (white arrows
in (C)). The discontinuity of the pial surface is also reflected in
immunohistochemical preparations, where a glial limiting membrane is only
demonstrable in regions of an intact meningeal surface (white arrows in
(D)), but is discontinuous or absent in fusion zones (remnants marked by
white arrowheads). Magnifications in A-C x 58, D x 110.

laminated structure, granule cells are irregularely spread out in the
dentate area, covering the region of the granule cell layer as well as the
entire hilus and part of the molecular zone, that is reduced in width to
about two thirds of the control value, since the commissural and
associational afferents are integrated into the granule cell cluster. A
major pathological gradient of cell deposition as in the neocortex is not
observed (Caviness and Rakic 1978; Stanfield and Cowan 1979 a,b).

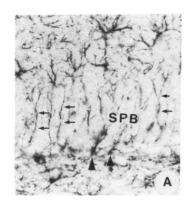 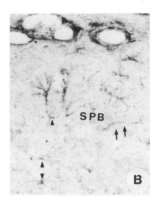

Fig. 8. The reeler defect of the dentate gyrus is associated with a
defective orientation and differentiation of monopolar radial glial cells.
A section of the suprapyramidal blade (SPB) of an control animal is shown
in (A), the same region of a mouse homozygous for the reeler allele in
(B). The regular glial scaffold (arrows in A) of the granule cell layer,
which arises from cell somata in the subgranular zone (arrowheads in A) is
replaced by scattered cells with various oblique orientations (arrows),
most of which have not developed their elongated basal processes
(arrowheads). Note the reduction of the number of GFAP-positive cells.
Magnification x 462.

     The most important feature distinguishing the reeler pathomorphology
in the dentate gyrus from the defects observed in the neocortex is the
effect of this mutation on the morphology and orientation of radial glial
cells. The secondary radial glial cells of the dentate gyrus, that in
contrast to the previously formed scaffold in the neocortex normally
differentiate during the formation of the granule cell layer, are not
formed in mutants. Instead, irregularly oriented astrocytes are
interspersed between the granule cells (see also Stanfield and Cowan 1979
a,b), only in rare cases exhibiting a somewhat elongated process, that
resembles a misshaped radial glial fiber (Fig. 8 A,B). In addition, the
overall density of GFAP - positive cells in the reeler dentate gyrus seems
to be considerably reduced.
     Thus, by contrast to the 'primordial' radial glial scaffold in the
isocortex, the late-differentiating secondary radial glial cells in the
dentate gyrus are apparently dependent on an intact neuron-glia
interaction not only for a proper positioning of migrating neurons into
their definitive laminae, but also for the establishment of their own
mature morphology. These findings support our concept of an interactive
mode of radial glia formation and neuronal lamination in the establishment
of the granule cell layer from the local proliferative matrices, which is
clearly distinct from the neuron-glia interaction during neocortical
ontogenesis.

SUMMARY

The development of the dentate gyrus differs in several aspects from the pattern of neocortical ontogenesis. Instead of the establishment of a primordial isocortical lamination featuring a cortical plate, proliferating neuronal and glial cells translocate from the dentate ventricular zone into secondary proliferative matrices, the most conspicuous of which lies underneath the pial surface within the marginal zone of the ventralmost portion of the cerebral hemisphere. Here, both cell types establish direct contacts to the basal lamina, which is only incompletely covered by typical glial endfeet. The assembly of the primordial granule cell layer is the result of a 'collateral aggregation' of columns of granule cells and unipolar 'secondary' radial glial cells which arise from the subpial and hilar dentate matrices. Radial growth of this primordial granule cell layer is attributable to the addition of neuronal and glial cells from the hilar dentate matrix and the subgranular zone which becomes predominant at the end of the first postnatal week in most rodents.

The unusual contacts of the cells within the subpial dentate matrix to the overlying basal lamina and thus to the mesenchyme have a profound influence on the differentiation of secondary radial glial cells and thereby on granule cell layer formation. Meningeal cell destruction during the period of existence of the subpial matrix inhibits the formation of the infrapyramidal blade, which is only able to partly regenerate after the reconstitution of the pia mater. A similar influence of meningeal lesions on the differentiation of bipolar radial glial cells and cortical plate formation in the neighbouring cornu ammonis or isocortex has not been observed.

Our concept, that the radial glial scaffold of the dentate gyrus differentiates locally during the integration of cells into the granular layer is further substantiated by a comparison of the pathomorphology of the reeler defect in the isocortex and dentate gyrus. In contrast to the isocortex, this genetic defect of neuron-glia-interaction is able to completely inhibit the formation of differentiated radial glial cells associated with the stratum granulosum.

REFERENCES

Altman, J. and Bayer, S.A., 1975, Postnatal development of the hippocampal dentate gyrus under normal and experimental conditions. in: "The Hippocampus", Vol. 1, pp. 95-122, Isaacson, R.L. and Pribram, K.H., eds., Plenum Press, New York

Altman, J. and Bayer, S. A., 1990 a, Mosaic organization of the hippocampal neuroepithelium and the multiple germinal sources of dentate granule cells. J. Comp. Neurol. 301:325

Altman, J. and Bayer, S.A., 1990 b, Prolonged sojourn of developing pyramidal cells in the intermediate zone of the hippocampus and their settling in the stratum pyramidale. J. Comp. Neurol. 301:343

Altman, J. and Bayer, S.A., 1990 c, Migration and distribution of two populations of hippocampal granule cell precursors during the perinatal and postnatal periods. J. Comp. Neurol. 301:365

Altman, J. and Das, G.D., 1965, Autoradiographic and histological evidence of postnatal hippocampal neurogenesis in rats. J. Comp. Neurol. 126:337

Altman, J. and Das, G.D., 1966, Autoradiographic and histological studies of postnatal neurogenesis. I. A longitudinal investigation of the kinetics, migration and transformation of cells incorporating tritiated thymidine in neonate rats, with special reference to postnatal neurogenesis in some brain regions. J. Comp. Neurol, 126:337

Angevine, J.B., 1965, Time of neuronal origin in the hippocampal region. Exp. Neurol 2:1

Angevine, J.B., 1975, Development of the hippocampal region. in: "The Hippocampus", Vol. 1, pp. 61-94, Isaacson, R.L.; Pribram, K.H., eds., Plenum Press, New York

Bayer, S.A., 1980 a, Development of the hippocampal region in the rat. I. Neurogenesis examined with (3)H-thymidine autoradiography. J. Comp. Neurol. 190:87

Bayer, S.A., 1980 b, Development of the hippocampal region in the rat. II. Morphogenesis during embryonic and and early postnatal life. J. Comp. Neurol. 190:115

Bayer, S.A. and Altman, J., 1974, Hippocampal development in the rat: Cytogenesis and morphogenesis examined with autoradiography and low-level X-irradiation. J. Comp. Neurol. 158:55

Bayer, S.A. and Altman, J., 1975, Radiation-induced interference with postnatal hippocampal cytogenesis in rats and its long-term effects on the acquisition of neurons and glia. J. Comp. Neurol. 163:1

Bayer, S.A., Yackel, J.W. and Purl, P.S., 1982, Neurons in the rat dentate gyrus granular layer substantially increase during juvenile and adult life. Science 216:890

Caviness, V.S., 1973, Time of neuron origin in the hippocampus and dentate gyrus of normal and reeler mice: An autoradiographic analysis. J. Comp. Neurol. 151:113

Caviness, V.S. and Rakic, P., 1978, Mechanisms of cortical development: A view from mutations in mice. Annu. Rev. Neurosci. 1:297

Caviness, V.S., Crandall, J.E. and Edwards, M.A., 1988, The reeler malformation. Implications for neocortical histogenesis. in: "Cerebral Cortex", Vol. 7, Development and Maturation of Cerebral Cortex, pp. 59 - 89, Peters, A. and Jones, E.G., eds., Plenum Press, New York

Cowan, W.M., Stanfield, B.B. and Kishi, K., 1980, The development of the dentate gyrus. in: "Current Topics in Developmental Biology", Vol. 15, pp. 103-157, Moscona, A. and Monroy, A., eds., Academic Press, New York

Cowan, W.M., Stanfield, B.B. and Amaral, D.G., 1981, Further observations on the development of the dentate gyrus. in: "Studies in Developmental Neurobiology", pp. 395435, Cowan, W.M., ed., Oxford University Press, Oxford

Crespo, D., Stanfield, B.B. and Cowan, W.M., 1986, Evidence that late-generated granule cells do not simply replace earlier formed neurons in the rat dentate gyrus. Exp. Brain Res. 62:541

Eckenhoff, M.F. and Rakic, P., 1984, Radial organization of the hippocampal dentate gyrus: A Golgi, ultrastructural and immunocytochemical analysis in the developing rhesus monkey. J. J. Comp. Neurol. 223:1

Eckenhoff, M.F. and Rakic, P., 1988, Nature and fate of proliferative cells in the hippocampal dentate gyrus during the life span of the rhesus monkey. J. Neurosci. 8:2729

Falconer, D.S., 1951, Two new mutants, 'trembler' and 'reeler' with neurological actions in the house mouse. J. Genet. 50:192

Gaarskjaer, F.B., 1985, The development of the dentate area and the hippocampal mossy fiber projection of the rat. J. Comp.Neurol. 241:154

Gaarskjaer, F.B., 1986, The organization and development of the hippocampal mossy fiber system. Brain Res. Rev. 11:335

Gall, C. and Lynch, G., 1980, The regulation of fiber growth and synaptogenesis in the developing hippocampus. in: "Current Topics in Developmental Biology", Vol. 15, pp 159 - 180, Moscona, A.A. and Monroy, A., eds., Academic Press, New York

Goffinet, A.M., 1984, Events governing organization of postmigratory neurons. Studies on brain development in normal and reeler mice. Brain Res. Rev. 7:261

Hartmann, D., Sievers, J., Pehlemann, F.W. and Berry, M., 1992,
Destruction of meningeal cells over the medial cerebral hemisphere of
newbom hamsters prevents the formation of the intrapyramidal blade of the
dentate gyrus- J. Comp. Neuro. 320:33

Hausmann, B. and Sievers, j., 1985, Cerebellar extemal granule cells are
attached to the basal lamina from the onset of migration up to the end of
their proliferative activity. J. Comp. Neurol. 241:50

Hausmann, B., Hartmann, D. and Sievers, J., 1987, Secondary euroepithelial
stem cells of the cerebellum and the dentate gyrus are attached to the
basal lamina during their migration and proliferation in: "Mesenchymal
Epithelial Interactions in Neural Development. pp. 279-292, Wolff,
J.R., Sievers, J. and Berry, m., eds., Springer, Berlin

Humphrey, T., 1966, The development of the human hippocampal formation
correlated with some aspects of its phylogenetic history. in: "Evolution
of the Forebrain. Phylogenesis and Ontogenesis of the Forebrain", pp. 104-
116, Hassler, R. and H. Stephen, eds., Thieme, Stuttgart

Humphrey, T., 1967, The development of the human hippocampal fissure. J.
Anat. 101:655

Jacobson, M., 1991, "Developmental Neurobiology", Third edition, Plenum
Press, New York

Kaplan, M.S. and Bell, D.H., 1983, Neuronal proliferation in the 9-month-
old rodent. Radioautographic study of granule cells in the hippocampus.
Exp. Brain Res. 52:1

Kaplan, M.S. and Bell, D.H., 1984, Mitotic neuroblasts in the 9-day-old
and 1 1-month-old rodent hippocampus. J. Neurosci. 4:1429

Kaplan, M.S. and Hinds, J.W., 1977, Neurogenesis in the adult rat:
Electron microscopic analysis of light autoradiographs. Science 197:1092

Marin-Padilla, M., 1978, Dual origin of the mammalian neocortex and
evolution of the cortical plate. Anat. Embryol. 152:109

Marin-Padilla, M., 1988, Early ontogenesis of the human cerebral cortex.
in: "Cerebral Cortex", Vol. 7, Development and Maturation of Cerebral
Cortex, pp. 1-34, Peters, A. and Jones, E.G. (eds.) Plenum Press, New York

Misson, J.-P., Edwards, M.A., Yamamoto, M. and Caviness, V.S., 1988
a, Mitotic cycling of radial glial cells of the fetal murine cerebral
wall: A combined autoradiographic and immunohistochemical study. Dev.
Brain Res. 38:183

Misson, J.-P., Edwards, M.A., Yamamoto, M. and Caviness, V.S., 1988
b, Identification of radial glial cells within the developing murine
central nervous system: Studies based upon a new immunohistochemical
marker. Dev. Brain Res.   44:95

Misson, J.-P., Takahashi, T. and Caviness, V.S., 1991, Ontogeny of radial
and other astroglial cells in the murine cerebral cortex.   Glia 4:138

Nowakowski, R.S. and Rakic, P., 1981, The site of origin and route and
rate of migration to the hippocampal region in the rhesus monkey. J. Comp
Neurol. 196:125

Pehlemann, F.-W., Sievers, J. and Berry, M., 1985, Meningeal cells are
involved in foliation, lamination and neurogenesis of the cerebellum:
Evidence from 6-OHDA-induced destruction of meningeal cells. Dev. Biol.
110:136

Pinto-Lord, M.C., Evrard, P. and Caviness, V.S., 1982, Obstructed neuronal
migration along radial glial fibers in the neocortex of the reeler mouse:
A Golgi-EM analysis. Dev. Brain Res. 4:379

Rakic, P., 1988 a, Defects of neuronal migration and the pathogenesis of
cortical malformations.   Prog. Brain Res. 73:15

Rakic, P., 1988 b, Specification of cerebral cortical areas: The radial
unit model. Science 241:170

Rakic, P. and Nowakowski, R.S., 1981, The time of origin of neurons in the
hippocampal region of the rhesus monkey.   J. Comp. Neurol. 196:99

Rickmann, M., Amaral, D.G. and Cowan, W.M., 1987, The organization of
radial glial cells during the formation of the dentate gyrus of the rat.
J. Comp. Neurol. 264:449

Habenular Innervation of the Interpeduncular Nucleus

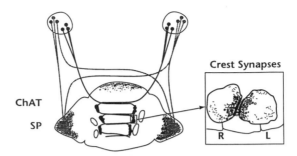

Fig. 1. Organization of cholinergic and peptidergic components of the habenular-interpeduncular system in the rat. SP and ChAT positive neurons are located in different portions of the habenulae and project to different subnuclei in the IPN. The intermediate subnucleus, identifiable by a system of penetrating blood vessels, contains dense accumulations of ChAT staining, some localized to terminals comprising the crest synapses.

however, is followed by replacement of both SP and ChAT staining by the contralateral habenular neurons.[5] The cholinergic and peptidergic systems therefore differ; the peptidergic system retains the capacity to sprout throughout life, while the cholinergic habenular cells manifest this ability only during a limited stage in their postnatal development, a period which coincides with the development of the cholinergic projection.[5,6]

The developmental regulation of both normal innervation and reactive reinnervation could imply developmental changes in the IPN target cells or changes in the cholinergic habenular neurons which limit the ability of cholinergic habenular cells to form projections to the IPN. One way to test these hypotheses is through use of transplants of fetal habenular neurons placed into host animals at different developmental stages following deafferentation of the IPN by FR lesions. If the habenular cells lose their ability to innervate IPN targets because of changes associated with their maturation, then fetal habenular cells transplanted to adult animals should still be competent to innervate their adult-denervated targets. On the other hand, if it is maturation of the target that limits competence to accept innervation, then transplanted fetal habenular cells should be incapable of innervating adult host cells. In contrast to the cholinergic system, the more plastic SP system should show transplant mediated recovery of staining whether the transplants are placed in neonatal or adult hosts.

In order to assess the functional significance of transplant mediated innervation, it is necessary to apply tests that distinguish between innervated and denervated nuclei. The functions of the habenulo-interpeduncular system have, however, remained obscure. The system is highly conserved evolutionarily[7,8,9,10,11] but lesions and stimulation experiments have heretofore produced a pattern of behavioral results that does not readily imply any known specific function.[12] This could indicate a comprehensive regulatory role for this system. Recent work has focused on the possibility that the system regulates endogenous levels of arousal and/or the degree of responsiveness to stimuli.[13,14,15,16] As a first attempt to explore this possibility, we chose to examine the integrity of sleep cycles under conditions of mild disruption in normal and FR-

Sprouting

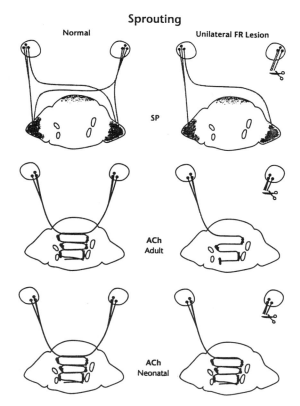

Fig. 2. Diagram summarizing effects of unilateral FR lesions on SP and ChAT staining in the IPN. Restoration of SP staining in the main portion of the lateral subnuclei occurs after unilateral lesions in adults and neonates. Restoration of cholinergic staining occurs only after unilateral lesions in the neonate.

denervated animals, with and without fetal transplants, to test the possibility that normal sleep cycles depend on the presence of normal projection patterns in the IPN.

METHODS

1. Surgery

a. <u>FR Lesions.</u> Stereotaxic thermal lesions of the FR were made in deeply anesthetized neonatal or adult female Sprague-Dawley rats.[3,5,17] Most of these rats were used as hosts for transplants, but some served as lesion-only controls.

b. <u>Transplant methods.</u> Pregnant rats at 14-15 days of gestation were deeply anesthetized, laparotomized, and the fetuses removed and placed on ice. For habenular excision, the cortex was reflected, exposing the two habenulae which were then excised. Ventral portions of the thalamus were excised from the diencephalic vesicle exposed by a midsagittal cut through the fetal brain. Each habenula or thalamus explant was then cultured for 5 days in a supplemented Ham's F-10 medium, following established procedures.[18,19] Following the culturing period, the tissue was dissociated using a mixture of trypsin and collagenase/dispase.[19] From each cell suspension, a sample was assayed for viability and cell concentration by counting cells that exclude trypan blue on a hemocytometer. The volume of cell suspension transplanted was then adjusted so that approximately the same number of viable cells (6-8 x 10⁴) was placed into each host.[20] Injections were made using a 10 ul Hamilton syringe fitted with a specially prepared micropipette tip.[19]

All host rats had received a bilateral FR lesion either 7 to 10 days (adult host) or 3 to 6 days (neonatal host) prior to transplantation. The host rat was then anesthetized, placed in the stereotaxic apparatus, and the needle was lowered into the brain according to predetermined coordinates localizing the degenerated FR pathway. The cells were injected slowly over 5-10 minutes, the needle was removed, the wound sutured, and the rat allowed to recover before being returned to its home cage.

All animals survived 2-3 months post transplantation before behavioral testing began.

2. Behavioral Testing

Sleep-cycle assay. The length and completeness of the animals, sleep cycles were assayed behaviorally using a variation of the standard pedestal or "flower-pot" technique[21,22,23] (Fig. 3). Each animal was placed on the pot beginning at the same time each day (10 a.m. or 11 a.m.), with the length of time gradually increasing over the first three acclimation days (.5hr, 1hr, and 3hr per day respectively). On the fourth day the animal was placed on the pot for 3 hrs, the last hour of which was the test period.

The principal measures were number and duration of sleep episodes during the test period, and the number of times a sleep episode ended with water contact by any part of the animal's body.

All measures were obtained by four separate observers over the course of this study, all of whom were unaware of the surgical history of the tested animals. Each observer tested animals from each of the groups in the study.

3. Anatomical Methods

Following behavioral testing, the animals were overdosed with chloral hydrate and perfused intracardially with normal saline, followed by 4% paraformaldehyde. Brains were removed and postfixed at least 24 hours. The blocks containing the transplant site and IPN were dissected out, cryoprotected in 30% sucrose, and frozen. 30mm sections were collected serially and every fourth section was stained with cresyl violet to localize the transplant site. The remaining sections were processed for immunocytochemistry using antibodies to SP or ChAT.[1,3] The analysis of immunocytochemical staining was unambiguous as the FR lesions eliminate SP and ChAT from the target subnuclei and there is normally very low background; transplant-induced restoration of specific staining was therefore readily apparent. Sections with IPN also contained substantia nigra, which stains densely for SP, and the occulomotor nuclei, which stain densely for ChAT. These two nuclei, which are independent of the medial habenulo-IPN system, served as internal controls for immunocytochemical staining intensity in lesion only and transplanted animals.

RESULTS

1. Recovery of Staining Patterns

a. <u>Normal habenulo-interpeduncular system.</u> The distribution of SP and
ChAT staining in IPN is shown in Figs. 4-5. Since bilateral FR lesions
permanently eliminate all SP and ChAT staining from the target subnuclei
in the IPN, any staining in these target subnuclei after bilateral lesions
in host brains can be attributed to the presence of the transplanted
cells.

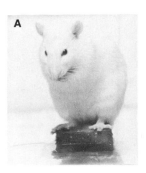 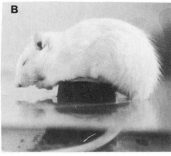 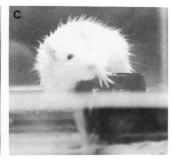

Fig. 3. Behavioral test. (A) The rat is placed on a small base inverted
flower pot affixed to the bottom of a glass fish tank. The top of the pot
extends 1 cm above water level. To avoid water contact, most animals
remain perched on the pot for several hours during their normal sleep
period. (B) From 13-17 times per hour, an intact animal will close its
eyes and hunch over, behaviors that correlate with EEG measures of mREM
sleep.[23,24] As REM-stage sleep begins, muscle tone becomes flaccid and
the animal either leans to one side or falls forward before (sometimes)
"catching" itself and resuming a more upright posture, usually accompanied
by at least a partial reopening of its eyes. However for normal animals,
a majority of these sleep episodes end when the muscle atonia (indicative
of REM sleep) is extensive enough to result in the animal coming in
contact with water (C).

b. <u>Transplants of habenular cells into adult FR lesioned host.</u> All
transplants were positioned in the ventral tegmentum, 1-2 mm from the
denervated IPN. The transplants survived and integrated well, the cells
were similar morphologically to normal habenular cells and
immunocytochemical staining revealed that SP and ChAT stained cells
aggregate (Fig. 6a,b), resembling in this respect the normal organization
of the habenula.

     Habenular transplants into adult hosts did not restore cholinergic
staining in the IPN, despite the presence of ChAT positive cells in the
transplant. The same transplants did, however, mediate some restoration
of SP staining in the habenular target subnuclei in the IPN (Fig. 7a). The
extent of the restored staining was variable, although always less than
normal, and was always restricted to subnuclei which are normal targets of
habenular SP neurons, e.g. the lateral subnuclei. Recovery of staining
was therefore specific and transplant dependent.

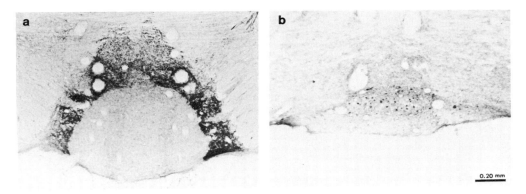

Fig. 4. Immunocytochemical staining for SP in normal IPN. 4a. SP staining in caudal IPN. Note extremely dense staining in lateral and dorsal subnuclei and faint staining, of non-habenular origin, in central subnucleus. 4b. SP staining in rostral IPN. Note very faintly staining population of intrinsic SP neurons in ventral sector of rostral subnucleus.

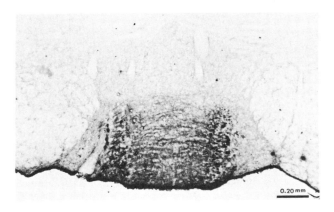

Fig. 5. Immunocytochemical staining for ChAT in normal IPN. Note extremely dense staining in central portion of the nucleus, including the central and intermediate nuclei.

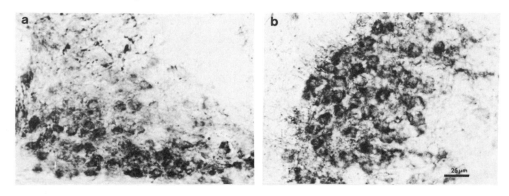

Fig. 6. Immunocytochemically stained cells in habenular transplants placed in the ventral tegmental area near host IPN. 6a. SP stained cells aggregated in transplant. 6b. ChAT stained cells aggregated in a different portion of the same transplant.

The transplants also mediated a consistent and marked enhancement of staining of the intrinsic SP neurons and their processes in the rostral subnucleus (Fig. 7b). The staining associated with the intrinsic cells was also restricted to their normal position in the ventral portion of the rostral subnucleus. Careful examination indicated no projection of these processes into the habenular SP target subnuclei, suggesting that these cells are not responsible for restoration of SP staining in the lateral subnuclei.

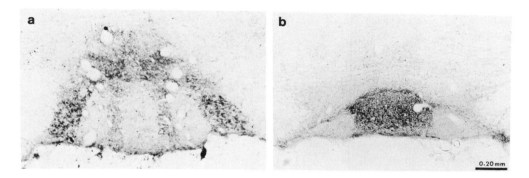

Fig. 7. Restoration of SP staining mediated by habenular transplants in IPN denervated by FR lesions. 7a. Note restoration of moderately dense staining in lateral subnucleus of IPN caudally and enhanced staining of non-habenular origin in the central subnucleus. 7b. Enhanced staining of intrinsic cells mediated by habenular transplants in denervated IPN.

c. _Transplants of habenular cells into neonatal FR lesioned host_. The habenular cells transplanted into neonatal lesioned hosts were also well integrated and contained aggregates of SP and ChAT positive cells.

SP staining in the lateral subnuclei was partially restored after transplants into neonatal brains; the extent of recovery of staining was similar to that seen after transplantation into adult hosts. Staining of the intrinsic cells was also enhanced by the transplants to an extent similar to that seen in adult hosts.

In contrast to the adult-lesioned host, ChAT staining was partially restored in the IPN of neonatal hosts with FR lesions (Fig. 8). Innervation of host targets by transplanted cholinergic neurons, like reinnervation by sprouting neurons, is thus developmentally regulated. Staining was found in cholinergic target subnuclei, the intermediate subnuclei and the central subnucleus.

Interestingly, ChAT staining was also present in the lateral subnuclei where it is normally never found. The staining in the lateral subnuclei therefore represents an aberrant projection of cholinergic habenular afferents.

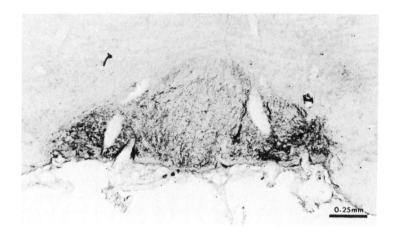

Fig. 8. Cholinergic staining in IPN of neonatal FR lesioned, habenular transplanted rat. Note moderately dense staining in intermediate subnucleus and extending into the lateral subnuclei.

d. <u>Transplants of thalamic cells into adult FR lesioned host.</u> Since the only SP and ChAT staining seen in adult thalamus is of extra-thalamic origin, we used transplants of fetal thalamic tissue into FR lesioned adult host brains to serve as a control for nonspecific effects of the introduction of fetal tissue into adult FR lesioned brains. These transplants also integrated well. As expected, SP staining showed no SP positive neurons in these transplants, and the staining pattern in the IPN was identical to that seen after FR lesions alone, i.e., an absence of staining in the lateral subnuclei and extremely faint staining of the intrinsic SP neurons in the rostral subnucleus.

Surprisingly, however, numerous ChAT positive neurons were found in all thalamic transplants (Fig. 9). Immunocytochemical staining of the diencephalic vesicle in normal E14 and E15 embryos revealed the presence of a transient population of ChAT positive neurons. Thus transplantation of E14/15 thalamic cells into the FR denervated host appears to have the unexpected effect of supporting the survival or continued expression of ChAT in this population of embryonic thalamic neurons. These thalamic transplants containing ChAT positive neurons also support the restoration of ChAT staining in the IPN (Fig. 9). The restored staining is primarily present in the intermediate subnuclei but also extends in some cases into the lateral subnuclei, the habenular SP targets, and therefore resembles the staining pattern mediated by habenular ChAT neurons implanted into neonatal hosts. The fact that this restoration occurred when thalamic cells were implanted into adult brains indicates that the mature IPN retains the ability to accept cholinergic innervation.

e. <u>Summary of anatomical observations.</u> Our lesion and transplant paradigms permit us to modify the staining pattern in the IPN: (1) Normal IPN contains dense accumulations of SP and ChAT staining; (2) FR lesioned IPN contains no ChAT or SP staining in habenular SP targets; (3) habenular transplants in neonatal animals partially restore both SP and cholinergic staining to habenular targets; (4) habenular transplants in adults restore only SP staining; and (5) thalamic transplants in adults restore only ChAT staining. This dissociation of cholinergic and SP staining in the IPN by

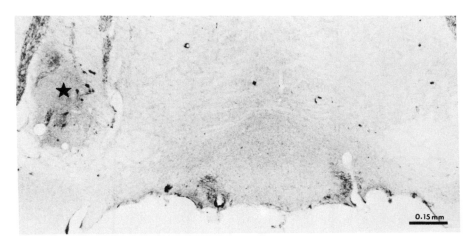

Fig. 9. Cholinergic staining in IPN of adult FR lesioned, thalamic transplanted rat. Note transplant containing ChAT positive neurons (*) and ChAT staining in intermediate subnucleus of denervated IPN.

the use of specific lesion-transplant paradigms allows us to examine the functions of these two systems.

2. Recovery of function

a. Normal sleep cycles. We used the "flower-pot test", originally designed as a way to eliminate REM sleep, to assess the integrity of sleep patterns during the animal's normal sleep period (Fig. 3). In this assay, the nREM stage of the sleep cycle ends just before the end of the sleep episode itself, the latter being truncated by the animal's restricted movement at the onset of muscle atonia. Therefore the duration of this behaviorally measured sleep episode is predominantly a measure of the duration of the nREM stage.

The REM stage of the sleep episode is characterized behaviorally by muscle atonia, accompanied by loss of balance, often culminating in water contact. The frequency of water contact therefore indicates the degree of completeness of the REM stage sleep.

b. FR Lesion. FR lesioned animals show marked reduction in both parameters (Figs. 10,11). These data indicate that integrity of the habenulo-interpeduncular system is necessary for normal functioning of the sleep cycles.

c. Effects of transplants on restoration of sleep cycles. Transplants of fetal habenular neurons into neonatal hosts, which restore both SP and ChAT staining in the IPN, also restore normal patterns of both the REM and nREM components of the sleep cycle (Figs. 10,11). Adult animals which received transplants of fetal habenular neurons, which restore only SP staining, have a normal frequency of REM-associated atonia (Fig. 11) but sleep episode duration remains shorter (Fig. 10). Adult animals that received transplants of fetal thalamic neurons, which restore ChAT staining in the IPN, show normal duration of nREM sleep (Fig. 10) but diminished frequency of REM sleep (Fig. 11). The behavioral data thus support an association of restoration of normal frequency of REM sleep with restoration of SP staining, and of normal duration of nREM sleep with restoration of ChAT staining (Table I).

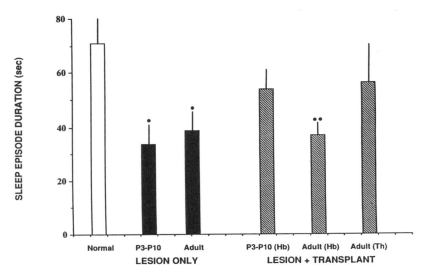

Fig. 10. Sleep episode duration. FR lesions result in a significantly shorter mean duration of sleep episodes (33.5 ± 7.5 secs when lesions are made between postnatal days 3 and 10; 38.7 ± 6.8 secs when lesions are made in the adult), compared to normal (71.1 ± 9.2 secs). Animals with lesions plus transplants that mediate cholinergic reinnervation of the IPN have sleep episode times that are similar to normals (53.9 ± 7.4 secs in perinatal hosts with habenular (Hb) transplants, 56.3 ± 13.1 secs in adult hosts with thalamic (Th) transplants). Duration remains significantly less than normal for animals with transplants that do not support cholinergic reinnervation (36.8 ± 4.6 secs in adult hosts with Hb transplants). Statistics and n's as in Fig. 11.

DISCUSSION

Restoration of innervation

Fetal diencephalic neurons survive when transplanted into midbrains of neonatal or adult hosts whose FRs have been sectioned bilaterally, and these transplanted neurons can mediate both partial recovery of staining patterns in the IPN and recovery of normal sleep patterns. SP staining recovered partially when cell suspensions of E14/15 habenulae were placed in neonatal or adult brains, while ChAT staining mediated by habenular transplants recovered only when these cells were placed in neonatal hosts. The restoration of staining by transplanted habenular cells thus appears subject to the same developmental regulation as restoration mediated by sprouting after unilateral FR lesions. Surprisingly ChAT staining also recovered when suspensions of fetal thalamic cells containing cholinergic neurons were implanted in adult FR lesioned brains. An aberrant source of cholinergic innervation was thus more successful in innervating the adult IPN than the normal source.

We attribute the recovered staining in the host IPN to cholinergic and peptidergic neurons contained within the transplants. In the case of the cholinergic system, there is no other source of ChAT within the IPN or near the IPN and there is no recovery of ChAT staining after FR lesions in the absence of transplanted fetal tissue containing cholinergic cells. In the case of the SP staining the issue is more ambiguous and the transplant may have both direct and indirect effects on staining in the IPN. The presence of intrinsic SP cells and the sparing of some SP staining from

258

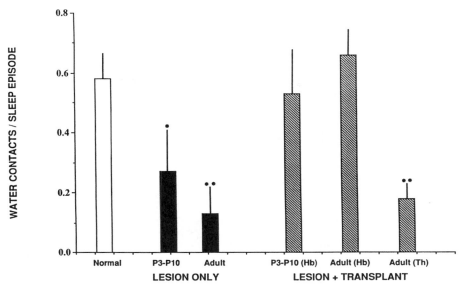

Fig. 11. Water contacts. A significantly smaller mean fraction of sleep
episodes end in REM-associated water contact by animals with FR lesions,
when the lesion is made in P3-P10 animals (.27 ± .14) or in adults (.13 ±
.09), compared to normals (.58 ± .08). Animals with FR lesions plus
transplants that mediate SP reinnervation of the IPN show normal
frequencies (.53 ± .15 in P3-P10 hosts with habenular transplants, .66 ±
.08 in adult hosts with habenular transplants). However, mean water
contact frequency remains significantly reduced from normal in hosts with
transplants that do not support SP reinnervation. (.18 ± .05 in adults
with thalamus cell transplants [Th]). Means are ± s.e.m.; P<.05; p<.01 by
Kruskal-Wallis test, compared to normals. N = 7 for all groups except
normal (n = 10), lesion + Hb transplant, adult host (n = 10) and P3-P10
lesion-only (n 6).

Table 1. Summary of the relationship between SP and ChAT staining in
habenular targets and sleep related behavior.

| | IPN INNERVATION | | SLEEP - RELATED BEHAVIOR | |
	SP	ACh	REM state	NREM state
CONTROL	+	+	+	+
FR LESION	-	-	-	-
FR LESION + HABENULA TP (Neonate)	+	+	+	+
FR LESION + HABENULA TP (Adult)	+	-	+	-
FR LESION + THALAMUS TP (Adult)	-	+	-	+

259

non-habenular sources after FR lesions suggests the possibility that the restoration of host IPN staining is mediated by these non-habenular sources. The most robust effect of the habenular transplants, placed either in adult or neonatal hosts, is, in fact, the greatly enhanced staining of the intrinsic SP containing cells in the ventral sector of the rostral subnucleus; the effect of the habenular transplant on these cells appears to be specific since enhanced staining of the intrinsic SP system is not seen in animals with thalamic transplants. The specificity of the effect suggests that the enhancement of staining of these host cells may be due to diffusible factors arising from those transplants that contain SP cells. These SP containing intrinsic cells are logical candidates for restoration of SP staining in the habenular targets, but they do not restore SP staining after FR lesions alone.[6,10] Moreover, close examination of staining patterns shows that the boundaries of the area occupied by these intrinsic host cells are strictly maintained following lesions and transplants. It therefore seems unlikely that these cells provide the SP staining seen in the lateral subnucleus of transplant-containing animals. The enhanced staining of the intrinsic SP cells may however be associated with the behavioral recovery.

Most studies in which fetal transplants have been used to reinnervate denervated structures have emphasized the restoration of normal patterns of projections and therefore, by extension, of normal innervation.[25,26,27,28,29,30] Transmitter specific reinnervation may take place regardless of whether the neurons are appropriate or inappropriate. For example, an appropriate pattern of cholinergic staining in the hippocampus is restored by implanted septal neurons, the normal source, and also by implanted habenular or striatal neurons, abnormal sources of cholinergic input.[25,26,29]

The pattern of restoration of SP staining in the IPN shows a recovery limited to normal habenular target areas and thus supports a transmitter-specific regulation of innervation mediated by the transplanted cells. The ease with which staining is restored by sprouting or by reinnervation with transplanted neurons in both adult and neonatal hosts indicates that the denervated target cells remain receptive to appropriate innervation.

The restoration of ChAT staining shows interesting differences from the SP system. In animals with FR lesions and transplants, there is clear evidence of restoration of staining within normal targets (the intermediate subnuclei), but also of extension of the ChAT staining into the lateral subnuclei which are normally innervated by habenular SP neurons. This extension of ChAT staining into an aberrant target occurs with both habenular transplants into neonatal hosts and thalamic transplants into adult hosts, and indicates that the neurons in the lateral subnuclei retain the capability of accepting cholinergic innervation throughout life even though they normally do not receive such innervation. The SP system develops before the cholinergic innervation[5] and its occupation of the lateral subnuclei may normally limit cholinergic innervation; the disruption of the temporal order of innervation by FR lesions and habenular transplants may eliminate the advantage normally enjoyed by the SP cells. Similarly when SP is eliminated by FR lesions and transplants provide only cholinergic input, the lateral subnuclei receive cholinergic innervation. A limitation on cholinergic innervation by the presence of the contralateral SP projection to the lateral subnuclei would explain the normal pattern of innervation achieved by sprouting of cholinergic projections after unilateral lesions in the neonate.[5]

The cholinergic innervation in hosts with the two types of

transplants had unpredicted results. Both appropriate habenular and inappropriate thalamic neurons mediated a similar pattern of cholinergic innervation, consistent with the findings of others that transmitter specific innervation occurs even by cells that normally do not project to the denervated host.[26,28,29,31] What was surprising was the finding that thalamic but not habenular cholinergic neurons could mediate innervation of adult IPN. Our hypothesis, based on studies of sprouting and development of the habenular cholinergic system, had suggested that a temporal limitation exists on cholinergic innervation of the IPN which could be due to changes in the target, e.g. cessation of release of adequate amounts of trophic substances, or to changes in the afferents, e.g. cessation of synthesis of adequate types or numbers of receptors for the trophic substances. The evidence of innervation of adult host IPN by thalamic transplants containing cholinergic neurons indicates that the host target cells remain receptive. The failure of embryonic habenular transplants containing cholinergic cells to innervate adult host targets suggested that innervation might be dependent on features associated with the immature afferents. However, others have shown that fetal habenular cells transplanted into adult hosts can restore staining patterns to denervated hippocampus, an anomalous target.[25,29] Taken together, these results lead to the conclusions that (1) habenular neurons retain the capability of forming new projections even in an adult and when forced to traverse foreign territory and (2) adult IPN neurons retain the capability of accepting cholinergic innervation. Additional factors must therefore be involved in the establishment of the appropriate habenular-IPN cholinergic projection. The habenular cholinergic projection does have the peculiar feature of innervating the system of crest synapses (Fig. 1) that densely populate the intermediate subnuclei. These synapses are complex structures, in which one terminal arises from cells in the left habenula and the other terminal arises from cells in the right habenula.[4,17,33] This left-right organization is established during postnatal development and indicates an additional constraint on the formation of synaptic complexes involving habenular neurons which may not operate in the formation of synapses by other cholinergic neurons.

Recovery of function

The behavioral assay that we used, the flower pot test of sleep-cycle patterns, proved to be an accurate indicator of the staining patterns in the habenulo-interpeduncular system. The frequency of normal REM-associated atonia and the duration of largely nREM sleep episodes were markedly decreased after bilateral FR lesions, but were restored to normal after transplants which mediated recovery of SP and ChAT staining. The use of different types of transplants further enabled us to distinguish functionally between (1) reinnervation of the SP habenular targets and enhanced staining in intrinsic SP cells, which are associated with restoration of normal REM atonia, and (2) reinnervation of ChAT habenular targets, which is associated with restoration of nREM sleep duration.

The muscle atonia component of REM-stage sleep, and the modulation of nREM-stage sleep, are thought to be under the control of dorsal tegmental/rostral pontine and dorsal raphe areas respectively,[34] areas that are principal efferent targets of the IPN.[35] The IPN is thus well positioned to have a functional role in the coordination of REM and nREM stages of sleep; our results further suggest that this coordination may be mediated between two distinct neurotransmitter systems.

REFERENCES

1. Artymyshyn, R. and Murray, M. (1985) Substance P in the

interpeduncular nucleus of the rat: normal distribution and the effects of deafferentation. J. Comp. Neurol. 231:78-90.

2. Contestabile, A., Villani, L., Fasolo, A., Franzoni, M.F., Gribaudo, L., Oktedalen, O. and Fonnum, F. (1987) Topography of cholinergic and substance P pathways in the habenulo-interpeduncular system of the rat. Neurosc. 21:253-270.

3. Eckenrode, T.C., Barr, G.A., Battisti, W.P. and Murray, M. (1987) Acetylcholine in the interpeduncular nucleus of the rat: normal distribution and effects of deafferentation. Brain Res. 418:273-286.

4. Lenn, N.J. and Bayer, S.A. (1986) Neurogenesis in the subnuclei of the rat interpeduncular nucleus and medial habenula. Brain Res. Bull. 16:219-224.

5ª Barr, G.A., Eckenrode, T.C. and Murray, M. (1987) Normal development and the effects of early deafferentation in choline acetyltransferase, substance P and serotonin like immunoreactivity in the interpeduncular nucleus. Brain Res. 418:301-313.

6. Contestabile, A., Virgili, M. and Barnabei, O. (1990) Developmental profiles of cholinergic activity in the habenulae and IPN of the rat. Int. J. Devl. Neurosc. 8:561-564.

7. Herrick, C.J., "The Brain of the Tiger Salamander," University of Chicago Press, Chicago, (1965) pp.247-264.

8. Kappers, C.U.A., Huber, G.C. and Crosby, E.C., "The Comparative Anatomy of the Nervous System of Vertebrates, including Man," Hafner Co., New York (1967).

9. Sharma, S.C., Berthoud, V.M. and Breckwoldt, R. (1989) Distribution of SP-like immunoreactivity in the goldfish brain. J. Comp. Neurol. 279:104-116.

10. Villani, L., Battistini, S., Bissole, R. and Contestabile, A. (1987) Cholinergic projections of the telencephalo-habenulo-interpeduncular system of the goldfish. Neurosc. Lett. 76:263-268.

11. Villani, L., Guarnieri, T., Salsi, U. and Bollini, D. (1991) Substance P in the habenulo-interpeduncular system of the goldfish. Brain Res. Bull. 26:225-228.

12. Sutherland, R.J. (1982) The dorsal diencephalic conduction system: a review of the anatomy and functions of the habenular complex. Neurosc. and Bio. Op. Beh. Reviews 6:1-13.

13. Herkenham, M. (1981) Anesthetics and the habenulo-interpeduncular system: selective sparing of metabolic activity. Brain Res. 210:461-466.

14. Lisoprawski, A., Blanc, G. and Glowinski, J. (1981) Activation by stress of the habenulointerpeduncular substance P neurons in the rat. Neurosc. Lett. 25:57-66.

15. Nishikawa, T., Fage, D. and Scatton, B. (1986) Evidence for, and nature of, the tonic inhibitory influence of habenulo-interpeduncular pathways upon cerebral dopaminergic transmission in the rat. Brain Res. 373:324-336.

16. Thornton, E.W. and Bradbury, G.E. (1989) Effort and stress influence the effect of lesion of the habenula complex on one-way active avoidance learning. Physiol. & Behav. 45:929-935.

17. Murray, M., Zimmer, J. and Raisman, G. (1979) Quantitative electron microscopic evidence for reinnervation in the adult rat interpeduncular nucleus after lesions of the fasciculus retroflexus. J. Comp. Neurol. 187:447-468.

18. Cunningham, T.J., Haun, F., and Chantler, P.D. (1987) Diffusible proteins prolong survival of dorsal lateral geniculate neurons following occipital cortex lesions in newborn rats. Dev. Brain Res. 37:133-141.

19. Haun, F. and Cunningham, T.J. (1987) Specific neurotrophic interactions between cortical and subcortical visual structures in developing rat. J. Comp. Neurol. 256:561-569.

20. Brundin, P., Issaccson, O. and Bjorklund, A. (1985) Monitoring of cell viability in suspensions of embryonic CNS tissue and its use as a criterion for intracerebral graft survival. Brain Res. 331:251-259.

21. McGrath, M.J. and Cohen, D.B. (1978) REM sleep facilitation of adaptive waking behavior: a review of the literature. Psych. Bull. 85:24-57.

22. Mendelson, W.B., Guthrie, R.D., Frederick, G. and Wyatt, R.J. (1974) The flower pot technique of rapid eye movement (REM) sleep deprivation. Pharm. Bioch. and Beh. 2:553-556.

23. Rideout, B.E. (1979) Non-REM sleep as a source of learning deficits induced by REM sleep deprivation. Physiol. and Behav. 22:1043-1047.

24. Swisher, J.E. (1972) Manifestations of "activated" sleep in the rat. Science 138:1110.

25. Anderson, K.J., Gibbs, R.B. and Cotman, C.W. (1988) Transmitter phenotype is a major determinant in the specificity of synapses formed by cholinergic neurons transplanted to the hippocampus. Neurosc. 25:19-25.

26. Clarke, D.J., Nilsson, O.G., Brundin, P. and Biorklund, A. (1990) Synaptic connections formed by grafts of different types of cholinergic neurons in the host hippocampus. Exp. Neurol. 107:11-22.

27. Freund, T.F., Bolam, J.P., Bjorklund, A., Stenevi, U., Dunnett, S.B., Powell, J.F. and Smith, A.D. (1985) Efferent synaptic connections of grafted dopaminergic neurons reinnervating the host neostriatum: a tyrosine hydroxylase immunocytochemical study. J. Neurosc. 5:603-616.

28. Gage, F.H. and Bjorklund, A. (1986) Enhanced graft survival in the hippocampus following selective denervation. Neurosc. 17:89-98.

29. Gibbs, R.B., Anderson, K.J. and Cotman, C.W. (1986) Factors affecting innervation in the CNS: comparison of three cholinergic cell types transplanted to the hippocampus of the rat. Brain Res. 383:362-366.

30. Zhou, C-F., Raisman, G. and Morris, R.J. (1985) Specific patterns of fibre outgrowth from transplants to host mice hippocampi, shown immunohistochemically by the use of allelic forms of thy-1. Neurosc. 16:819-833.

31. Dunnett, S.B., Whishaw, I.Q., Bunch, S.T. and Fine, A. (1986) Acetylcholine-rich neuronal grafts in the forebrain of rats: effects of environmental enrichment, neonatal adrenaline depletion, host transplantation site and regional source of embryonic donor cells on graft size and acetylcholinesterase-positive fibre outgrowth. Brain Res. 378:357-373.

32. Lenn, N.J. (1976) Synapses in the interpeduncular nucleus. J. Comp. Neurol. 166:73-100.

33. Lenn, N.J., Wong, V. and Hamill, G.S. (1983) Left-right pairing at the crest synapses of rat IPN. Neurosc. 9:383-389.

34. Vertes, R.P. Brainstem mechanisms of slow-wave and REM sleep. In: "Brainstem Mechanisms of Behavior," W.R. Kyemm and R.P. Vertes, eds., John Wiley & Sons, New York, (1990) pp. 535-583.

35. Groenewegen, H.J., Ahlenius, S., Haber, S.N., Kowall, N.W. and Nauta, W.J.H. (1986) Cytoarchitecture, fiber connections, and some histochemical aspects of the interpeduncular nucleus in the rat. J. Comp. Neurol. 249:65-102.

DEVELOPMENT OF DESCENDING PROJECTION NEURONS TO THE SPINAL CORD OF THE
GOLDFISH, Carassius auratus

S.C. Sharma and V.M. Berthoud

Department of Ophthalmology
New York Medical College
Valhalla, NY 10595

The descending supra-spinal projection neurons, especially certain
reticulospinal neurons, have been implicated in the integration of spatial
and temporal aspects of certain sensory modalities such as taste in
teleost (Kanwal & Finger, '88). In addition it has been postulated that
reticulospinal neurons are involved in modulating the locomotion behavior
in fish (Bando, '75; McClellan & Grillner, '84). Furthermore, sexual
behavior in goldfish is controlled by preoptico-spinal pathway (Demski &
Sloane, '85). Mauthner cells (reticulospinal neurons) are involved in
eliciting the startle response (Eaton & Bompardieri, '78). These few
examples attest to the varied influences of supra-spinal projection
neurons onto the behavior of fish.

The role of descending spinal projections in modulating spinal
neurons has been extensively studied in higher vertebrates. In fish, the
detailed anatomy of these projection neurons has advanced appreciably in
recent years (Smeets & Timerick, '81, Kimmel et al., '82, Prasada Rao et
al., '87). As discussed by Prasada Rao et al., ('87) the supra-spinal
projection nuclei in both midbrain and brain stem, amongst the vertebrate
species studied so far remain rather constant. Efforts has been made
previously to correlate the genesis of behavior with the ontogeny of
nervous system (Coghill, '29; Hamburger '73; Robert & Khan, '82).
However, comparatively fewer studies exist to date which deal with fish
nervous system development and behavior (Leghissa, '42; Whiting, '48;
Harris, '62; Gideiri, '66). Recent studies on the developing nervous
system of fish (Kuwada, '86; Kimmel et al., '82; Metcalfe et al., '86;
Mendelson et al., '86 a,b) have provided impetus for using fish embryos
for to study both nervous system development and behavior. Since Prasada
Rao et al., '87 have described the descending projection neurons in common
goldfish (Carassius auratus), an animal commonly used in many
neurobiological studies, the present study describing the development of
supra-spinal projection was undertaken in order to delineate the
developmental stages at which these projections to the spinal cord emerge
and the sequence of their maturation.

Fertilized goldfish (Carassius auratus) eggs were obtained from
Mount Parnall fisheries, Pennsylvania or Hunting Creek fisheries,
Maryland. Eggs were separated from the spawn and were washed in several
changes of distilled water and were transferred to the goldfish ringer
solution (Foster & Taggard, '50). Embryos were staged according to Sharma

Development of the Central Nervous System in Vertebrates
Edited by S.C. Sharma and A.M. Goffinet, Plenum Press, New York, 1992

265

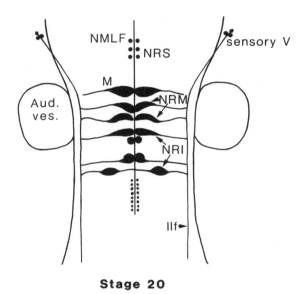

Stage 20

Fig. 1. Diagram summarizing labelled cells found at stage 20. Labelled cells are found in sensory nuclei of V nerve; presumptive NMLF and NRS, M neuron, NRM and NRI; llf formed by the descending axons of the sensory nucleus of V is distinguishable.

and Unger ('80). In general, stage 20 is the early tail bud stage and it occurs about 33 hrs. after fertilization when the eggs are maintained at 18°C ± 1°C. Stage 21 is at 36 hrs. after fertilization and stage 22 is at 50 hrs., stage 23 is at 60 hrs., stage 24 is at 80 hrs. after fertilization. Embryos hatch at stage 25 which is at 100 hrs after spawning. After hatching, larvae were staged by the number of days.

Embryos from stage 20 onwards were anesthetized with 0.1% MS-222 (Sigma) prepared in goldfish ringer solution. The spinal cord was bilaterally cut at the level of 3rd or 5th spinal segment and a small pledget of gelfoam soaked in 30% HRP (Sigma type VI) in phosphate buffer (pH 7.4) was inserted at the cut end. The embryos were allowed to recover and they transferred to fresh goldfish ringer solution. In prehatched embryos, 30 minutes to 4 hours were allowed for HRP transport whereas, in hatched larvae, an average of 12-24 hrs were allowed for the enzyme transport. 50 μm sections of the embryo were cut at coronal, longitudinal or horizontal planes.

HRP was reacted using Hanker Yates' modified method (Bell et al., '81). HRP labelled cells were seen at all stages studied. In younger embryos, labelled axons were not revealed consistently. Only those stages showing changes either in position or number of labelled neurons as compared with the previous stage are included. Labelled cells were designated belonging to a particular nucleus after considering their position relative to major land marks such as the optic and auditory vesicles, and their position in later developmental stages. The terminology used in the present study was adapted from Prasada Rao et al. ('87) who described the projection nuclei to the spinal cord in adult goldfish.

The labelled cells in the brain, following HRP application to the spinal cord, were recognized at embryonic stage 20. Most labelled cells were sequestered near the midline immediately rostral to and in the vicinity of the auditory vesicle and extended caudal to it (Fig. 1). Hence, rostralmost labelled cells were either the cells of the nucleus of the medial longitudinal fascicle (NMLF) or perhaps the nucleus of the reticular formation (NRS). These cell bodies usually were rounded with no apparent dendritic elaborations. Distinct lateral longitudinal fascicles (llf) were evident at this stage. Fibers in this tract emerged from the peripherally situated sensory nuclei of the trigeminal and extend their axons into the brain and run caudally to the spinal cord.

The posterior labelled neurons corresponding to the medial and inferior reticular formation (NRM and NRI) and the Mauthner neurons (M) were paired and they extended from the rostral end of the auditory vesicles to the caudal end of the brain. Most paired neurons had fusiform somas. The Mauthner neuron cell bodies were the largest in size even at this early stage and they occupied a dorsal position.

Proliferation of new cells continued at stage 23. The first signs of heart pulsations are evident at this stage. The labelled reticular formation neurons were positioned laterally, due perhaps to their displacement by newly generated cells. At stage 23, Mauthner neurons were more prominent; their somas were located at the rostralmost level of the auditory vesicle; their lateral dendritic processes extended to the level of the lateral longitudinal fascicle and the crossed axonal pattern was clearly distinguishable (Fig. 2). Rostral to the Mauthner neurons, at the level of the posterior portion of the eye, a few paired neurons in the midline were evident. These cells represented the future nucleus of the medial longitudinal fascicle (NMLF, Fig. 2). Laterally displaced neurons, slightly caudal to the NMLF, represented the scattered cells of the

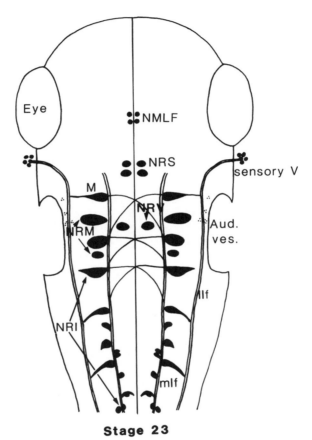

Stage 23

Fig. 2. Diagram summarizing labelled cells found at stage 23. Labelled
cells are found in NMLF, NRS, M neuron, NRM, NRI and NRV; labelled fibers
in llf and mlf are distinguishable. Presumptive neurons of the octaval
area are labelled (arrow). The decussating axons of M neuron, one pair of
NRM and one of NRI neurons are seen. Displacement of neurons to more
lateral locations can be noticed (compare with stage 20); displacement has
also occurred along the rostrocaudal axis.

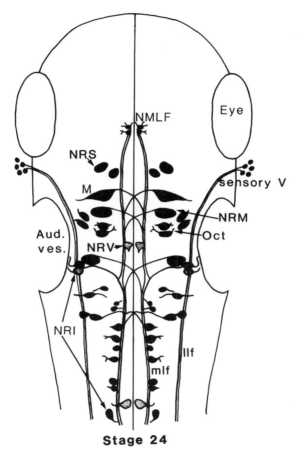

Stage 24

Fig. 3. Diagram of a horizontal section through the brain of an embryo at
stage 24, summarizing all labelled neurons. Labelled neurons can be seen
at the NMLF, NRS, NRM, M neurons, octaval area, NRV and NRI. Another pair
of NRI neurons show decussating axons; mlf and llf are distinguished; mlf
has become more medial in location (compare with stage 23). Dendrites
begin to develop at this stage. The neuron with bifurcating axons extends
it dendrites towards the otic vesicle. Octaval nuclei appear to be formed
by two clusters of cells. Ventrally positioned cells are indicated by the
stippling.

superior reticular formation (NRS). Dendritic processes, other than those of Mauthner neurons were still indistinguishable at this stage. A few neurons in the octaval area were labelled. No subdivisions of the octavial area were evident at this stage. The labelled neurons positioned immediately caudal to the Mauthner neurons were designated as medial and inferior reticular formation neurons (NRM and NRI, respectively; Fig. 2). Labelled cells near the midline were designated as ventromedial reticular formation neurons (NRV). The majority of labelled spinal projecting neurons (9 pairs) at this stage belonged to the NRI. These cells were mostly fusiform in shape. Some NRI somas were so laterally located that they touched the lateral longitudinal fascicle. One rostral pair of NRI cells showed a clear contralateral projection (Fig. 2).

At stage 24, the number of labelled cells in the NMLF increased, and dendritic elaborations were apparent. Rostral to the M neuron, superior reticular formation (NRS) neurons had enlarged somas. The NRS neurons were laterally positioned.

Two clusters of cells were observed at the octaval area and were placed at the midlevel between dorsally located M neuron and more ventrally placed NRV. These cellular groups were situated caudal to the M neurons and rostral to NRI (Fig. 3). We designated the lateral cell group as descending octaval nucleus (DON).

The cells belonging to NRM, NRI and raphae nucleus (NR) neurons appeared consolidated in distinct groups immediately caudal to the M neuron. M neuron axons assumed a more medial position (Fig. 3). The NRV cells were ventrally located. The rostralmost NRI cells were laterally located; those in a dorsal position had contralateral projections wereas cells located in a ventral position had bifurcated axons which extended rostrocaudally. The later axons traversed ipsilaterally in the medial longitudinal fascicle (mlf). Further caudally, another NRI neuron pair projected their axons contralaterally and travelled in the vicinity of the mlf. The medially located caudalmost NRI cells were ventral in position.

The formation of cellular clusters and the dendritic elaborations continued at stage 25 (hatching).

One day post hatched larvae

Within 24 hours of hatching, the pattern and positioning of the neurons in the lower brainstem which gave rise to the descending projections were somewhat similar to those of the adult. The M neuron extended its dendritic arbor toward the auditory vesicle (Fig. 4). Two clusters of 8-10 neurons were found on each side of the midline rostrally and comprised the nucleus of the medial longitudinal fascicle. A medial and lateral group of NMLF neurons on each side was evident. Two clusters of cells were also evident in the NRS. Rostrally and caudally situated cell groups were recognized in the NRM, and were located slightly ventral to the M neuron. The rostralmost cell group was situated anteriorly to the M neuron. One caudal cell group, consisting of 7 labelled cells on each side, is shown in Fig. 4B. Four groups of cells belong to the NRI as seen at this level of the section.

As the number of neurons increased, the llf and mlf showed a distinct character. Contralateral descending axons arising from NRM and NRI neurons were easily recognized at 3 locations extending rostrocaudally.

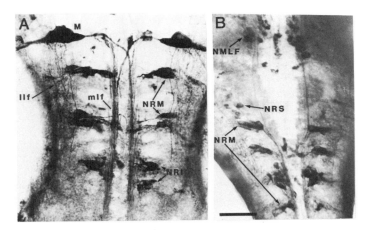

Fig. 4. A. Horizontal section of the brain of a one day-old larva.
Labelled cells and fiber bundles can be seen. M neurons, NRM, NRI are
labelled. The bar represents 29.0 μm. B. Horizontal section of the
brain of a one day-old larva. The increase in number of cells in the
NMLF, NRS, and NRM neurons can be appreciated. The level of sectioning is
ventral to the M neuron (Fig. 5A). The bar represents 54 μm.

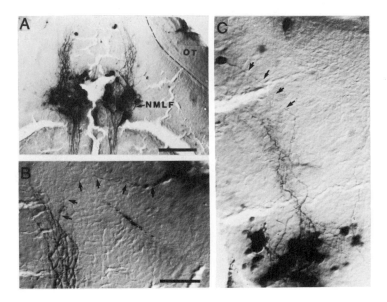

Fig. 5. A. Photograph of a horizontal section of 7 day-old larvae
illustrating the extensive dendritic network of NMLF neurons. Optic
tectum (OT) boundries are demarcated with dashed lines. Bar represents
104 μm. B. High power photograph of another horizontal section from a
different animal of the same age showing an axon leaving the tectum
(extreme right upper corner). This axon (labelled with small arrows)
leaves the tectum and merges with the dentric branches of NMLF neurons.
Bar represent 45 μm. C. Photograph of a horizontal section of a 7 day-
old embryo showing a labelled NPO neuron (upper left hand corner) with its
axon (arrows) descending caudally. Axon can be traced for a distance and
it merges with the dendrites of the NMLF neurons bottom. Magnification is
same as in B.

271

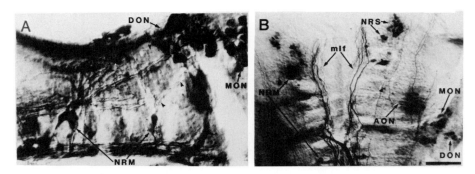

Fig. 6. A. Horizontal section of a 9 day-old larvae. This photograph shows in detail DON, MON and the projecting axons of DON which are in the vicinity of NRM neurons (arrowheads). The bar represents 45 μm. B. Horizontal section of a 23 days-old larvae. This picture shows the almost adult pattern of projections present at this stage. The bar represents 104 μm.

2-4 days post hatched larvae

At this stage in the development extensive dendritic elaboration was noticed in neurons of the NMLF and the reticular formation neuronal clusters. The M neuron showed extensive ventrally oriented dendrites which extended almost to the ventral margin of the brain.

5-7 day-old larvae

Labelled neurons in the preoptic nucleus (NPO) and in the rostral tectal layers were observed for the first time. At this stage in development, the rostrally extended dendrites of neurons in the NMLF (Fig. 5A) reached the level of the rostral tectum and the preoptic area. The axons of the labelled NPO cells and the tectal cells were seen to mingle with the rostrally directed dendrites of NMLF neurons (Fig. 5B and C).

8-10 day-old larvae

The lateral NMLF had extensive rostral dendritic branches whereas medial cells extended their dendrites to the contralateral nucleus. The axons of the octaval neurons descended obliquely and reached the mlf (Fig. 6A). A tentative designation of DON and magnocellular octaval nucleus (MON) was given to the octaval neurons at this stage (Fig. 6A). Some of the labelled axons of cells in the DON were traceable but were lost in the extensive dendritic arbor of giant NRM neurons (Fig. 6A). Cell clusters were seen in the rostrocaudal extent of NRM and NRI. Contralaterally projecting neurons were scattered on the dorsal level within the boundaries of NRM and NRI. The mlf and llf were well developed.

15-16 post hatched larvae

The earliest labelled neurons in the ruber nucleus were seen at this stage. In all other aspects, most of the descending projection neurons were similar to those seen in the adult (not shown).

21-23 day-old larvae

Reduced dendritic arbors of the NMLF neurons were seen between 21-23 days-old larvae as compared to 8-10 day-old larvae (Fig. 7). Two clusters of cells formed the NRS. The rostral cluster showed axons entering the llf whereas axons of the caudal cluster ran in the mlf (Fig. 6B, 7). Rostrolaterally located NRM neurons sent axons towards the mlf (Fig. 7-9). In the octaval area, three distinct cellular clusters were apparent. They were designated as anterior octaval nucleus (AON), MON and DON (Fig. 6B, 7). However, we were unable to discern any definite posterior octaval nucleus (PON) in these preparations. Ventral to the M neurons, a few cells belonging to NRM were easily distinguishable (Fig. 9). Caudal to M neuron, NRM neurons were found at two locations, whereas NRI neurons were scattered at least at 5 locations (Fig. 7-9) and had either ipsilaterally or contralaterally projecting axons. Scattered among the mlf in the midline level were labelled raphe neurons (NR, Fig. 7) whose pattern of labelling was similar to that seen in the adult.

29-30 day-old fish

The pattern of labelled cells in most projecting cell groups resembled that of the adult. However, neurons in the nucleus ventromedialis of the rostral thalamus (NVMD), vagal motor nucleus and facial lobe neurons which project to the spinal cord in the adult (Prasada Rao et al., '87) were not labelled. In addition, a clear distinction of PON in the octaval area was still obscure.

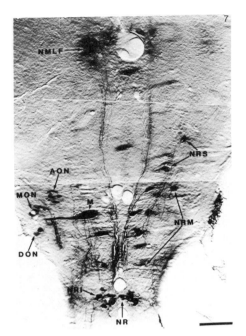

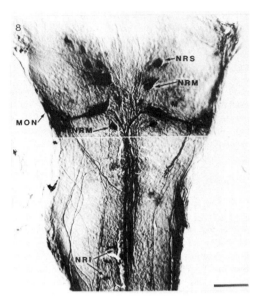

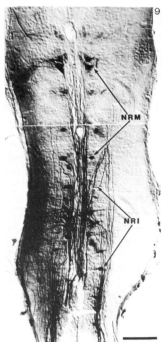

Fig. 7-9. Horizontal sections through the brain of a 23 days-old larvae.
Fig. 7. Dorsal level. Labelled cells are seen in NMLF, M, NRS, NRM, NRI
and NR, as well as in AON, MON and DON. Fig. 8. Middle level (ventral
with respect to that in Fig. 7). M, NRS, NRM, some NRI and MON neurons
are labelled. Fig. 9. Ventralmost level. Labelled neurons can be seen
in NRM and NRI. Fibers running in the ventral portion of the brain can be
observed. The bar represents 104 μm.

The time course of the appearance of supraspinal projecting neurons in goldfish can be summarized as follows. By embryonic stage 20, the earliest NMLF, NRS, NRM, M and NRV axons had arrived at the spinal cord. Cellular clustering was evident at stage 24. Nuclear groupings in the octaval area were evident at stage 24. In 5-7 day old larvae, axons of the NPO neurons and rostral tectal neurons were seen in the vicinity of the dendrites of the NMLF neurons. In 15-22 day old larvae, DON and ruber nucleus cells were labelled. In one month old fish, the oldest stage studied, no labelled cells were seen in the facial lobe, vagal motor nucleus or in the NVMD nucleus. These results suggest that later three nuclei either develops much later or that cells do not project to the spinal cord at this stage. In a separate series of unlabelled tissue of all stages studied showed that the facial lobe primordium developed after hatching and at 1 month old animal when all other projection neurons to the spinal cord had developed, the facial lobe was not yet fully developed. An adult-like pattern of supra-sinal projection neurons was evident in 21-23 day old larvae.

Descending projection neurons in the ventral portion of the brainstem developed earlier. Neurons develop on the ventral surface and are displaced dorsally. Hence, dorsal neurons are the oldest (Mendelson, '86 a&b). This dorsoventral sequence of the emergence of labelled neurons seen in the present study supports similar observations in zebrafish (Mendelson, '86 a&b); chick (Okado and Oppenheim, '85) and North American opossum (Cabana and Martin, '82). In general, the appearance of supraspinal projection neurons in goldfish is similar to that of most vertebrates studied so far (Cabana and Martin, 1982; Okado and Oppenheim, 1985; Mendelson, '86 a&b). However, differences in the time of the appearance of reticular neurons, and NMLF neurons are evident (Cabana and Martin, '84; Nordlander et al., '85; Okado and Oppenheim, '85). Raphae neurons in the present study were not distinguishable till 21-23 days after hatching.

Studies on the zebrafish (Kimmel et al., '82) showed a limited projection of octaval area neurons, whereas in the goldfish the majority of nuclear groups in the octaval area projected to the spinal cord. This discrepancy can be attributed to the fact that the present study encompassed a longer developmental period than the earlier studies on zebrafish (Kimmel et al., '82). It is clear from the present study that descending octaval neurons develop over a longer time period.

One of the first projection neurons to appear during development in goldfish is the M neuron which is involved in the startle response. At about the same time, reticular formation neurons appear to project to the cord and are, perhaps, involved in the control of swimming movements. Late in development the descending neurons involved in mating behavior emerge (Demski and Sloan, '85). A correlative developmental sequence in the spinal cord has been shown to exist in mammals. In the North American opossum, study of the development of the hind-limb movement shows that immature brainstem axons are present within the marginal zone of the lumbosacral cord before the initiation of hind-limb movements (Martin et al., '78). Similar observations were made in amphibian (Forehand and Farel, '82).

Mendelson ('86 a&b) utilized different terminologies for the neurons in the brain stem nuclei especially the reticulospinal neurons in developing zebrafish. He named identifiable neurons individually and these names differed from the conventional names used to identify reticulospinal neurons in other fish (Sweet & Timerick, '81; Prasada Rao et al., '87) and Agnathan fish (Ronan, '89). Since in earlier studies of adult goldfish reticulospinal projection we followed the conventional name

(Prasada Rao et al., '87), we have used similar conventions in the present study. Nevertheless, to our best abilities, zebrafish neurons (Mendelson et al., '86 a&b) correspond to the followings: MEM and MEL neurons in zebrafish correspond to the neurons in the nucleus of the medial longitudinal fascicle in the present study. Similarly, ROL_1, ROM_1C, ROM_2 and ROL_2 neurons correspond to neurons in the superior reticular formation. ROM_3, MiM_1, MiV_1 and MiD_3Cl neurons correspond to the medial reticular formation neurons of goldfish. Furthermore, zebrafish CaD, CaV and ic neurons correspond to the cells in the nucleus of inferior reticular formation of the present study.

The clustering of various neurons at later developmental stages as seen in the present study confirms similar observations in anurans (Forehand and Farel, '82; Nordlander et al., '85), teleosts (Mendelson, '86b), and chick (Okado and Oppenheim, '85).

Another notable observation in the present study is the late appearance of dendritic processes, whereas the soma is differentiated much earlier with the axonal processes extending down to the spinal cord. This situation is similar to that observed in Xenopus (Nordlander, '84). Similar observations have been reported in the development of retinal ganglion cell dendritic arbors in chick (Fraley, '87).

In the present study, extensive dendritic outgrowth continued in larvae of 8-10 days old; however, in later stages remodeling of arbor occurred which perhaps involved retraction of dendrites. This process brought the dendritic arbor of a particular cell to its adult pattern. This dendritic pruning effect seems to be present in both vertebrate and invertebrate neuronal development (Goodman and Spitzer, '79; Sherman, '85; Rakic, '86) and perhaps is part of the general mechanism by which neuronal population establish their final terminations. Extensive dendritic elaboration is thought to be the outcome of early developing neurons where extra space is available. The retraction or pruning phenomenon is thought to be a consequence of dendritic interactions with the newly formed dendrites of later generated neurons competing for the available space. Earlier extensive dendritic elaboration may have a crucial role by providing a substrate for the guidance of later developing axons.

Okado and Oppenheim ('85) showed the existance of transitory projection neurons to the spinal cord in developing chick. These neurons were confined to an area immediately dorsal to the optic chiasm and in an area of the lateral wall of the ventral hypothalamus. Both of these cell groups do not project to the spinal cord in newly hatched chick. In goldfish we were unable to locate any labelled neuron in the ventral hypothalamus.

In conclusion, the development of supraspinal projections in the goldfish may involve the following sequence: (a) differentiation of presumptive neurons by stage 20; growth cones of these cells may extend in close contact with the neuroepithelial cell, preferably, those of dorsal and anterolateral marginal cells as proposed by Nordlander ('84). However, it is possible that some transitory neurons may form the initial mlf which most of reticulospinal neurons seems to follow. This transitory pathway would be analogous to the pioneer axonal pathway as has been recently described by McConnell et al., ('89) in the developing cat cortex.

REFERENCES

Bando, T. (1975) Synaptic organization in teleost spinal motor neurons. JAP. J. Physiol. 25:317-331.

Bell, C.C., Finger, T.E. and Russel, C.J. (1981) Central connections of the posterior lateral line lobe in mormyrid fish. Exp. Brain Res. 42: 9-22.

Cabana, T. and Martin, G.F. (1982) The origin of brainstem-spinal projections at different stages of development in the North American opossum. Dev. Brain Res. 2: 163-168.

Cabana, T. and Martin, G.F. (1984) Developmental sequence in the origin of descending spinal pathways. Studies using retrograde transport techniques in the North American opossum (Didelphis virginiana). Dev. Brain Res. 15: 247-263.

Coghill, G.E. (1929) Anatomy of the problem of behavior. Cambridge Univ. Press.

Demski, L.S. and Sloan, H.E. (1985) A direct magnocellular-preoptic spinal pathway in goldfish. Implication for control of sexual behavior. Neuroscience Lett. 55:283-288.

Eaton, R.C. and Bompardieri, R.A. (1978) Behavioral function of the Mauthner neuron. In Neurobiology of Mauthner cells: D.S. Faber and H. Korn (eds.). New York, Raven Press, pp. 212-244.

Forehand, C.J. and Farel, P.B. (1982) Spinal cord development in anuran larvae: II ascending and descending pathways. J. Comp. Neurol. 209: 395-408.

Fraley, S.M. (1987) Dendritic development of chick retinal ganglion cells. Soc. Neurosci. Abst. 13: 1297.

Goodman, C.S. and Spitzer, N.C. (1979) Embryonic development of identified neurones: differentiation from neuroblast to neurone. Nature 280: 208-214.

Guideiri, Y.B.A. (1966) The behavior and neuroanatomy of some developing teleost fishes. J. Zool. 149:215-241.

Hamburger, V. (1973) Anatomical and physiological basis of embryonic motility in buds and mammals. In: Studies on the development of behavior and the nervous system. G. Gotlieb, ed., New York, Academic Press, 1:51-76.

Harris, J.E. (1962) Early embryonic movements. J. Obst. Gynaecol. Br. Commonw. 69:818-821.

Kanwal, J.S. and Finger, T.E. (1988) Spatial and temporal integration of taste and tactile information in the reticular formation of a teleost. Soc. Neurosci. Abstr. 14:691.

Kimmel, C.B., Power, S.L. and Metcalfe, W.K. (1982) Brain neurons which project to the spinal cord in young larvae of the zebrafish. J. Comp. Neurol. 205: 112-127.

Kuwada, J. (1986) Cell recognition by neuronal growth cones in a simple vertebrate embryo. Science 233:740-746.

Lamborghini, J.E. (1980) Rohon-Beard cells and other large neurons in Xenopus embryos originate during gastrulation. J. Comp. Neurol. 189: 323-333.

Leghissa, S. (1942). Le basi anatomiche wella jevolazione del 'compartments' durante lo svilappo embrionale e post embryonale di Trota (Salmo fario, irideus e lacustris). Z. Ant. Etw Gesch. III, 601-675.

Martin, G.F., Beals, J.K., Culberson, J.L., Dom, R., Goode, G. and Humbertson, A.O. (1978) Observations on the development of brainstem-spinal systems in the North American opossum. J. Comp. Neurol. 181: 271-290.

McClellan, A.D. and Grillner, S. (1984) Activation of "fictive swimming" by electrical microstimulation of brainstem locomotor region in an "in vitro" preparation of the lamprey central nervous system. Brain Res. 300:357-361.

McConnell, S.K., Ghosh, A. and Shatz, C.J. (1989) Subplate neurons pioneer the first axon pathway from the cerebral cortex. Science 245:978-989.

Mendelson, B. (1986a) Development of reticulospinal neurons of the zebrafish. I. Time of origin. J. Comp. Neurol. 251: 160-171.

Mendelson, B. (1986b) Development of reticulospinal neurons of the zebrafish. II. Early axonal outgrowth and cell body position. J. comp. Neurol. 251: 172-184.

Metcalfe, W.K., Mendelson, B. and Kimmel, C.B. (1986) Segmental homologies among reticulospinal neurons in the hindbrain of the zebrafish larva. J. Comp. Neurol. 251: 147-159.

Nordlander, R.H. (1984) Developing descending neurons of the early Xenopus tail spinal cord in the caudal spinal cord of early Xenopus. J. Comp. Neurol. 228: 117-128.

Nordlander, R.H., Baden, S.T. and Ryba, T.M.J. (1985) Development of early brainstem projections to the tail spinal cord of Xenopus. J. Comp. Neurol. 231: 519-529.

Okado, N. and Oppenheim, R.W. (1985) The onset and development of descending pathways to the spinal cord in the chick embryo. J. Comp. Neurol. 232: 143-161.

Prasada Rao, P.D., Jadhao, A.G. and Sharma, S.C. (1987) Descending projection neurons to the spinal cord of the goldfish, (Carassius auratus). J. Comp. Neurol. 285: 96-108.

Rakic, P. (1986) Mechanism of ocular dominance segregation in the lateral geniculate nucleus: competitive elimination hypothesis. TINS 9: 11-15.

Rhines, R. and Windle, W.F. (1941) The early development of the fasciculus longitudinalis medialis and associated secondary neurons in the rat, cat and man. J. Comp. Neurol. 75: 165-189.

Roberts, A. and Khan, J.A. (1982) Intracellular recordings from spinal neurons during swimming in paralysed amphibian embryos. Phil. Trans. R. Soc. Lond. B. 296: 213-228.

Ronan, M. (1989) Origin of descending spinal projection in petromyzontid and myxinoid Agnathans. J. comp. Neurol. 281:54-68.

Sharma, S.C. and Unger, F. (1980) Histogenesis of the goldfish retina. J. Comp. Neurol. 191: 373-382.

Sherman, S.M. (1985) Development of retinal projections to the cat's lateral geniculate nucleus. TINS 8: 350-355.

Sweet, W.J.A.J. and Timerick, S.J.B. (1981) Cell of origin of pathways descending to the spinal cord in chondichtyans, the shark, Scyliorhinus canicula and the ray Raja clavata. J. Comp. Neurol. 202:473-491.

Whiting, H.P. (1948) Nervous structure of the spinal cord of the young larval brook lamprey. Q.J. Miros. Sci. 89:359-383.

INDEX